Lowering Cholesterol: Concerns and Challenges

Lowering Cholesterol: Concerns and Challenges

Edited by Mia Norris

hayle
medical

New York

Hayle Medical,
750 Third Avenue, 9th Floor,
New York, NY 10017, USA

Visit us on the World Wide Web at:
www.haylemedical.com

ISBN: 978-1-63241-870-8

Cataloging-in-Publication Data

Lowering cholesterol : concerns and challenges / edited by Mia Norris.
   p. cm.
Includes bibliographical references and index.
ISBN 978-1-63241-870-8
1. Cholesterol. 2. Hypercholesteremia--Treatment. 3. Low-cholesterol diet.
4. Coronary heart disease--Prevention. I. Norris, Mia.
QP752.C5 L69 2020
612.12--dc23

Table of Contents

Permissions

List of Contributors

Index

Preface

This book has been a concerted effort by a group of academicians, researchers and scientists, who have contributed their research works for the realization of the book. This book has materialized in the wake of emerging advancements and innovations in this field. Therefore, the need of the hour was to compile all the required researches and disseminate the knowledge to a broad spectrum of people comprising of students, researchers and specialists of the field.

Cholesterol is a sterol that is biosynthesized by all animal cells. It is an important structural component of animal cell membranes. It also acts as a precursor for the biosynthesis of steroid hormones, vitamin D and bile acid. The cholesterol ingested is esterified but it is poorly absorbed by the body. It compensates for the absorption of additional cholesterol by reducing further synthesis. The liver excretes cholesterol in a non-esterified form into the digestive tract. About half of this cholesterol is reabsorbed back into the bloodstream at the small intestine. High levels of cholesterol are associated with a high risk of atherosclerosis, cardiovascular disease, stroke, heart attack, etc. The risk of acquiring these conditions is dependent on the quantity of cholesterol one consumes and also the kind of cholesterol in blood. The management of cholesterol does not necessarily resolve with dietary control alone, but also requires exercise and medication. This book covers in detail some existing theories and innovative concepts revolving around the management of cholesterol. The topics covered herein deal with the concerns and challenges of high cholesterol. With state-of-the-art inputs by acclaimed experts of this field, this book targets students and professionals.

At the end of the preface, I would like to thank the authors for their brilliant chapters and the publisher for guiding us all-through the making of the book till its final stage. Also, I would like to thank my family for providing the support and encouragement throughout my academic career and research projects.

Editor

Cholesterol Lowering in Cancer Prevention and Therapy

Chunfa Huang and Carl E. Freter

Abstract

The accumulation of cholesterol in cancer cells and tumor tissues promotes cell growth, proliferation, and migration as well as tumor progression. Cholesterol synthesis is catalyzed by a series of enzymatic reactions. Regulation of these key enzymes can control cholesterol synthesis and modulate cellular cholesterol levels in the cells. Meanwhile, controlling cholesterol transportation, absorption, and depletion could also significantly reduce cellular cholesterol levels. The current evidence supports that cholesterol lowering agents, beyond the expected cholesterol-lowering properties, also display an important anticancer activity in reducing cancer cell growth, proliferation and migration, and inducing apoptosis in a variety of cancer cells. Understanding the mechanisms of cholesterol metabolism and cholesterol lowering could potentially benefit cancer patients in cancer prevention and treatment.

Keywords: cholesterol metabolism, cholesterol-lowering agents, cancer, prevention, therapy

1. Introduction

Cholesterol is an essential component of cellular membrane. It serves as a spacer between the hydrocarbon chains, functions as dynamic glue during membrane assembly, and plays a crucial role in the stability, architecture, dynamics, and function of cellular membrane [1, 2]. In addition, cholesterol is involved in vesicle trafficking and transmembrane receptor signaling [3–6]. Meanwhile, cholesterol itself is also as a precursor of steroid hormones and sterols in the steroidogenesis [6–8]. The vesicle trafficking, receptor-mediated signaling, and steroidogenesis further lead to specific biological responses and regulate different cellular functions such as membrane biogenesis, cell growth, proliferation, apoptosis and migration, as well as tumor progression [6–8].

Due to the key physiological roles that cholesterol plays, the circulating and cellular cholesterol levels in our body are tightly regulated by a physiological balance of cholesterol biosynthesis, cholesterol catabolism, cholesterol transportation (influx and efflux), dietary cholesterol absorption, and cholesterol depletion. Higher cholesterol, also known as hypercholesterolemia, is a risk factor for a variety of human diseases such as cardiovascular diseases, dyslipidemia, Alzheimer's disease, HIV dyslipidemia, chronic inflammation, and developing diabetes. Earlier data also indicates that accelerated cholesterol metabolism and elevated cholesterol levels contribute to the hallmarks of cancer development and malignant transformation [9–15]. Cancer cells need excess cholesterol and intermediates of the cholesterol biosynthetic pathway to maintain a high level of cell growth and proliferation. Meanwhile, cholesterol is capable of regulating multiple signaling pathways involved in carcinogenesis, cancer cell migration, and tumor progression and is also involved in chemosensitivity and chemotherapy resistance of cancer cells [9–19]. It is very important to understand cholesterol as an important factor contributing to carcinogenesis and tumor progression and to elucidate the regulation of cholesterol metabolism as a new strategy for searching cancer prevention and therapy drugs.

2. Cell biology of cholesterol

2.1. De novo cholesterol biosynthesis

Cholesterol is a 27-carbon and tetracyclic ring steroid that is catalyzed by a series of more than 26 separate enzymatic reactions in several subcellular compartments [20, 21]. The de novo biosynthesis can be considered as five major steps: (1) From acetyl-CoA to 3-hydroxy-3-methylglutaryl coenzyme A (HMG-CoA): the acetyl-CoA can be derived from the oxidation of fatty acids or synthesized from cytosolic acetate precursors (metabolites or taken up from dietary or exogenous sources), and three acetyl-CoAs condense to form acetoacetyl-CoA by acetoacetyl-CoA acetyltransferases or thiolase and then HMG-CoA by HMG-CoA synthase. (2) The formation of mevalonate: HMG-CoA is reduced to mevalonate by HMG-CoA reductase, a rate-limiting and irreversible step in the metabolic pathway that produces cholesterol and other isoprenoids. (3) From mevalonate to isopentenyl pyrophosphate (IPP): mevalonate is further converted to IPP through two phosphorylation steps and one decarboxylation step. This conversion is involved in seven different enzymes (mevalonate-3-kinase, mevalonate-5-kinase, mevalonate-3-phosphate-5-kinase, phosphomevalonate kinase, mevalonate-5-phosphate decarboxylase, mevalonate pyrophosphate decarboxylase, and isopentenyl phosphate kinase) via different avenues. (4) From IPP to squalene: three molecules of IPP further condense to form a farnesyl pyrophosphate (FPP) and two molecules of FPP then condense to form squalene. The enzymes involved in the process are IPP isomerase, farnesyl-diphosphate synthase, and squalene synthase. (5) From squalene to lanosterol to cholesterol: the oxidation of squalene by squalene epoxidase forms 2,3-oxidosqualene which is further cyclized to lanosterol by squalene oxidocyclase. Lanosterol is finally converted to cholesterol by a series of demethylations, desaturations, isomerizations, and reductions. Demethylation reactions produce zymosterol as an intermediate and further converted to cholesterol by at least two pathways that differ in the order of the desaturations, isomerizations, and reductions (**Figure 1**) [22–27].

Acetyl-CoA ———1———►Acetoacetyl-CoA

2   2

3-Hydroxyl-3-methylglutary-CoA

↓ 3

Mevalonic acid

↓ 4

Mevalonate-5-phosphate

↓ 5

Mevalonate-5-pyrophosphate

↓ 6,7,8

Isopentenyl pyrophosphate

↓ 8,9,10

Geranyl pyrophosphate

↓ 10

Farnesyl pyrophosphate

↓ 11

Squalene

↓ 12

2,3-Oxidosqualene

↓ 12

Lanosterol

19 reactions ⋮

↓

Cholesterol

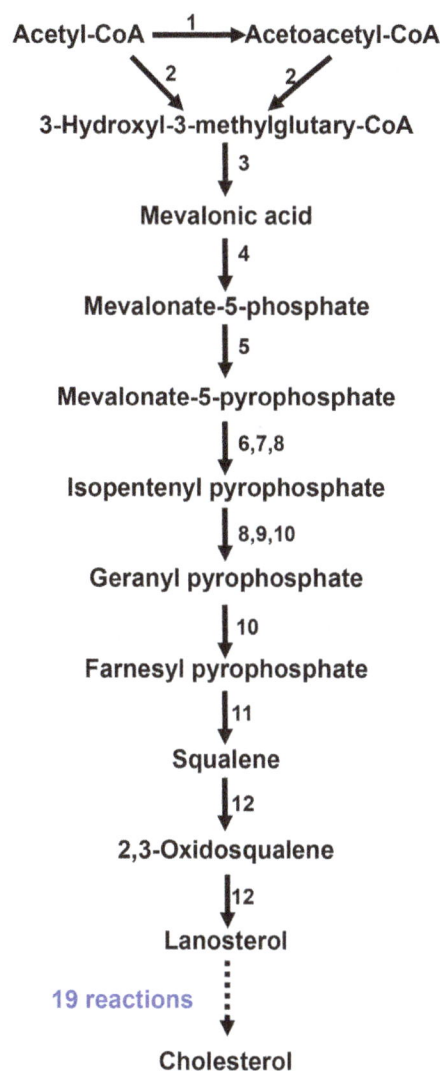

Figure 1. Scheme of the cholesterol biosynthesis pathway. (1) Thiolases or acetyl-coenzyme A acetyltransferases, (2) hydroxy-3-methylglutaryl-CoA synthase, (3) hydroxy-3-methylglutaryl-CoA reductase, (4) mevalonate-3-kinase or mevalonate-5-kinase, (5) mevalonate-3-phosphate-5-kinase or phosphomevalonate kinase, (6) mevalonate-5-phosphate decarboxylase, (7) mevalonate pyrophosphate decarboxylase, (8) isopentenyl phosphate kinase, (9) isopentenyl pyrophosphate isomerase, (10) farnesyl-diphosphate synthase, (11) squalene synthase, (12) squalene monooxygenase or squalene epoxidase, and 19 reactions are included multiple demethylations, desaturations, isomerizations, and reductions.

2.2. Cholesterol homeostasis

Cholesterol is a vital lipid and plays well-described biochemical roles and diverse functions at cellular level [1–3]. The homeostasis of cholesterol is among the most intensely regulated processes in our body. High cholesterol is a risk factor to numerous pathologies such as cardiovascular disease, atherosclerosis, dyslipidemia, and neurodegenerative diseases and is associated with the development of diabetes and cancer. Cholesterol homeostasis is achieved through intricate mechanisms involving biosynthesis, catabolism, dietary absorption, transportation (influx or efflux), and depletion (**Figure 2**) [28–32]. Slightly less than half of cholesterol in our body derives from de novo biosynthesis every day. The liver is the dominant site of cholesterol biosynthesis, and in vivo liver cholesterol production has been estimated at 1–2 g/day. Cholesterol is synthesized in liver and then secreted as circulating lipoproteins into bloodstream. The intestine and skin are also very important for cholesterol synthesis [33–35]. Although the majority of cholesterol sources comes from cholesterol biosynthesis, it is under feedback regulation. The absorption of cholesterol mainly derives from three sources: diet, bile, and intestinal epithelial sloughing. The average intake of cholesterol in the Western diet is approximately 300–500 mg per day. Bile is estimated to contribute nearly 800–1200 mg of cholesterol per day to the intraluminal pool. A third source of intraluminal cholesterol comes from the turnover of intestinal mucosal epithelium, which provides roughly 300 mg of cholesterol per day [36]. In cholesterol catabolism, the conversion of cholesterol into excretable bile acids represents the most relevant mechanism of irreversible elimination of cholesterol from the body, which plays a key role in hepatic and systemic cholesterol homeostasis. Under physiological conditions, approximately 300–400 mg of cholesterol is disposed in the liver daily [37]. Because peripheral cells do not catabolize the cholesterol molecule, there are two distinct mechanisms for maintaining cellular cholesterol homeostasis. One is the nonspecific classical pathway mediated by physicochemical diffusion of cholesterol through the aqueous phase and the other is cholesterol esterification on high-density lipoprotein (HDL) by lecithin: cholesterol acyltransferase reaction [38, 39]. The reaction is initiated by the interaction of lipid-free or lipid-poor apolipoproteins with cellular surface resulting in the assembly of HDL particles with phospholipid and cholesterol as well as extracellular cholesterol esterification mainly on HDL [40]. Furthermore, changing dietary style to control cholesterol absorption and using pharmaceutical drugs to inhibit several key enzymes in cholesterol synthesis can also significantly reduce the level of cellular cholesterol. All of these pharmaceutical drugs and dietary style have been commonly used for keeping a healthy life and preventing heart disease [41–44].

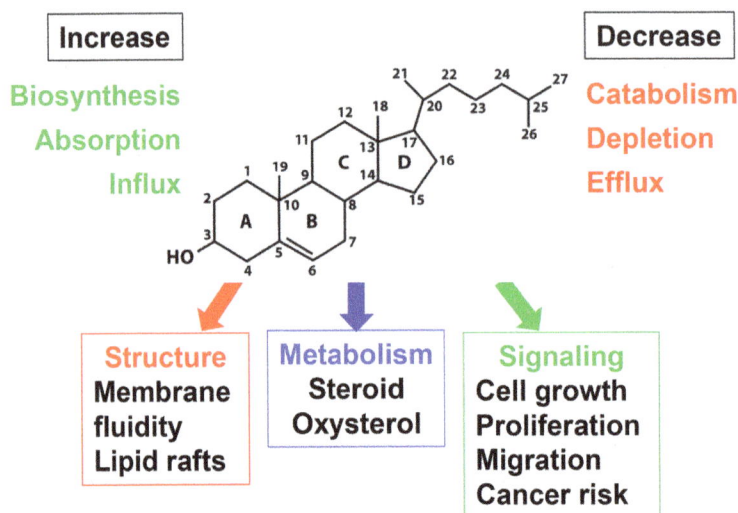

Figure 2. Cholesterol homeostasis and functions. Cholesterol homeostasis is tightly regulated in our body and can be achieved through intricate mechanisms involved in biosynthesis, dietary absorption, transportation (influx or efflux), catabolism, and depletion. The functions of cholesterol are composed of distinct membrane, control membrane fluidity and protein recruitment, produce steroid and oxysterol, and are involved in cell signaling to regulate cell growth, proliferation, and migration.

2.3. Biological functions of cholesterol

Disruption to cholesterol homeostasis leads to a variety of diseases such as coronary heart disease, atherosclerosis, and metabolic syndrome as well as cancer [9–19, 45–51]. This indicates that cholesterol plays a crucial role in the regulation of cellular function (**Figure 2**). In the cells, cholesterol is mandatory for cellular growth and serves as one of the necessary building blocks for new membranes demanded by dividing cells during proliferation. Cell membranes have been recognized as heterogeneous structures composed of distinct membrane microdomains with different proteins and lipids. Lipid rafts, cholesterol-rich domains, play an important platform as a signaling station for many cellular processes, including membrane sorting and trafficking, cell polarization, and signal transduction [52–56]. Cholesterol promotes cell proliferation by inducing the activation of the AKT and/or the ERK signaling pathway as well as Ca^{2+} channel [57–60] and cell migration by increasing the activity of calpain that is also Ca^{2+} dependent [61, 62] and is also involved in Hedgehog processing, diffusion, and reception [63, 64]. Cholesterol can be converted to steroid hormones which activate nuclear receptors and thus help to control metabolism, inflammation, immune functions, salt and water balance, the development of sexual characteristics, and the ability to withstand illness and injury [65, 66]. Meanwhile, the metabolites of cholesterol such as hydroxycholesterols play multiple biological functions in the body [67, 68]. Cholesterol also contributes to chemotherapy resistance which leads to treat failure [11–14]. Taken together, cholesterol is tightly associated with cancer cell growth, proliferation and therapy.

3. The balance of cholesterol and cancer

Cholesterol accumulation in cancer cells and tumor tissues was discovered in cancer cells and tumor tissues started in earlier 1900s [12, 69, 70]. Since then, researchers have studied the relationship between cellular cholesterol and cancer in depth. Recent epidemiological studies suggest the correlation between serum cholesterol level and the risk of certain types of cancer [15, 71–74]. It is difficult to draw conclusions from epidemiological studies on whether cholesterol is a key factor of cancer incidence because of of their intrinsic limitations. On the other hand, experimental evidence from cell and animal models indicates that cholesterol plays a promotional role in cancer cell growth and cancer development and progression [57–60]. These findings support the notion that lowering cholesterol level may be a useful and effective strategy for cancer prevention and a therapeutic potential for cancer treatment.

3.1. Lowering cholesterol level

As described above, cholesterol homeostasis is controlled by its biosynthesis, catabolism, dietary absorption, transportation, and depletion [28–32]. Among these, cholesterol biosynthesis and absorption with low-density lipoprotein (LDL) receptor (LDLR) which mediates the endocytosis of cholesterol-rich LDL are key to elevate cellular cholesterol. By contrast, there are also two common avenues to achieve cholesterol lowering: (1) pharmacological treatment which inhibits cholesterol biosynthesis [41–45] and (2) dietary control that reduces cholesterol absorption [36, 75]. Meanwhile, cholesterol metabolite, 27-hydroxycholesterol, and other oxysterols can activate the liver X receptors (LXR), resulting in a reduction of intracellular cholesterol [76–78]. Modulation of LXR and their downstream targets has appeared to be involved in cholesterol and lipid metabolism in response to changes in cellular cholesterol status [76–78]. This also draws attention to the therapeutic interest of developing LXR agonists as a bona fide therapeutic approach in cancer treatment. The cross talk of LDLR-SREBP (sterol regulatory element-binding protein) signaling and LXR signaling in the regulation of cholesterol metabolism is potential as a new strategy to develop cancer therapeutic drugs and treatment regimen.

3.2. Cholesterol-lowering drugs

There are many different agents that can inhibit cholesterol biosynthesis at different enzymatic steps or reduce cholesterol level by different regulation pathways. **Table 1** summaries the targets and effects of different cholesterol-lowering agents. Statins, first marketed in 1987, are the most common drugs to lower cholesterol level. As structural analogues of HMG-CoA, statins inhibit HMG-CoA reductase to block the conversion of HMG-CoA to mevalonic acid in a rate-limiting step of cholesterol biosynthesis. Up to date, a number of different compounds in this class drugs have been developed: atorvastatin (Lipitor), cerivastatin (Baycol; withdrawn from the market in 2001), fluvastatin (Lescol), lovastatin (Mevacor), mevastatin (Compactin), pitavastatin (Livalo), pravastatin (Pravachol or Selektine), rosuvastatin (Crestor), and simvastatin (Zocor). They are effective for treating cardiovascular disease, atherosclerosis, dyslipoproteinemia, and liver disease [79–81] and are also recommended for those who do not meet their lipid-lowering goals through diet and lifestyle changes. Statins are also considered as an anticancer agent to prevent and treat cancer patients [42–44]. Because of multiple side effects of statins, such as muscle pain, increased risk of diabetes mellitus, and abnormalities in liver enzyme tests, many other enzymes that are involved in cholesterol biosynthetic pathway beyond HMG-CoA reductase are also being considered as targets for developing cholesterol-lowering drugs. These drugs include bisphosphonates which inhibit farnesyl-diphosphate synthase [82] and lonafarnib (SCH66366) and tipifarnib (R115777) which inhibit farnesyltransferase [83]. YM-53601, RPR-107393, and TAK-475 (Lapaquistat) can inhibit squalene synthase [84–86], and Ro 48-8071, BIBB515, and terbinafine (Lamisil) are potent inhibitors of 2,3-oxidosqualene cyclase or squalene epoxidase [87–89]. These agents are used in clinic and in clinic trials.

In addition, several another classes of compounds which can lower cholesterol level via different molecular mechanisms have recently been developed. Ezetimibe (Zetia), a cholesterol uptake-blocking drug, prevents cholesterol absorption from dietary intake [90]. Fibrate drugs (Gemfibrozil, Tricor, Atromid-S), an activator of peroxisome proliferator-activated receptor α (PPARα), can reduce very-low-density lipoprotein (VLDL) - and LDL-containing apoprotein B and increase HDL-containing apoprotein AI and AII [91, 92]. Cholestyramine, colestipol, and colesevelam, bile acid sequestrants, can remove bile acids from the body and further convert more plasma cholesterol to bile acids to reduce cholesterol level [93, 94]. Some other cholesterol-lowering agents are also on the market or available for research. Acyl-CoA:cholesteryl acyltransferase inhibitor (avasimibe or CI-1011) induces cholesterol 7-α-hydroxylase and increases bile acid synthesis [95]. Green tea or catechins can inhibit the intestinal absorption of dietary lipids [96]. Lomitapide (Juxtapid) inhibits the microsomal triglyceride transfer protein required for VLDL assembly and secretion [97]. Mipomersen is a second-generation antisense oligonucleotide targeted to human apolipoprotein B-100 which is the structural core of LDL cholesterol [98]. Anacetrapib is a novel inhibitor of cholesteryl ester transfer protein [99]. Evolocumab (AMG145) and alirocumab are monoclonal antibodies which inactivate the proprotein convertase subtilisin/kexin type 9 (PCSK9) and lower LDL level [100, 101]. Dynasore reduces labile cholesterol in the plasma membrane [102]. Some of these cholesterol-lowering drugs have demonstrated their anticancer property and have the potential of cancer pharmacological prevention [41–45].

Agents	Targets	Effects	References
Statins	HMG-CoA reductase	Block the conversion of HMG-CoA to mevalonic acid	[79–81]
Bisphosphonate	FPP synthase	Attenuate the formation of FPP	[82]
SCH66366 R115777	Farnesyltransferase	Reduce adding a farnesyl group to proteins	[83]
YM-53601 RPR-107393 TAK-475	Squalene synthase	Inhibit the conversion of FPP to squalene	[84–86]
Ro 48-8071	2,3-Oxidosqualene synthase	Block the formation of 2,3 oxidosqualene	[87, 88]
BIBB515 Terbinafine	Squalene epoxidase		
Ezetimibe Catechins	Cholesterol absorption	Block cholesterol uptake in the small intestine	[89, 90]
Gemfibrozil Tricor Atromid-S	PPARα	Reduce VLDL and LDL level	[91, 92]
Cholestyramine Colesevelam and the conversion of cholesterol to bile acid Colestipol	Bile acid sequestrants	Increase bile acid removal	[93, 94]
Avasimibe CI-1011	ACAT	Increase cholesterol oxidation and bile acid synthesis	[95, 96]
Lomitapide	Triglyceride transfer protein	Reduce VLDL assembly and secretion	[97]
Mipomersen	Apolipoprotein B-100	Reduce LDL level	[98]
Evolocumab Alirocumab	PCSK9 antibody	Inactivate PCSK9 and lower LDL level	[99, 100]
Dynasore	Dynamin	Reduce membrane cholesterol	[101]

*PPARα, peroxisome proliferator-activated receptor α; ACAT, Acyl-CoA:cholesteryl acyltransferase.

Table 1. Targets and effects of different cholesterol-lowering agents.

3.3. Anticancer property of cholesterol-lowering drugs

Accumulating evidence supports that deregulation of any steps in cell growth, proliferation, and migration may result in cell malignant transformation. More than a century ago, cholesterol was observed to accumulate in malignant tissues [69]. Now, more and more evidence shows that cholesterol plays a critical role in the regulation of cancer cell growth and proliferation and tumor progression [8, 10–18, 70]. The key regulators in cholesterol metabolism attract many researchers around the world to search for novel anticancer agents. Based on cholesterol biofunctions and experimental data, the role of cholesterol-lowering drugs may not limit on the property of LDL-cholesterol lowering but may also be involved in the prevention or treatment of cancer. Statins are the most common cholesterol-lowering drugs and are also the most studied drugs. Whether statins exhibit anticancer properties is based on experimental studies, epidemiological studies, and clinical studies. In experimental studies, statins reduce a variety of cancer cell viability (**Figure 3**) [75, 103–105]. The epidemiologic data also support that statins reduce the incidence of gastric cancer, breast cancer, advanced prostate cancer, colorectal cancer, and cholangiocarcinoma [105–109]. However, there are also some studies that do not support the association of statin use with cancer risk [110, 111]. In clinical studies, statins can significantly reduce prostate cancer-specific mortality and reduce the risk of biochemical recurrence among the patients treated with radiation therapy [112] and are also associated with improved survival in patients with metastatic renal cell carcinoma [113]. So far, statins show some promising results in certain types of cancer. The potential of statins in modern cancer prevention and treatment is very promising. Meanwhile, it is also important to search other cholesterol-lowering agents that are more effective and reduce adverse side effects. Some of these agents have already been studied at the different stages [89, 114].

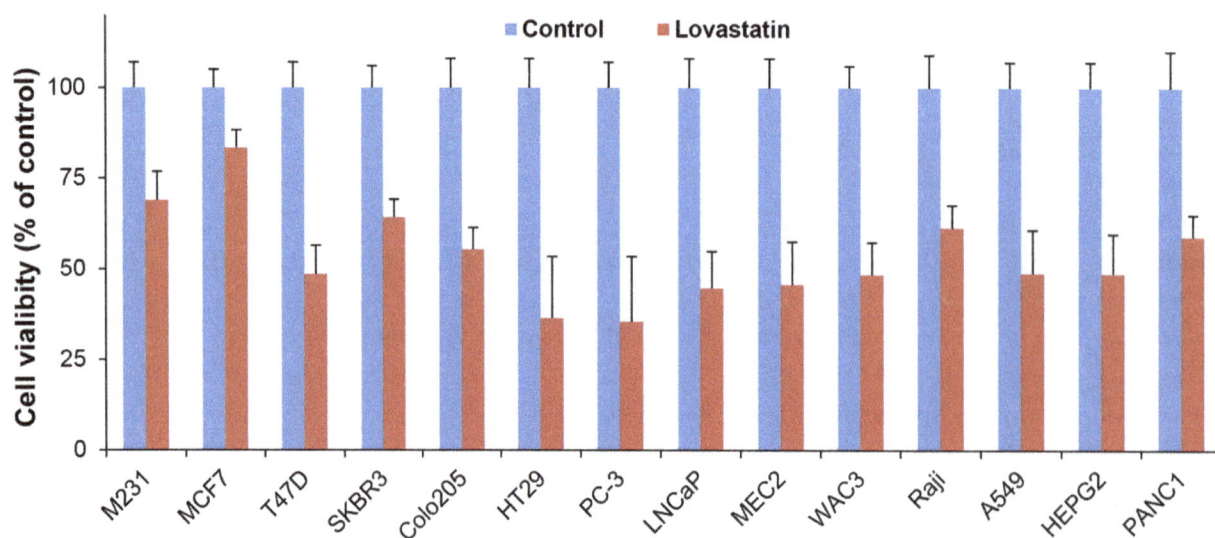

Figure 3. Treatment of lovastatin reduces cell viability in different cancer cell lines. Different cancer cells were cultured in 96-well plates and treated with 10 μM lovastatin for 3 days; the samples analyzed cell viability by MTT assay (n = 16). The values of lovastatin treatment were statistically different from the controls. $P < 0.05$. M231, MDA-MB-231.

3.4. Molecular mechanism of anticancer properties of cholesterol-lowering drugs

Expression of HMG-CoA reductase gene can be regulated by genetic or dietary interaction [115], in which it is transcriptionally regulated by endoplasmic reticulum-based transcription factor, SREBP-2 [116], or high-fat diet feeding [117]. Statins inhibit HMG-CoA reductase to block cholesterol biosynthesis which attenuate cell proliferation and arrest cell cycle progression by interrupting growth-promoting signals and involving in RAS/RAF/MEK/ERK, PI3K/AKT/mTOR and Wnt/β-catenin signaling cascades [118, 119]. Statins also selectively induce proapoptotic potential in tumor cells and synergistically enhance proapoptotic potential of several cytotoxic agents. The mechanism for this effect has been demonstrated by disrupted binding of RhoA inhibitor GDIα which leads to increased levels of GTP-bound forms of RhoA, Rac1, and cdc42 proteins. These proteins induce apoptosis 1) by suppression of anti-apoptotic proteins such as Bcl2 or activation of the superoxide-activated JNK pathway [120] or 2) by inhibiting Akt/mTOR pathway and inducing programmed cell death 4 expression in renal cell cancer cells [121]. Statins alter the angiogenic potential of cells by modulating apoptosis inhibitory effects of VEGF and decrease secretion of metalloproteases and suppress the rate of activation of multiple coagulation factors and thus prevent coagulation-mediated angiogenesis [122]. Statins suppress the Rho/Rho-associated coiled-coil-containing protein kinase pathways, thereby inhibiting cell migration, invasion, adhesion, and metastasis [123]. Other cholesterol-lowering agents have not been widely studied as statins. However, all cholesterol-lowering agents could affect membrane composition, in particular cholesterol-rich domain, termed lipid rafts. Membrane lipid rafts are highly ordered membrane domains that are enriched in cholesterol, sphingolipids, and gangliosides and selectively recruit certain classes of proteins (a large number of cancer-related signaling and adhesion molecules) and act as major modulators of membrane geometry, lateral movement of molecules, and traffic and signal transduction [52, 54]. Cholesterol-lowering drugs lead to membrane cholesterol depletion which could disrupt membrane lipid rafts, block the adhesion and migration processes of cancer cells, and induce cancer cell apoptosis [124, 125].

4. Cholesterol-lowering drugs in cancer prevention and therapy

A growing body of evidence from cell biology and animal models has strongly demonstrated the anticancer activity of cholesterol-lowering drugs such as statins [7, 83–89, 104–108]. Epidemiological studies also suggest an anticancer effect of statins evidenced by the reductions of cancer incidence and cancer-related mortality, although the association between statin use and cancer incidence based on different cancer remains controversial from different laboratories around the world. Statins as part of pharmacological cancer prevention and chemotherapy have generated interest in the oncology community and have been investigated in a variety of cancers at early and late stages and in the combination with chemotherapy and radiation therapy. Here, we summarize the current data that statin use affects cancer incidence and therapy.

Study	No. of subjects/ studies	Results	References
Bonovas, 2008	12 studies	No significant relationship between statins and pancreatic cancer risk	[129]
Khurana, 2007	483,733	Protective against the development of pancreatic cancer	[130]
Lin, 2016	19,727	Prevent *H. pylori*-associated gastric cancer	[105]
Singh, 2013	11 studies	Prevent gastric cancer risk in both Asian and Western population	[131]
Tsan, 2012	33,413	Reduce the risk for hepatocellular carcinoma in HBV-infected patients	[132]
Chen, 2015	2,053	Decrease hepatocellular carcinoma in diabetic patients	[133]
Zhang, 2013	13 studies	No association between statin use and risk of bladder cancer	[134]
Peng, 2015	3,174	Reduce the risk of cholangiocarcinoma	[108]
Yi, 2014	20 studies	Preventive effects against hematological malignancies	[135]
Pradelli, 2015	14 studies	Negatively associated with all hematological malignancies	[136]
Wang, 2013	20 studies	Nonsignificant association between statin users and lung cancer risk	[137]
Bansal, 2012	27 studies	Reduce the risk of total and advanced prostate cancer	[138]
Jacobs, 2007	55,454	Reduce the risk of advanced prostate cancer	[109]
Undela, 2012	24 studies	Do not support that statins have a protective effect against breast cancer	[139]
Lytras, 2014	40 studies	Do not support that statin users reduce the risk of colorectal cancer	[140]
Setoguchi, 2007	24,439	No effect in the risk of colorectal, lung, or breast cancer in older patients	[141]
Kuoppala, 2008	42 studies	No effect on the incidence of lung, breast, or prostate cancer Protect from stomach and liver cancer and from lymphoma Increase the incidence of both melanoma and nonmelanoma skin cancer	[142]

Table 2. Effect of statins on cancer incidence.

4.1. Cholesterol-lowering drugs in cancer prevention

Cholesterol is accumulated in different solid tumors and cancer cells [12, 69–71, 126, 127], raising questions concerning the role of cholesterol in cancer cell growth, proliferation, and migration as well as tumor progression [57–61]. Although cholesterol-lowering drugs have also been shown to possess an important antitumor activity that reduces cell growth, proliferation, and migration through ERK-mediated and Akt-mediated signaling pathways and is capable of inducing apoptosis through extrinsic and intrinsic pathways using different cancer cells as models [43–45, 75, 78, 104, 118–123], it is still unclear whether statins are suitable to prevent the incidence of cancer. More than a hundred of epidemiological studies around the world have been performed to evaluate the effect of statin on the risk of cancer incidence [105, 108, 109, 126–142]. These studies have been focused on statin type, potency, lipophilic or hydrophobicity status, and duration of use. Due to the limitation of epidemiological studies with the patients different in age, sex, living regions, and life style, the results are controversial. **Table 2** summarizes the association of cancer risk and statin use in pancreatic cancer, gastric cancer, liver cancer, lung cancer, bladder cancer, breast cancer, prostate cancer, colorectal cancer, blood cancer, and other malignancies. The clinical studies have provided conflicting data regarding whether statins may reduce or may be no effect on the risk of cancer. It is clear that current data cannot rule out the association of statin use with the risk of some cancers. Analyses of larger numbers of cases, subgroup design (participant ethnicity or confounder adjustment), randomized controlled trials, and high-quality cohort studies with longer duration of follow-up are needed to further confirm this association. Meanwhile, we also need to study cancer patient genetic mutations and determine whether the effect of statins on cancer prevention and therapy is associated with genetic mutation. It is clear that defining the underlying mechanisms of how cholesterol lowering contributes to cancer prevention and the search for other cholesterol-lowering agents with better outcome has emerged as future objectives. Whether cholesterol-lowering agents are used in cancer prevention will be based on the analysis of responses to these agents with cancer patient genetic information.

4.2. Cholesterol-lowering drugs in cancer treatment

Cholesterol is implicated in various cellular processes including the involvement of cell proliferation/apoptosis balance regulation in various types of cancers. Statins and other cholesterol-lowering agents are very common and effective medication used in preventing heart disease in those with high cholesterol, but no history of heart disease. The anticancer activity of these drugs has also attracted oncologists to consider whether cholesterol-lowering drugs can be a tool for cancer treatment. A variety of studies have focused on the effect of statins alone or in combination with other chemo- or/and immune-therapeutic drugs or radiation therapy on the treatment of different cancer patients. McKay et al. [113] showed some promising data that statin use improved survival in patients with metastatic renal cell carcinoma. Raval et al. found that statin significantly reduced the prostate cancer-specific mortality and improved the biochemical recurrence in certain subgroup of men with prostate cancer [112]. Song et al. found that statin use also reduces biochemical recurrence in men with prostate cancer after radical prostatectomy [143]. Statin use is related to reductions in overall and cancer-specific mortality [144] and associated with longer rates of survival [145] in colorectal cancer survivors. Two recent studies indicate that statin use is associated with improved overall survival in patients with resectable pancreatic ductal adenocarcinoma [146, 147]. Statin use also improves overall survival among patients undergoing resection for pancreatic cancer [148]. Lipophilic statins are associated with a reduced risk of breast cancer recurrence and inflammatory breast cancer [149]. Because statins negatively interfere with CD-20 and rituximab-mediated activity, statins have a negatively effect on clinical outcome in patients with rituximab-treated leukemia [150]. No association of statin use with patient survivals was also reported from colorectal cancer study [151]. Future studies are needed to further evaluate which cancer patients may benefit from statin treatment, what the best treatment is, and which cholesterol-lowering drugs are better to use in cancer treatment.

5. Concluding remarks and future perspectives

Cholesterol is tightly regulated by a physiological balance of cholesterol metabolism (biosynthesis and degradation), dietary absorption, transportation (efflux and influx), and depletion.

Importantly, cholesterol is accumulated in cancer cells and tumor tissues and is implicated in various cellular processes including cell growth, proliferation, and migration. The increase and decrease in cellular and circulating cholesterol levels have demonstrated the involvement of cell proliferation/apoptosis balance regulation. This chapter reviewed our current understanding of how cholesterol metabolism contributes to cancer development and progression and cholesterol-lowering drugs may be associated with the therapeutic potential of cancer prevention and treatment. Current evidence cannot exclude the relevance of cancer risk with statin use as seen in a variety of studies. Whether the genetic mutations of cancer patients are associated with the response of statins is also unknown. It is clear that more studies are needed to better characterize potential statin-mediated mechanisms that prevent cancer incidence. On the other hand, statins alone or used in combination with certain anticancer drugs or radiation therapy can improve survival in patients with several different tumors. Further research using large cohort studies in different cancers is needed to clarify these issues. In addition, searching for novel classes of cholesterol-lowering drugs with more effects and less side effects could provide new therapeutic options for cancer prevention and therapy.

Acknowledgements

Conflict of interest: The authors declare no conflict of interest.

Author details

Chunfa Huang* and Carl E. Freter

*Address all correspondence to: chunfahuang@slu.edu

Division of Hematology and Oncology, Department of Internal Medicine, and Cancer Center, Saint Louis University, Saint Louis, Missouri, United States of America

References

[1] Grouleff J, Irudayam SJ, Skeby KK, Schiøtt B. The influence of cholesterol on membrane protein structure, function, and dynamics studied by molecular dynamics simulations. Biochim Biophys Acta. 2015; 1848:1783-95.

[2] Mesmin B, Maxfield FR. Intracellular sterol dynamics. Biochim Biophys Acta. 2009; 1791:636-45.

[3] Wüstner D, Solanko K. How cholesterol interacts with proteins and lipids during its intracellular transport. Biochim Biophys Acta. 2015; 1848:1908-26.

[4] Sengupta D, Chattopadhyay A. Molecular dynamics simulations of GPCR-cholesterol interaction: an emerging paradigm. Biochim Biophys Acta. 2015; 1848:1775-82.

[5] Du X, Brown AJ, Yang H. Novel mechanisms of intracellular cholesterol transport: oxysterol-binding proteins and membrane contact sites. Curr Opin Cell Biol. 2015; 35:37-42.

[6] Papadopoulos V, Aghazadeh Y, Fan J, Campioli E, Zirkin B, Midzak A. Translocator protein-mediated pharmacology of cholesterol transport and steroidogenesis. Mol Cell Endocrinol. 2015; 408:90-8.

[7] Issop L, Rone MB, Papadopoulos V. Organelle plasticity and interactions in cholesterol transport and steroid biosynthesis. Mol Cell Endocrinol. 2013; 371:34-46.

[8] Simons K, Ikonen E. How cells handle cholesterol. Science. 2000; 290:1721-6.

[9] Cruz PM, Mo H, McConathy WJ, Sabnis N, Lacko AG. The role of cholesterol metabolism and cholesterol transport in carcinogenesis: a review of scientific findings, relevant to future cancer therapeutics. Front Pharmacol. 2013; 4:119.

[10] Nelson ER, Chang CY, McDonnell DP. Cholesterol and breast cancer pathophysiology. Trends Endocrinol Metab. 2014; 25:649-55.

[11] Danilo C, Frank PG. Cholesterol and breast cancer development. Curr Opin Pharmacol. 2012; 12:677-82.

[12] Krycer JR, Brown AJ. Cholesterol accumulation in prostate cancer: a classic observation from a modern perspective. Biochim Biophys Acta. 2013; 1835:219-29.

[13] Drabkin HA, Gemmill RM. Cholesterol and the development of clear-cell renal carcinoma. Curr Opin Pharmacol. 2012; 12:742-50.

[14] Jacobs RJ, Voorneveld PW, Kodach LL, Hardwick JC. Cholesterol metabolism and colorectal cancers. Curr Opin Pharmacol. 2012; 12:690-5.

[15] Murai T. Cholesterol lowering: role in cancer prevention and treatment. Biol Chem. 2015; 396:1-11.

[16] Silvente-Poirot S, Poirot M. Cancer. Cholesterol and cancer, in the balance. Science. 2014; 343:1445-6.

[17] Pelton K, Freeman MR, Solomon KR: Cholesterol and prostate cancer. Curr Opin Pharmacol 2012; 12:751-759.

[18] Gorin A, Gabitova L, Astsaturov I: Regulation of cholesterol biosynthesis and cancer signaling. Curr Opin Pharmacol. 2012; 12:710-716.

[19] Hilvo M, Denkert C, Lehtinen L, Muller B, Brockmoller S, Seppanen-Laakso T, Budczies J, Bucher E, Yetukuri L, Castillo S, Berg E, Nygren H, Sysi-Aho M, Griffin JL, Fiehn O,

Loibl S, Richter-Ehrenstein C, Radke C, Hyötyläinen T, Kallioniemi O, Iljin K, Oresic M: Novel theranostic opportunities offered by characterization of altered membrane lipid metabolism in breast cancer progression. Cancer Res 2011; 71:3236-3245.

[20]   Nelson DL and Cox MM eds. Lehninger Principles of Biochemistry. 6th edition, 2012, W.H. Freeman & Company, New York.

[21]   Berg JM, Tymockzo JL and Stryer L. Biochemistry. 7th edition, 2012, W.H. Freeman & Company, New York.

[22]   Porter FD, Herman GE. Malformation syndromes caused by disorders of cholesterol synthesis. J Lipid Res. 2011; 52:6-34.

[23]   Fu Z, Voynova NE, Herdendorf TJ, Miziorko HM, Kim JJ. Biochemical and structural basis for feedback inhibition of mevalonate kinase and isoprenoid metabolism. Biochemistry 2008; 47: 3715-24.

[24]   Gaylor JL. Membrane-bound enzymes of cholesterol synthesis from lanosterol. Biochem Biophys Res Commun 2002; 292:1139-46.

[25]   Goldstein JL, Brown MS. Regulation of the mevalonate pathway. Nature 1990; 343:425-30.

[26]   Miziorko HM. Enzymes of the mevalonate pathway of isoprenoid biosynthesis. Arch Biochem Biophys 2011; 505:131-43.

[27]   Houten SM, Frenkel J, Waterham HR. Isoprenoid biosynthesis in hereditary periodic fever syndromes and inflammation. Cell Mol Life Sci 2003; 60:1118-34.

[28]   Luu W, Sharpe LJ, Gelissen IC, Brown AJ. The role of signalling in cellular cholesterol homeostasis. IUBMB Life. 2013; 65:675-84.

[29]   van der Wulp MY, Verkade HJ, Groen AK. Regulation of cholesterol homeostasis. Mol Cell Endocrinol. 2013; 368:1-16.

[30]   Goedeke L, Fernández-Hernando C. Regulation of cholesterol homeostasis. Cell Mol Life Sci. 2012; 69:915-30.

[31]   Sharpe LJ, Cook EC, Zelcer N, Brown AJ. The UPS and downs of cholesterol homeostasis. Trends Biochem Sci. 2014; 39:527-35.

[32]   Malgrange B, Varela-Nieto I, de Medina P, Paillasse MR. Targeting cholesterol homeostasis to fight hearing loss: a new perspective. Front Aging Neurosci. 2015; 7:3.

[33]   Nestel PJ, Whyte HM, Goodman DS. Distribution and turnover of cholesterol in humans. J Clin Invest. 1969; 48:982-991.

[34]   Nestel PJ. Cholesterol turnover in man. Adv Lipid Res. 1970; 8:1-39.

[35]   Ho KJ, Taylor CB. Control mechanisms of cholesterol biosynthesis. Arch Pathol. 1970; 90:83-92.

[36] Wang DQ. Regulation of intestinal cholesterol absorption. Annu Rev Physiol. 2007; 69:221-48.

[37] Bertolotti M, Gabbi C, Anzivino C, Carulli L, Loria P, Carulli N. Nuclear receptors as potential molecular targets in cholesterol accumulation conditions: insights from evidence on hepatic cholesterol degradation and gallstone disease in humans. Curr Med Chem 2008; 15:2271–2284.

[38] Czarnecka H, Yokoyama S. Lecithin:cholesterol acyltransferase reaction on cellular lipid released by free apolipoprotein-mediated efflux. Biochemistry 1995; 34:4385-4392.

[39] Tomimoto S, Tsujita M, Okazaki M, Usui S, Tada T, Fukutomi T, Ito S, Itoh M, Yokoyama S. Effect of probucol in lecithin:cholesterol acyltransferase-deficient mice: inhibition of 2 independent cellular cholesterol-releasing pathways in vivo. Arterioscler Thromb Vasc Biol 2001; 21:394-400.

[40] Yokoyama S. Release of cellular cholesterol: molecular mechanism for cholesterol homeostasis in cells and in the body. Biochim Biophys Acta. 2000; 1529:231-44.

[41] Gumbs PD, Verschuren MW, Mantel-Teeuwisse AK, de Wit AG, de Boer A, Klungel OH. Economic evaluations of cholesterol-lowering drugs: a critical and systematic review. Pharmacoeconomics. 2007; 25:187-99.

[42] Alla VM, Agrawal V, DeNazareth A, Mohiuddin S, Ravilla S, Rendell M. A reappraisal of the risks and benefits of treating to target with cholesterol lowering drugs. Drugs. 2013; 73:1025-54

[43] Bardou M, Barkun A, Martel M. Effect of statin therapy on colorectal cancer. Gut. 2010; 59:1572-85.

[44] Sassano A, Platanias LC. Statins in tumor suppression. Cancer Lett. 2008; 260:11-9.

[45] Goldstein JL, Brown MS. A century of cholesterol and coronaries: from plaques to genes to statins. Cell. 2015; 161:161-72.

[46] Seo HS, Choi MH. Cholesterol homeostasis in cardiovascular disease and recent advances in measuring cholesterol signatures. J Steroid Biochem Mol Biol. 2015; 153:72-9.

[47] Varbo A, Nordestgaard BG. Remnant cholesterol and ischemic heart disease. Curr Opin Lipidol. 2014; 25:266-73.

[48] Tall AR, Yvan-Charvet L. Cholesterol, inflammation and innate immunity. Nat Rev Immunol. 2015; 15:104-16.

[49] Zhang J, Liu Q. Cholesterol metabolism and homeostasis in the brain. Protein Cell. 2015; 6:254-64.

[50] Leoni V, Caccia C. The impairment of cholesterol metabolism in Huntington disease. Biochim Biophys Acta. 2015; 1851:1095-105.

[51] Hannaoui S, Shim SY, Cheng YC, Corda E, Gilch S. Cholesterol balance in prion diseases and Alzheimer's disease. Viruses. 2014; 6:4505-35.

[52] Simons K, Toomre D. Lipid rafts and signal transduction. Nat Rev Mol Cell Biol. 2000; 1:31–39.

[53] Brown DA, London E. Functions of lipid rafts in biological membranes. Annu Rev Cell Dev Biol. 1998; 14:111–136.

[54] Mollinedo F, Gajate C. Lipid rafts as major platforms for signaling regulation in cancer. Adv Biol Regul. 2015; 57:130-46.

[55] Reeves VL, Thomas CM, Smart EJ. Lipid rafts, caveolae and GPI-linked proteins. Adv Exp Med Biol. 2012; 729:3-13.

[56] Lajoie P, Nabi IR. Lipid rafts, caveolae, and their endocytosis. Int Rev Cell Mol Biol. 2010; 282:135-63.

[57] Sun Y, Sukumaran P, Varma A, Derry S, Sahmoun AE, Singh BB. Cholesterol-induced activation of TRPM7 regulates cell proliferation, migration, and viability of human prostate cells. Biochim Biophys Acta. 2014; 1843:1839-50.

[58] dos Santos CR, Domingues G, Matias I, Matos J, Fonseca I, de Almeida JM, Dias S. LDL-cholesterol signaling induces breast cancer proliferation and invasion. Lipids Health Dis. 2014; 13:16.

[59] Xu F, Rychnovsky SD, Belani JD, Hobbs HH, Cohen JC, Rawson RB. Dual roles for cholesterol in mammalian cells. Proc Natl Acad Sci U S A. 2005; 102:14551-6.

[60] Chen BY, Wei JG, Wang YC, Yu J, Qian JX, Chen YM, Xu J. Effects of cholesterol on proliferation and functional protein expression in rabbit bile duct fibroblasts. World J Gastroenterol. 2004; 10:889-93.

[61] Franco SJ, Huttenlocher A. Regulating cell migration: calpains make the cut. J Cell Sci 2005; 118:3829-3838.

[62] Sukumaran P, Lof C, Pulli I, Kemppainen K, Viitanen T, Tornquist K. Significance of the transient receptor potential canonical 2 (TRPC2) channel in the regulation of rat thyroid FRTL-5 cell proliferation, migration, adhesion and invasion. Mol Cell Endocrinol 2013; 374:10–21.

[63] Riobo NA. Cholesterol and its derivatives in Sonic Hedgehog signaling and cancer. Curr Opin Pharmacol. 2012; 12:736-41.

[64] Callahan BP, Wang C. Hedgehog cholesterolysis: specialized gatekeeper to oncogenic signaling. Cancers (Basel). 2015; 7:2037-53.

[65] Sewer MB, Li D. Regulation of steroid hormone biosynthesis by the cytoskeleton. Lipids. 2008; 43:1109-15.

[66] Mani SK, Mermelstein PG, Tetel MJ, Anesetti G. Convergence of multiple mechanisms of steroid hormone action. Horm Metab Res. 2012; 44:569-76.

[67] Javitt NB. Biologic role(s) of the 25(R),26-hydroxycholesterol metabolic pathway. Biochim Biophys Acta. 2000; 1529:136-41.

[68] Ren S, Ning Y. Sulfation of 25-hydroxycholesterol regulates lipid metabolism, inflammatory responses, and cell proliferation. Am J Physiol Endocrinol Metab. 2014; 306:E123-30.

[69] White, C.P. On the occurrence of crystals in tumours. J Pathol Bacteriol. 1909; 13: 3-10.

[70] Clayman RV, Gonzalez R, Elliott AY, Gleason DE, Dempsey ME. Cholesterol accumulation in heterotransplanted renal cell cancer. J Urol. 1983; 129:621-4.

[71] Wang J, Wang WJ, Zhai L, Zhang DF. Association of cholesterol with risk of pancreatic cancer: a meta-analysis. World J Gastroenterol. 2015; 21:3711-9.

[72] Touvier M, Fassier P, His M, Norat T, Chan DS, Blacher J, Hercberg S, Galan P, Druesne-Pecollo N, Latino-Martel P. Cholesterol and breast cancer risk: a systematic review and meta-analysis of prospective studies. Br J Nutr. 2015; 114:347-57.

[73] Vílchez JA, Martínez-Ruiz A, Sancho-Rodríguez N, Martínez-Hernández P, Noguera-Velasco JA. The real role of prediagnostic high-density lipoprotein cholesterol and the cancer risk: a concise review. Eur J Clin Invest. 2014; 44:103-14.

[74] Freeman MR, Solomon KR. Cholesterol and prostate cancer. J Cell Biochem. 2004; 91:54-69.

[75] Kato S, Smalley S, Sadarangani A, Chen-Lin K, Oliva B, Brañes J, Carvajal J, Gejman R, Owen GI, Cuello M. Lipophilic but not hydrophilic statins selectively induce cell death in gynaecological cancers expressing high levels of HMGCoA reductase. J Cell Mol Med. 2010; 14:1180-93.

[76] Millatt LJ, Bocher V, Fruchart JC, Staels B. Liver X receptors and the control of cholesterol homeostasis: potential therapeutic targets for the treatment of atherosclerosis. Biochim Biophys Acta. 2003; 1631:107-18.

[77] Oosterveer MH, Grefhorst A, Groen AK, Kuipers F. The liver X receptor: control of cellular lipid homeostasis and beyond Implications for drug design. Prog Lipid Res. 2010; 49:343-52.

[78] Bovenga F, Sabbà C, Moschetta A. Uncoupling nuclear receptor LXR and cholesterol metabolism in cancer. Cell Metab. 2015; 21:517-26.

[79] Simon TG, Butt AA. Lipid dysregulation in hepatitis C virus, and impact of statin therapy upon clinical outcomes. World J Gastroenterol. 2015; 21:8293-303.

[80] Antoniou GA, Fisher RK, Georgiadis GS, Antoniou SA, Torella F. Statin therapy in lower limb peripheral arterial disease: systematic review and meta-analysis. Vascul Pharmacol. 2014; 63:79-87.

[81] Pang J, Chan DC, Watts GF. Critical review of non-statin treatments for dyslipoproteinemia. Expert Rev Cardiovasc Ther. 2014; 12:359-71.

[82] Szajnman SH, Ravaschino EL, Docampo R, Rodriguez JB. Synthesis and biological evaluation of 1-amino-1,1-bisphosphonates derived from fatty acids against Trypanosoma cruzi targeting farnesyl pyrophosphate synthase. Bioorg Med Chem Lett. 2005; 15:4685-90.

[83] Graaf MR, Richel DJ, van Noorden CJ, Guchelaar HJ. Effects of statins and farnesyl-transferase inhibitors on the development and progression of cancer. Cancer Treat Rev. 2004; 30:609-41.

[84] Ugawa T, Kakuta H, Moritani H, Matsuda K, Ishihara T, Yamaguchi M, Naganuma S, Iizumi Y, Shikama H. YM-53601, a novel squalene synthase inhibitor, reduces plasma cholesterol and triglyceride levels in several animal species. Br J Pharmacol. 2000; 131:63-70.

[85] Nishimoto T, Ishikawa E, Anayama H, Hamajyo H, Nagai H, Hirakata M, Tozawa R. Protective effects of a squalene synthase inhibitor, lapaquistat acetate (TAK-475), on statin-induced myotoxicity in guinea pigs. Toxicol Appl Pharmacol. 2007; 223:39-45.

[86] Amin D, Rutledge RZ, Needle SN, Galczenski HF, Neuenschwander K, Scotese AC, Maguire MP, Bush RC, Hele DJ, Bilder GE, Perrone MH. RPR 107393, a potent squalene synthase inhibitor and orally effective cholesterol-lowering agent: comparison with inhibitors of HMG-CoA reductase. J Pharmacol Exp Ther. 1997; 281:746-52.

[87] Chuang JC, Valasek MA, Lopez AM, Posey KS, Repa JJ, Turley SD. Sustained and selective suppression of intestinal cholesterol synthesis by Ro 48-8071, an inhibitor of 2,3-oxidosqualene:lanosterol cyclase, in the BALB/c mouse. Biochem Pharmacol. 2014; 88:351-63.

[88] Eisele B, Budzinski R, Müller P, Maier R, Mark M. Effects of a novel 2,3-oxidosqualene cyclase inhibitor on cholesterol biosynthesis and lipid metabolism in vivo. J Lipid Res. 1997; 38:564-75.

[89] Ryder NS. Terbinafine: mode of action and properties of the squalene epoxidase inhibition. Br J Dermatol. 1992; 126 Suppl 39:2-7.

[90] Nutescu EA, Shapiro NL. Ezetimibe: a selective cholesterol absorption inhibitor. Pharmacotherapy. 2003; 23:1463-74.

[91] Lee M, Saver JL, Towfighi A, Chow J, Ovbiagele B. Efficacy of fibrates for cardiovascular risk reduction in persons with atherogenic dyslipidemia: a meta-analysis. Atherosclerosis. 2011; 217:492-8

[92] Wierzbicki AS. Fibrates: no ACCORD on their use in the treatment of dyslipidaemia. Curr Opin Lipidol. 2010; 21:352-8.

[93] Corsini A, Windler E, Farnier M. Colesevelam hydrochloride: usefulness of a specifically engineered bile acid sequestrant for lowering LDL-cholesterol. Eur J Cardiovasc Prev Rehabil. 2009; 16:1-9.

[94] Hou R, Goldberg AC. Lowering low-density lipoprotein cholesterol: statins, ezetimibe, bile acid sequestrants, and combinations: comparative efficacy and safety. Endocrinol Metab Clin North Am. 2009; 38:79-97.

[95] Llaverías G, Laguna JC, Alegret M. Pharmacology of the ACAT inhibitor avasimibe (CI-1011). Cardiovasc Drug Rev. 2003; 21:33-50.

[96] Koo SI, Noh SK. Green tea as inhibitor of the intestinal absorption of lipids: potential mechanism for its lipid-lowering effect. J Nutr Biochem. 2007; 18:179-83.

[97] Perry CM. Lomitapide: a review of its use in adults with homozygous familial hypercholesterolemia. Am J Cardiovasc Drugs. 2013; 13:285-96.

[98] Ricotta DN, Frishman W. Mipomersen: a safe and effective antisense therapy adjunct to statins in patients with hypercholesterolemia. Cardiol Rev. 2012; 20:90-5.

[99] Gutstein DE, Krishna R, Johns D, Surks HK, Dansky HM, Shah S, Mitchel YB, Arena J, Wagner JA. Anacetrapib, a novel CETP inhibitor: pursuing a new approach to cardiovascular risk reduction. Clin Pharmacol Ther. 2012; 91:109-22.

[100] Tavori H, Melone M, Rashid S. Alirocumab: PCSK9 inhibitor for LDL cholesterol reduction. Expert Rev Cardiovasc Ther. 2014; 12:1137-44.

[101] Cicero AF, Tartagni E, Ertek S. Efficacy and safety profile of evolocumab (AMG145), an injectable inhibitor of the proprotein convertase subtilisin/kexin type 9: the available clinical evidence. Expert Opin Biol Ther. 2014; 14:863-8.

[102] Preta G, Cronin JG, Sheldon IM. Dynasore - not just a dynamin inhibitor. Cell Commun Signal. 2015; 13:24.

[103] Gbelcová H, Lenícek M, Zelenka J, Knejzlík Z, Dvoráková G, Zadinová M, Poucková P, Kudla M, Balaz P, Ruml T, Vítek L. Differences in antitumor effects of various statins on human pancreatic cancer. Int J Cancer. 2008; 122:1214-21.

[104] Benakanakere I, Johnson T, Sleightholm R, Villeda V, Arya M, Bobba R, Freter C, Huang C. Targeting cholesterol synthesis increases chemoimmuno-sensitivity in chronic lymphocytic leukemia cells. Exp Hematol Oncol. 2014; 3:24.

[105] Lin CJ, Liao WC, Lin HJ, Hsu YM, Lin CL, Chen YA, Feng CL, Chen CJ, Kao MC, Lai CH, Kao CH. Statins attenuate Helicobacter pylori CagA translocation and reduce incidence of gastric cancer: in vitro and population-based case-control studies. PLoS One. 2016; 11:e0146432.

[106] Bjarnadottir O, Romero Q, Bendahl PO, Jirström K, Rydén L, Loman N, Uhlén M, Johannesson H, Rose C, Grabau D, Borgquist S. Targeting HMG-CoA reductase with statins in a window-of-opportunity breast cancer trial. Breast Cancer Res Treat. 2013; 138:499-508.

[107] Sehdev A, O'Neil BH. The role of aspirin, vitamin D, exercise, diet, statins, and metformin in the prevention and treatment of colorectal cancer. Curr Treat Opt Oncol. 2015; 16:43.

[108] Peng YC, Lin CL, Hsu WY, Chang CS, Yeh HZ, Tung CF, Wu YL, Sung FC, Kao CH. Statins are associated with a reduced risk of cholangiocarcinoma: a population-based case-control study. Br J Clin Pharmacol. 2015; 80:755-61.

[109] Jacobs EJ, Rodriguez C, Bain EB, Wang Y, Thun MJ, Calle EE. Cholesterol-lowering drugs and advanced prostate cancer incidence in a large U.S. cohort. Cancer Epidemiol Biomark Prev. 2007; 16:2213-7.

[110] Vinogradova Y, Hippisley-Cox J, Coupland C, Logan RF. Risk of colorectal cancer in patients prescribed statins, nonsteroidal anti-inflammatory drugs, and cyclooxyge- nase-2 inhibitors: nested case-control study. Gastroenterology. 2007; 133:393-402.

[111] Jacobs EJ, Rodriguez C, Brady KA, Connell CJ, Thun MJ, Calle EE. Cholesterol-lowering drugs and colorectal cancer incidence in a large United States cohort. J Natl Cancer Inst. 2006; 98:69-72.

[112] Raval AD, Thakker D, Negi H, Vyas A, Salkini MW. Association between statins and clinical outcomes among men with prostate cancer: a systematic review and meta- analysis. Prostate Cancer Prostatic Dis. 2016; doi: 10.1038/pcan.2015.58.

[113] McKay RR, Lin X, Albiges L, Fay AP, Kaymakcalan MD, Mickey SS, Ghoroghchian PP, Bhatt RS, Kaffenberger SD, Simantov R, Choueiri TK, Heng DY. Statins and survival outcomes in patients with metastatic renal cell carcinoma. Eur J Cancer. 2016; 52:155-62.

[114] Freeman SR, Drake AL, Heilig LF, Graber M, McNealy K, Schilling LM, Dellavalle RP. Statins, fibrates, and melanoma risk: a systematic review and meta-analysis. J Natl Cancer Inst. 2006; 98:1538-46.

[115] Hwa JJ, Zollman S, Warden CH, Taylor BA, Edwards PA, Fogelman AM, Lusis AJ. Genetic and dietary interactions in the regulation of HMG-CoA reductase gene expression. J Lipid Res. 1992; 33:711-25.

[116] Horton JD, Goldstein JL, Brown MS. SREBPs: activators of the complete program of cholesterol and fatty acid synthesis in the liver. J Clin Invest 2002; 109:1125–31.

[117] Wu N, Sarna LK, Hwang SY, Zhu Q, Wang P, Siow YL, O K. Activation of 3-hydroxy-3- methylglutaryl coenzyme A (HMG-CoA) reductase during high fat diet feeding. Biochim Biophys Acta. 2013; 1832:1560-8.

[118] Martínez-Botas J, Suárez Y, Ferruelo AJ, Gómez-Coronado D, Lasuncion MA. Cholesterol starvation decreases p34(cdc2) kinase activity and arrests the cell cycle at G2. FASEB J. 1999; 13:1359-70.

[119] Tsubaki M, Yamazoe Y, Yanae M, Satou T, Itoh T, Kaneko J, Kidera Y, Moriyama K, Nishida S. Blockade of the Ras/MEK/ERK and Ras/PI3K/Akt pathways by statins reduces the expression of bFGF, HGF, and TGF-β as angiogenic factors in mouse osteosarcoma. Cytokine. 2011; 54:100-7.

[120] Zhu Y, Casey PJ, Kumar AP, Pervaiz S. Deciphering the signaling networks underlying simvastatin-induced apoptosis in human cancer cells: evidence for non-canonical activation of RhoA and Rac1 GTPases. Cell Death Dis 2013; 4:e568.

[121] Woodard J, Sassano A, Hay N, Platanias LC. Statin-dependent suppression of the Akt/ mammalian target of rapamycin signaling cascade and programmed cell death 4 up-regulation in renal cell carcinoma. Clin Cancer Res 2008; 14:4640-4649.

[122] Weis M, Heeschen C, Glassford AJ, Cooke JP. Statins have biphasic effects on angio-genesis. Circulation. 2002; 105:739-45.

[123] Kidera Y, Tsubaki M, Yamazoe Y, Shoji K, Nakamura H, Ogaki M, Satou T, Itoh T, Isozaki M, Kaneko J, Tanimori Y, Yanae M, Nishida S. Reduction of lung metastasis, cell invasion, and adhesion in mouse melanoma by statin-induced blockade of the Rho/ Rho-associated coiled-coil-containing protein kinase pathway. J Exp Clin Cancer Res. 2010; 29:127.

[124] Murai T. The role of lipid rafts in cancer cell adhesion and migration. Int J Cell Biol. 2012; 2012:763283.

[125] Jeon JH, Kim SK, Kim HJ, Chang J, Ahn CM, Chang YS. Lipid raft modulation inhibits NSCLC cell migration through delocalization of the focal adhesion complex. Lung Cancer. 2010; 69:165-71.

[126] Coleman PS. Membrane cholesterol and tumor bioenergetics. Ann N Y Acad Sci. 1986; 488:451-67.

[127] Swyer G. The cholesterol content of normal and enlarged prostates. Cancer Res 1942; 2:372–375.

[128] Singer SJ, Nicolson GL. The fluid mosaic model of the structure of cell membranes. Science 1972; 175:720-731.

[129] Bonovas S, Filioussi K, Sitaras NM. Statins are not associated with a reduced risk of pancreatic cancer at the population level, when taken at low doses for managing hypercholesterolemia: evidence from a meta-analysis of 12 studies. Am J Gastroenterol. 2008 103:2646-51.

[130] Khurana V, Sheth A, Caldito G, Barkin JS. Statins reduce the risk of pancreatic cancer in humans: a case-control study of half a million veterans. Pancreas. 2007; 34:260-5.

[131] Singh PP, Singh S. Statins are associated with reduced risk of gastric cancer: a systematic review and meta-analysis. Ann Oncol. 2013; 24:1721-30.

[132] Tsan YT, Lee CH, Wang JD, Chen PC. Statins and the risk of hepatocellular carcinoma in patients with hepatitis B virus infection. J Clin Oncol. 2012; 30:623-30.

[133] Chen HH, Lin MC, Muo CH, Yeh SY, Sung FC, Kao CH. Combination therapy of metformin and statin may decrease hepatocellular carcinoma among diabetic patients in Asia. Medicine (Baltimore). 2015; 94:e1013.

[134] Zhang XL, Geng J, Zhang XP, Peng B, Che JP, Yan Y, Wang GC, Xia SQ, Wu Y, Zheng JH. Statin use and risk of bladder cancer: a meta-analysis. Cancer Causes Control. 2013; 24:769-76.

[135] Yi X, Jia W, Jin Y, Zhen S. Statin use is associated with reduced risk of haematological malignancies: evidence from a meta-analysis. PLoS One. 2014; 9:e87019.

[136] Pradelli D, Soranna D, Zambon A, Catapano A, Mancia G, La Vecchia C, Corrao G. Statins use and the risk of all and subtype hematological malignances: a meta-analysis of observational studies. Cancer Med. 2015;4(5):770-80.

[137] Wang J, Li C, Tao H, Cheng Y, Han L, Li X, Hu Y. Statin use and risk of lung cancer: a meta-analysis of observational studies and randomized controlled trials. PLoS One. 2013; 8:e77950.

[138] Bansal D, Undela K, D'Cruz S, Schifano F. Statin use and risk of prostate cancer: a meta-analysis of observational studies. PLoS One. 2012; 7:e46691.

[139] Undela K, Srikanth V, Bansal D. Statin use and risk of breast cancer: a meta-analysis of observational studies. Breast Cancer Res Treat. 2012; 135:261-9.

[140] Lytras T, Nikolopoulos G, Bonovas S. Statins and the risk of colorectal cancer: an updated systematic review and meta-analysis of 40 studies. World J Gastroenterol. 2014; 20:1858-70.

[141] Setoguchi S, Glynn RJ, Avorn J, Mogun H, Schneeweiss S. Statins and the risk of lung, breast, and colorectal cancer in the elderly. Circulation. 2007; 115:27-33.

[142] Kuoppala J, Lamminpää A, Pukkala E. Statins and cancer: a systematic review and meta-analysis. Eur J Cancer. 2008; 44:2122-32.

[143] Song C, Park S, Park J, Shim M, Kim A, Jeong IG, Hong JH, Kim CS, Ahn H. Statin use after radical prostatectomy reduces biochemical recurrence in men with prostate cancer. Prostate. 2015 75:211-7.

[144] Cai H, Zhang G, Wang Z, Luo Z, Zhou X. Relationship between the use of statins and patient survival in colorectal cancer: a systematic review and meta-analysis. PLoS One. 2015; 10:e0126944.

[145] Cardwell CR, Hicks BM, Hughes C, Murray LJ. Statin use after colorectal cancer diagnosis and survival: a population-based cohort study. J Clin Oncol. 2014; 32:3177-83.

[146] Kozak MM, Anderson EM, von Eyben R, Pai JS, Poultsides GA, Visser BC, Norton JA, Koong AC, Chang DT. Statin and metformin use prolongs survival in patients with resectable pancreatic cancer. Pancreas. 2016; 45:64-70.

[147] Jeon CY, Pandol SJ, Wu B, Cook-Wiens G, Gottlieb RA, Merz CN, Goodman MT. The association of statin use after cancer diagnosis with survival in pancreatic cancer patients: a SEER-medicare analysis. PLoS One. 2015; 10:e0121783.

[148] Wu BU, Chang J, Jeon CY, Pandol SJ, Huang B, Ngor EW, Difronzo AL, Cooper RM. Impact of statin use on survival in patients undergoing resection for early-stage pancreatic cancer. Am J Gastroenterol. 2015; 110:1233-9.

[149] Lacerda L, Reddy JP, Liu D, Larson R, Li L, Masuda H, Brewer T, Debeb BG, Xu W, Hortobágyi GN, Buchholz TA, Ueno NT, Woodward WA. Simvastatin radiosensitizes differentiated and stem-like breast cancer cell lines and is associated with improved local control in inflammatory breast cancer patients treated with postmastectomy radiation. Stem Cells Transl Med. 2014; 3:849-56.

[150] Winiarska M, Bil J, Wilczek E, Wilczynski GM, Lekka M, Engelberts PJ, Mackus WJ, Gorska E, Bojarski L, Stoklosa T, Nowis D, Kurzaj Z, Makowski M, Glodkowska E, Issat T, Mrowka P, Lasek W, Dabrowska-Iwanicka A, Basak GW, Wasik M, Warzocha K, Sinski M, Gaciong Z, Jakobisiak M, Parren PW, Golab J. Statins impair antitumor effects of rituximab by inducing conformational changes of CD20. PLoS Med. 2008; 5:e64.

[151] Hoffmeister M, Jansen L, Rudolph A, Toth C, Kloor M, Roth W, Bläker H, Chang-Claude J, Brenner H. Statin use and survival after colorectal cancer: the importance of comprehensive confounder adjustment. J Natl Cancer Inst. 2015; 107:djv045.

2

Structural Basis and Functional Mechanism of Lipoprotein in Cholesterol Transport

Zhiwei Yang, Dongxiao Hao, Yizhuo Che,
Lei Zhang and Shengli Zhang

Abstract

Lipoprotein transports lipids in circulation and is primary driver/modulator of athero-sclerosis. Highly dynamics of lipoprotein conformations are crucial to lipid transport along the cholesterol transport pathway, where high-density lipoprotein (HDL), low-density lipoprotein (LDL) and cholesteryl ester transfer protein (CETP) are major players in lipid digestion & transport and the plasma cholesterol metabolism. This chapter covered how do HDL, LDL and CETP induce the metabolisms during cholesterol transport, and summarized recent process in the spatial information of the three lipoproteins, especially the elevations of plasma HDL and LDL, and shine a light on the assembly processes of lipoprotein particles and the substrates dynamics exchanges, for an in-depth understanding on the correlation between various lipoprotein classes and cardiovascular risk.

Keywords: lipoproteins, structure–function relationship, cholesterol transport, reverse cholesterol transport (RCT), lipoprotein particle metabolism

1. Introduction

Cardiovascular disease (CVD), a leading cause of mortality in many developed and developing countries [1], roots in the evolvement of atherosclerosis which is associated with profound disturbances of cholesterol metabolism. To some degree, these metabolism disturbances attribute to the net movement of cholesterol among blood and peripheral tissues. For instance, cellular cholesterol uptake is increased in atherosclerosis, while cholesterol efflux is downregulated [2]. Lipoproteins (consists of apolipoproteins, phospholipid and cholesterol) play an important role in the transport of cholesterol [3]. Based on density and size, lipoproteins can be classified as ultra-low- (chylomicrons), very low- (VLDL), intermediate- (IDL), low- (LDL), and high- density lipoproteins (HDL) [4]. The last two might be the significant sections of cholesterol transport and metabolism: (1) LDL could transfer lipids into the blood vessel walls, and contribute to the atherosclerosis, which causally be associated with CVD and all-cause mortality; (2) HDL could remove the lipids and carry them back to the liver, being regarded as "good" one [5, 6]. Hence, the lipoprotein-mediated cholesterol metabolism (cholesterol transport) has aroused great attention and showed the benefit for the in-depth understanding of CVDs, as well as the prevention and treatment of CVDs.

As shown in **Figure 1**, the lipoprotein-mediated cholesterol metabolism can be divided into exogenous and endogenous pathways [7]. Exogenous pathway is one of crucial ways to transport cholesterol to the body tissues (chylomicrons → VLDL → IDL → LDL) [8, 9], under the co-action of lipoprotein lipase (LPL) and hepatic lipase (HL) [10, 11]. While the higher plasma LDL level might drive the process of atherosclerosis [12]. Endogenous pathway delivers cholesteryl esters back to the liver, working cooperatively in a concurrent manner with ATP-binding cassette transporter A1 (ABCA1) [13], enzyme lecithin-cholesteryl acyltransferase (LCAT) [14], as well as HDL receptors scavenger receptor B1 (SR-BI) [15] or other unidentified HDL receptor (HDLR) [16]. It is widely accepted that HDL protein particles alleviate atherosclerosis with better cardiovascular health (reverse cholesterol transport, RCT) [6, 17, 18]. Besides, cholesteryl ester transfer protein (CETP) does a heteroexchange of triglycerides and cholesteryl esters between VLDL/ LDL and HDL, with the lessen of cholesterol eliminations [19, 20]. Therefore, the functions of HDL, LDL and CETP play the important roles during the cholesterol transport (lipoprotein particle metabolism), and pharmacological inhibition of CETP is being regarded as a way to prevent CVDs [19, 20].

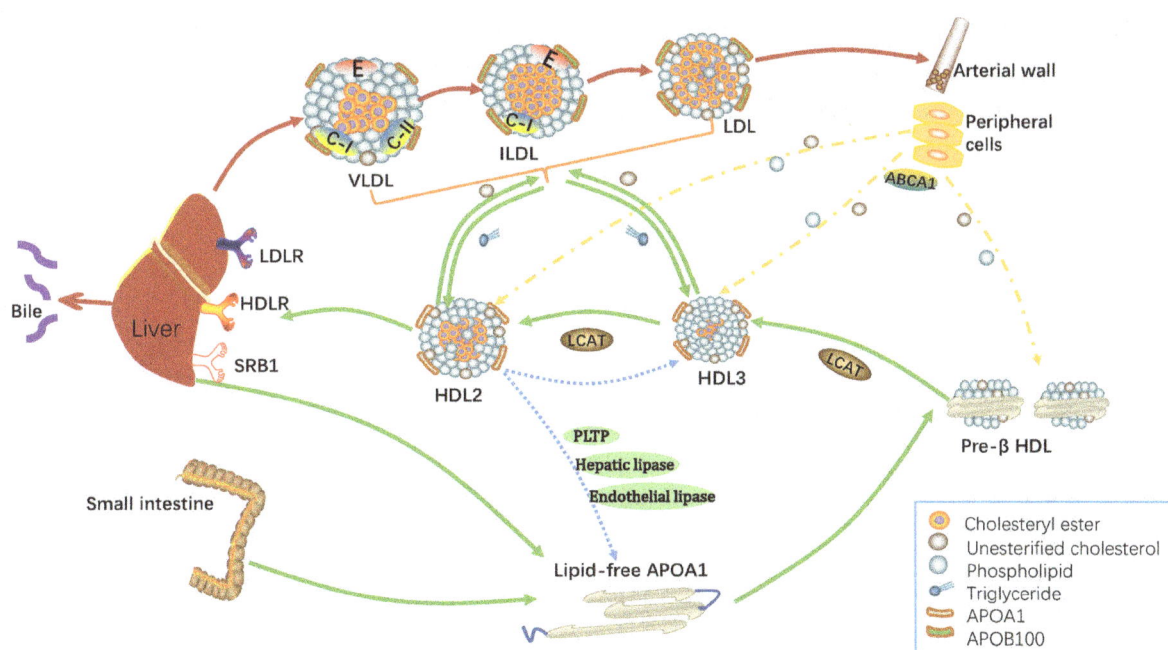

Figure 1. Lipoprotein-mediated cholesterol metabolism in human body.

To best of our knowledge, there are scant reviews elaborating the structure–function relationship of lipoproteins albeit the schematic illustrating is oncoming clear. A comprehensive understanding in this regard was endeavored, and then bioavailability that is closely related with cholesterol transport was discussed. In this chapter, we will summarize the recent achievements towards the structural basis and functional mechanism of lipoproteins in cholesterol transport, mainly focusing on functions of HDL, LDL and CETP, conformation dynamics of lipoprotein particles, and substrates dynamics exchanges.

2. Structure and function of HDL

HDL, a plasma lipoprotein, plays an important role in cholesterol metabolism [21–23], with several potentially anti-atherogenic properties (remove cholesterol from macrophages) [24–26]. Knowing the assembly mechanism and spatial information is of great importance to mediate cholesterol transport. HDLs exit three main steadier state during the cholesterol transport process: lipid-free apoA-I (apoA-I, the major protein component of HDL particles), discoidal and spherical HDL, with highly heterogeneous and differences of density, size, shape, as well as composition of lipid and protein.

2.1. Lipid-free apoA-I

Structure of full-length lipid-free apoA-I (28-kD, 243 residues) at native states still remains unclear due to its high flexibility. The initial X-ray crystal structure revealed that N-terminal truncated (Δ(1–43)) lipid-free apoA-I features "horseshoe-shape" antiparallel helical dimers [27], being regarded as a vital initial model ("double-belt" model) for comprehending the structure of apoA-I on HDL subclasses (**Figure 2b**) [28]. Subsequent crystal organization of lipid-free Δ(1–43)apoA-I accommodated a four-helix bundle [29–31]. However, the structural information is out of step with some physical biochemical measurements, hinting the conformation dynamics of lipid-free apoA-I. The crystal structures of the N- and C-terminally truncated

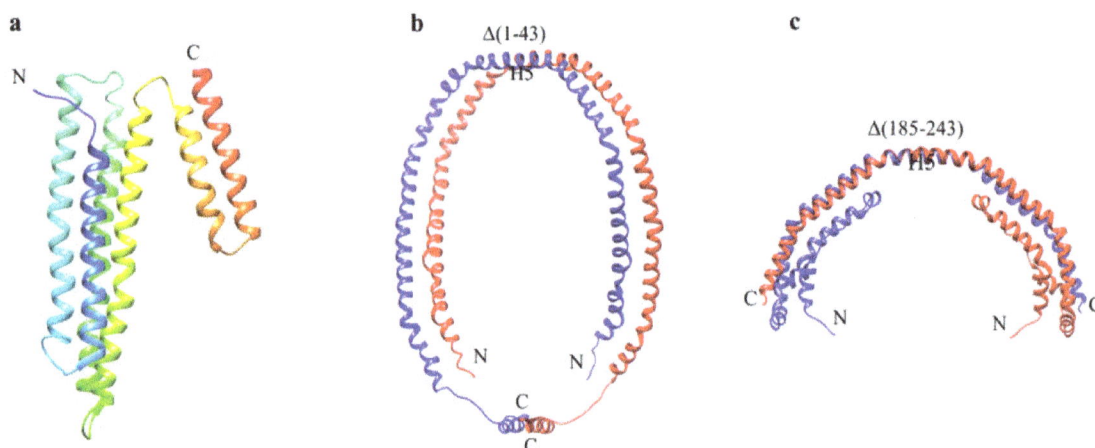

Figure 2. Three structures of lipid-free apoA-I: (a) full-length lipid-free apoA-I, [36] (b) N-terminal truncated Δ(1–43) apoA-I dimer, [27] and (c) C-terminal truncated Δ[185–243] apoA-I dimer [32].

proteins presented antiparallel helical dimers, with inherent properties (e.g., 5/5 repeat register, **Figure 2b** and **c**) in the lipid-bound and intermediate states [27, 32]. Amphipathic α-helix enables apoA-I to stabilize all HDL subclasses via the conformation change, and N-terminal two thirds constitute a dynamic, four-helix bundle, and the helical segments unfold and refold in seconds. While the C-terminal third, an intrinsically disordered domain, mediates initial binding to phospholipid surfaces. These structural motifs are important for the remodeling of apoA-I during the formation of various HDL particles. Nowadays, there remains some confusions for the structure of full length free apoA-I, especially the dynamic conformations in solutions. The dynamic helical structure is unfolding and refolding in seconds, and the helices bundle at the N-terminal of apoA-I is far more stable than could be achieved in isolation, with mutually stabilizing interactions [33, 34]. The highly dynamic apoA-I molecules are capable of adopting an array of conformations through remodeling HDL that is crucial to lipid transport during the RCT process. Further studies show that mutations in apoA-I induce varied types of dyslipidemias [35].

2.2. Discoidal HDL

Human plasma HDL is high heterogeneous, and exists as a short-lived heterogeneous substrate for LCAT in human plasma. Hence, reconstituted HDL particle (rHDL) is a powerful in vivo model system to study its structure and function, with most of the properties of native lipoprotein complexes (e.g., LCAT activation, lipid transfer, and receptor binding) [37–39]. Based on the crystal structure of Δ(1–43)apoA-I, [27] the original double-belt model features two antiparallel monomers, where each helix 5 segments directly oppose each other [40, 41], and the closely contact involved hydrophobic face of amphipathic α-helix with the fatty acid acyl chains [42]. In refined "looped belt" model, N- and C-terminal 40–50 residues doubled back as the "belt and buckle" [43], and residues 134–145 were coincide with a looping region, resulting in partial opening of the parallel belts. It is consistent with the accession between LCAT and the cholesterol and phospholipid acyl chains [44], With the aid of mass spectrometry (MS) and rHDL, lipid-free and lipid-bound apoA-I structures were solved at 104 Å resolution, and resulted in a "solar flares" model, where C-terminal of both apoA-I molecules interacted with each other, and 159–178 loop might be the LCAT binding site, with reduced deuterium exchange [45, 46], Different from normal discoidal shape, double super-helix (DSH) apoA-I model [47] has an open helical shape, with the similar interface interaction between two apoA-I molecules (5/5 double-belt). While, the DSH model is not stable, and could rapidly collapse to a disc-shaped structure during the molecular dynamics (MD) simulations [48].

In according to the rapid growth of transmission electron microscopy (EM) technique, the directly imaging particle's structure can be performed on individual particles, in order to preferably investigate lipoprotein structures. Negative stain EM combined with cryo-EM tomography have been applied to uncover the discoidal shape of apoA-I/HDL particles (both plasma HDL and 7.8, 8.4, 9.6 nm of rHDLs) [49, 50]. In these rHDL particles, the double belt was formed in an antiparallel fashion, with a gross "right-to-right" rotation of the helices after lipidation. The nonhelical regions in lipid-free apoA-I (residues 45–53, 66–69, 116–146, and 179–236) change conformation from random coil to α-helix, to adjust a hydrophobic interior

[34, 46]. Above descriptions were further confirmed by the structures of reconstituted discoidal HDL particles via nuclear magnetic resonance (NMR), electron paramagnetic resonance (EPR) and transmission electron microscopy (TEM) methods [51]. Based on the structures of lipid-free and lipid-bound apoA-I, we can speculate that the monomeric apoA-I forms a helix bundle in which the C-terminal domain binds the lipid to form a helical structure (**Figure 3**). Discoidal HDL are stabilized by two apoA-I molecules wrapped around the edge of the disc in an antiparallel, double-belt arrangement so that the hydrophobic PL acyl chains are protected from exposure to water [52]. These apoA-I molecules are in a highly dynamic state and adapt to discs of different sizes by certain segments forming loops that detach reversibly from the particle surface.

2.3. Spherical HDL

Due to the complexity of spherical HDL particles in human plasma, the spherical HDL structures are rarely known compared with lipid-free apoA-I and discoidal HDL. Recent developments in native and reconstituted spherical HDL supported a trefoil model, using by the elegant chemical cross-linking and mass spectrometry [53]. In this model, half of each apoA-I molecule in the double-belt arrangement is bent 60° out of the plane of the particle, suggesting the hinging of the Δ(1–43)apoA-I molecule is occur near residues 133 and 233 [53] which is different from the hinging of the full-length protein conformation, meanwhile, trefoil model is assumed to occur near residues 65 and 185 [54]. Determined by small angle neutron scattering method, the helical dimer with a hairpin (HdHp) model was proposed, associated with the intramolecular interactions within the hairpined apoA-I [55].

The first LpA-I HDL model at molecular level was proposed, with only apoA-I fractions isolated from human plasma [56]. These isolated human plasma HDL particles range in diameter from 8.8 to 11.2 nm and contain 3–5 apoA-I molecules. It was found that apoA-I adopts intermolecular interactions in plasma HDL which is very similar to those of the double-belt and trefoil models derived from reconstituted systems. Thus, apoA-I might adopt a common structural organization, characterized by distinct intermolecular contacts, regardless of size and shape or natural versus synthetic method of production [57]. Furthermore, circulating

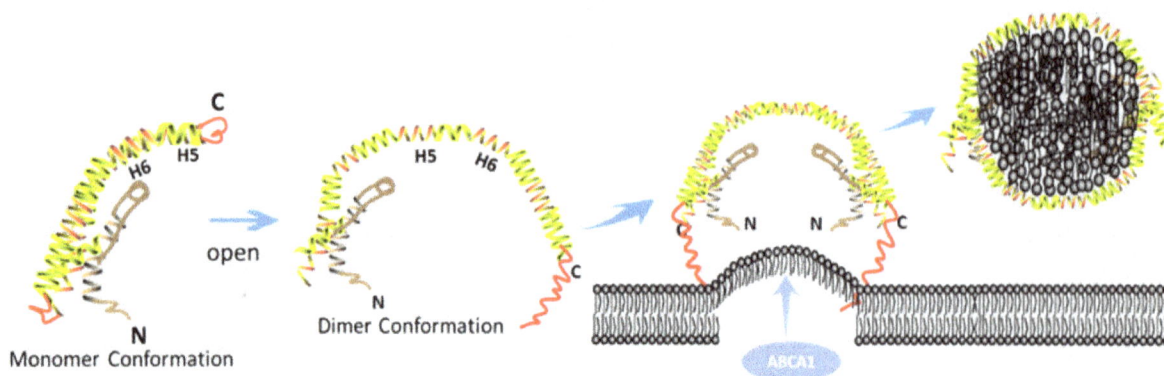

Figure 3. The monomer open conformation transfer to dimer conformation of apoA-I (intermediate state) and final HDL state in solution regulated by the H5 region.

sHDL contains similar amount of core lipid in reconstituted sHDL and has obviously less surface lipid monolayers, indicating that the apoA-I package on native spheres is much closer than the typical recombinant particles [46]. When a HDL disc alters to a sphere (LCAT converts free cholesterol to cholesteryl ester), global apoA-I conformation does not change significantly between particles of different shapes or origins, with similar protein–protein contacts.

3. Structure and function of LDL

In normal human body, there are about 70% plasma cholesterol contained in LDLs, and the endocytosis of cholesterol-rich LDLs is mediated by LDL Receptor (LDL-R) on the surface of body cell. Hence, LDLs work as the vehicle for cholesterol transportation between liver and cells to maintain a constant cholesterol supply in human body [58, 59]. In some abnormal conditions, LDL might induce over-accumulation of cholesterol to form foam cells, resulting in the development of atherosclerosis [60]. The apo-B48 (apoprotein B48) and apo-B100 (apoprotein B100) located in surface of LDL particles tend to interact with extracellular material, which make LDL particles easy to bind with blood vessel intima [61]. The oxidation-LDL can promote lipoproteins aggregation [62, 63] and provoke inflammation by recruiting the circulating monocytes to the site followed invade the vessel wall and differentiate into macrophages, to finally produce atherosclerotic plaque [62, 64–66]. Cryo-EM combined with single particle technology and small angle scattering model reconstruction technology have been effectively applied to analyze the LDL structures, and molecular components [67]. LDLs include difference in density (~1.019–1.063), shape, size (diameter ~18–25 nm), surface charge and chemical composition [68]. A general consensus is that LDLs particles all have two compartments, an amphipathic surface phospholipid monolayer which surrounded by one single copy of apoB-100, and a hydrophobic lipid-cholesteryl esters core [69]. The structure and physical function of LDLs predominantly depend on the core-lipid composition and the conformation of the apoB-100 [70, 71].

3.1. Lipid core of LDL

Lipid core of LDL mainly consists of cholesteryl esters, some triglycerides, and some free-cholesterol. Structural changes of LDL are strikingly related to physiological temperature [72]. Lipids located in core show order arranged to a liquid-crystalline phase below the critical temperature, indicated by the results of X-ray and neutron small angle scattering technology, with the transition temperature of 15~35°C [73, 74]. Besides, the overall structure of LDL is a classical spherical particle when core structure is composed of radial cholesteryl esters arranged into a concentric spherical shell [75, 76]. However, the core-located lipids present in the liquid-crystalline state within an ellipsoidal shape particle revealed by the cryo-EM data [76, 77]. It seems reasonable to speculate that the change of temperature might indirectly change the shape of LDL particles from roughly spherical to ellipsoid [67]. Many efforts have been made to explore the structure of LDL at different temperatures, such as 4, 6 [77–79] and 37°C [80].

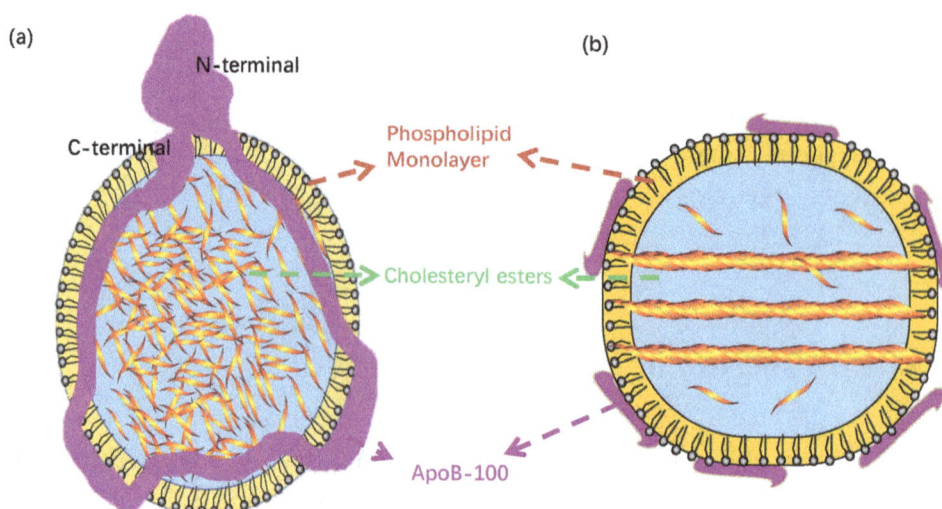

Figure 4. Overall structure and core structure of LDL above (a) or below (b) the critical temperature.

3.2. apoB-100 in LDL

ApoB-100 (4536 residues, ~20% of overall LDL) is the only protein component of LDL, and wrapped around the phospholipid monolayer on the surface of LDL particle, with an irregular ring shape. N- and C-terminus of apoB-100 touch each other, with the formation of a protruding globular structure at N-terminal [81]. A more generally accepted structural model of apoB-100 is "pentapartite" structure, which generated by molecular simulations. In this model, apoB-100 has five consecutive functional domains, NH2-βα1-β1-α2-β2-α3-COOH [79]. As shown in **Figure 4**, a new LDL reconstruction in which lipid core is revealed an organized three-layer structure by using the single particle approach, including a pair of "paddles" configurations with several long "fingers" extensions which have similar length and interval [82].

4. Structure and function of CETP

CETP acts as a medium between lipoproteins for elevating plasma LDL-C (or VLDL-C) level and lowering HDL-C level [19]. A series of CETP inhibitors have been investigated in clinical, such as torcetrapib, dalcetrapib, evacetrapib, and anacetrapib [83–85]. However, current inhibitors represent the turbulent beginning of CETP inhibition and an increased mortality rate related to off-target effects and lack of efficacy [86–88]. Accompanying adverse effects call for a deeper exploration of the mechanism for CETP-mediated lipid transfer.

CETP is a hydrophobic transfer protein composed of 476 amino acids and reveals a so-called banana-shape (the size is 135 × 30 × 35 Å, see **Figure 5**) [20]. Its crystal structure includes two different β-barrel structures in N- and C- terminal respectively, and a central β-sheet with an ~60 Å-long hydrophobic central cavity, which can hold two phospholipids and two cholesterol molecules. Moreover, the two phospholipid molecules that located in two pores near the central domain expose the hydrophilic terminal to the aqueous environment and hydrophobic terminal to the hydrophobic cavity. Because of its special function to transfer cholesterol

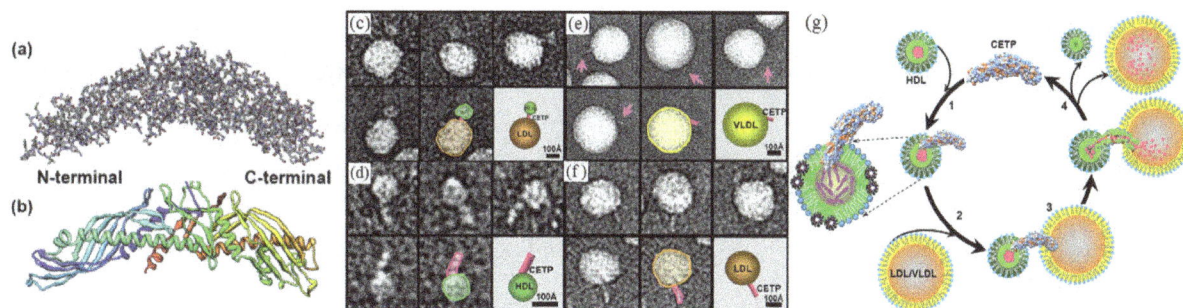

Figure 5. The crystal structure of CETP (PDB: 2OBD) and three-dimensional density maps of CETP binging lipoproteins. (a) Atom figure of CETP. (b) Secondary structure of CETP. (c) Ternary complexes of HDL-CETP-LDL in cryo-EM micrographs. (d)~(f) the CETP insert into HDL, VLDL, LDL respectively in cryo-EM micrographs. (g) (color online) the tunnel model of CETP-mediated lipid transfer [89].

esters between HDL and LDL (or VLDL), the way of CETP interacts with lipoproteins is extremely essential. CETP shows a high binding affinity for nascent HDL and other lipoproteins to cover the lipoproteins surfaces owing to its proper curvature radius. They proposed a lipid transport mechanism, shuttle model. In this mechanism, the CETP in turn covers the surface of LDL (or VLDL) and HDL to swap LDL-cholesterol esters (or VLDL-cholesterol esters) with HDL-triglycerides. These steps are constantly recycled until the completion of the transport process, in which cholesterol esters move from LDL (or VLDL) to HDL [20]. This model based on the hydrophobic cavity of CETP and its feasibility of binding to lipoproteins, explains the mechanism of CETP-mediate lipid transfer reasonably, but there are not complex of CETP binding to lipoproteins in the cryo-EM micrographs intuitively to verify the authenticity of the model.

Zhang et al. [89] studied human recombinant CETP with cryo-EM by using an optimized negative-staining (OpNS) EM protocol [49, 90]. Applied the single-particle techniques, they obtained the 3D structure of CETP and the complexes of CETP binging to lipoproteins. In the 3D-map of complexes, they discovered the HDL-CETP binding structure which appears to be formed by N-terminal of CETP insert into HDL and the HDL-LDL (or HDL-VLDL) is formed by C-terminal of CETP insert into HDL (or LDL) (**Figure 5c~f**). This conclusion was later confirmed by Geraldine et al. by using large-scale atomistic molecular dynamics [91]. The measurement of the protrusion from the lipoproteins surface shows that ~48 Å of the tapered N-terminal end of CETP penetrates the HDL surface and ~25 Å of the C-terminal end of CETP penetrates the LDL surface (~20 Å of the C-terminal end of CETP penetrates the VLDL surface) reaching the lipid–rich, lipoproteins core. Furthermore, Zhang et al. proposed the tunnel model of lipid transfer mediated by CETP [89, 92, 93]. In this model, both CETP terminals finish penetrating surface sites on lipoproteins, N-terminal to HDL and C-terminal to LDL (or VLDL). Then neutral lipids, including cholesterol esters and triglycerides, transfer through the hydrophobic tunnel at the core of the CETP (**Figure 5**).

However, there are some discrepancies with the tunnel model mentioned above. Matthias et al. used the experiments which involve three monoclonal antibodies to demonstrate that the antibodies binding on both ends of CETP do not inhibit CETP's function of transshipment cholesterol esters, but the antibodies on the middle does [94]. In their research they supposed that the formation of the ternary tunnel complexes is not a mechanistic prerequisite by CETP to perform its functions. Hence, the real mechanism of CETP-mediated lipid transfer still remains to be studied and verified.

5. Conclusion

In this chapter, we briefly summarized the functional mechanism and structural basis of lipoproteins (e.g., HDL, LDL and CETP) in cholesterol transport, as well as their structural dynamics during the transport process. Furthermore, the latest developments in the plasma lipoprotein (HDL and LDL) elevations were summarized, especially the conformational changes of lipoprotein particles. Due to the incapability of the current assays and highly heterogeneous of lipoprotein particles, the function of lipoprotein in cholesterol transport remains elusive with regard to many important questions, such as how the lipoprotein particle assembles and how the assembly modulates the neutral lipids dynamic exchanges at the molecular level. Cryo-EM coupled with MD simulations have revealed several important mechanisms of CETP-mediated lipid exchange and metabolism with all-atom detail [89, 95]. Further researches could pay more attention to simultaneously monitor the dynamic structural change of lipoproteins and the dynamic mechanism of lipid transfer, especially the internal motivation of physical mechanism during the process of lipid transport.

Acknowledgements

Project supported by the National Natural Science Foundation of China under Grant No. 11374237, 11504287, 11774279 and 11774280, Fundamental Research Funds for the Central Universities (xjj2017029), China Postdoctoral Science Foundation (2017 M613147) and Shaanxi Province Postdoctoral Science Foundation (2017).

Author details

Zhiwei Yang[1,2,3], Dongxiao Hao[1], Yizhuo Che[1], Lei Zhang[1] and Shengli Zhang[1*]

*Address all correspondence to: zhangsl@xjtu.edu.cn

1 Department of Applied Physics, School of Science, Xi'an Jiaotong University, Xi'an, Shaanxi, China

2 Department of Applied Chemistry, School of Science, Xi'an Jiaotong University, Xi'an, China

3 School of Life Science and Technology, Xi'an Jiaotong University, Xi'an, China

References

[1] Yamashita T et al. Anti-inflammatory and immune-modulatory therapies for preventing atherosclerotic cardiovascular disease. Journal of Cardiology. 2015;**66**(1):1

[2] Chistiakov DA et al. Mechanisms of foam cell formation in atherosclerosis. Journal of Molecular Medicine. 2017;**95**(11):1153-1165

[3] Lusis AJ, Pajukanta P. A treasure trove for lipoprotein biology. Nature Genetics. 2008; **40**(2):129-130

[4] Fredrickson DS, Levy RI, Lees RS. Fat transport in lipoproteins--an integrated approach to mechanisms and disorders. Nutrition Reviews. 1967;**276**(1):34

[5] Kannel WB et al. Risk factors in coronary HEART disease. An evaluation of several serum lipids as predictors of coronary heart disease; the Framingham study. Annals of Internal Medicine. 1964;**61**(1):888-899

[6] Glomset JA et al. Role of plasma lecithin: Cholesterol acyltransferase in the metabolism of high density lipoproteins. Journal of Lipid Research. 1966;**7**(5):638

[7] Kingwell BA et al. HDL-targeted therapies: Progress, failures and future. Nature Reviews. Drug Discovery. 2014;**13**(6):445-464

[8] Tatami R et al. Intermediate-density lipoprotein and cholesterol-rich very low density lipoprotein in angiographically determined coronary artery disease. Circulation. 1981; **64**(6):1174-1184

[9] Superko HR, Nejedly M, Garrett B. Small LDL and its clinical importance as a new CAD risk factor: A female case study. Progress in Cardiovascular Nursing. 2002;**17**(4):167-173

[10] Bilheimer DW, Eisenberg S, Levy RI. The metabolism of very low density lipoprotein proteins I. Preliminary in vitro and in vivo observations. Biochimica et Biophysica Acta (BBA)-Lipids and Lipid Metabolism. 1972;**260**(2):212-221

[11] Eisenberg S, Bilheimer DW, Levy RI. The metabolism of very low density lipoprotein proteins: II. Studies on the transfer of apoproteins between plasma lipoproteins. Biochimica et Biophysica Acta (BBA)-Lipids and Lipid Metabolism. 1972;**280**(1):94-104

[12] Lusis AJ. Atherosclerosis. Nature. 2000;**407**(6801):233

[13] Parks JS, Chung S, Shelness GS. Hepatic ABC transporters and triglyceride metabolism. Current Opinion in Lipidology. 2012;**23**(3):196

[14] Rousset X et al. Lecithin: Cholesterol acyltransferase: From biochemistry to role in cardio-vascular disease. Current Opinion in Endocrinology, Diabetes, and Obesity. 2009;**16**(2):163

[15] Hoekstra M, Van Berkel TJ, Van Eck M. Scavenger receptor BI: A multi-purpose player in cholesterol and steroid metabolism. World Journal of Gastroenterology: WJG. 2010; **16**(47):5916

[16] Martinez LO et al. Ectopic β-chain of ATP synthase is an apolipoprotein AI receptor in hepatic HDL endocytosis. Nature. 2003;**421**(6918):75-79

[17] Fielding CJ, Fielding P. Molecular physiology of reverse cholesterol transport. Journal of Lipid Research. 1995;**36**(2):211-228

[18] Schaefer EJ, Anthanont P, Asztalos BF. High-density lipoprotein metabolism, composition, function, and deficiency. Current Opinion in Lipidology. 2014;**25**(3):194-199

[19] Barter PJ et al. Cholesteryl ester transfer protein – A novel target for raising HDL and inhibiting atherosclerosis. Arteriosclerosis Thrombosis & Vascular Biology. 2003;**23**(2): 160-167

[20] Qiu X et al. Crystal structure of cholesteryl ester transfer protein reveals a long tunnel and four bound lipid molecules. Nature Structural & Molecular Biology. 2007;**14**(2):106

[21] Badimon JJ, Badimon L, Fuster V. Regression of atherosclerotic lesions by high density lipoprotein plasma fraction in the cholesterol-fed rabbit. Journal of Clinical Investigation. 1990;**85**(4):1234

[22] Rubin EM et al. Inhibition of early atherogenesis in transgenic mice by human apolipoprotein AI. Nature. 1991;**353**(6341):265-267

[23] Tangirala RK et al. Regression of atherosclerosis induced by liver-directed gene transfer of apolipoprotein A-I in mice. Circulation. 1999;**100**(17):1816-1822

[24] Rosenson RS et al. Translation of high-density lipoprotein function into clinical practice. Circulation. 2013;**128**(11):1256-1267

[25] Rader DJ et al. The role of reverse cholesterol transport in animals and humans and relationship to atherosclerosis. Journal of Lipid Research. 2009;**50**(Supplement):S189-S194

[26] Lewis GF, Rader DJ. New insights into the regulation of HDL metabolism and reverse cholesterol transport. Circulation Research. 2005;**96**(12):1221-1232

[27] Borhani DW et al. Crystal structure of truncated human apolipoprotein AI suggests a lipid-bound conformation. Proceedings of the National Academy of Sciences. 1997;**94**(23): 12291-12296

[28] Brouillette CG et al. Structural models of human apolipoprotein AI: A critical analysis and review. Biochimica et Biophysica Acta (BBA)-Molecular and Cell Biology of Lipids. 2001;**1531**(1):4-46

[29] Rogers DP et al. Structural analysis of apolipoprotein AI: Effects of amino-and carboxy-terminal deletions on the lipid-free structure. Biochemistry. 1998;**37**(3):945-955

[30] Brouillette CG et al. Förster resonance energy transfer measurements are consistent with a helical bundle model for lipid-free apolipoprotein AI. Biochemistry. 2005;**44**(50): 16413-16425

[31] Borhani DW, Engler JA, Brouillette CG. Crystallization of truncated human apolipoprotein AI in a novel conformation. Acta Crystallographica Section D: Biological Crystallography. 1999;**55**(9):1578-1583

[32] Mei X, Atkinson D. Crystal structure of C-terminal truncated apolipoprotein AI reveals the assembly of high density lipoprotein (HDL) by dimerization. Journal of Biological Chemistry. 2011;**286**(44):38570-38582

[33] Chetty PS et al. Helical structure and stability in human apolipoprotein AI by hydrogen exchange and mass spectrometry. Proceedings of the National Academy of Sciences. 2009;**106**(45):19005-19010

[34] Chetty PS et al. Apolipoprotein AI helical structure and stability in discoidal high-density lipoprotein (HDL) particles by hydrogen exchange and mass spectrometry. Proceedings of the National Academy of Sciences. 2012;**109**(29):11687-11692

[35] Zannis VI, Chroni A, Krieger M. Role of apoA-I, ABCA1, LCAT, and SR-BI in the biogenesis of HDL. Journal of Molecular Medicine. 2006;**84**(4):276

[36] Ajees AA et al. Crystal structure of human apolipoprotein AI: Insights into its protective effect against cardiovascular diseases. Proceedings of the National Academy of Sciences of the United States of America. 2006;**103**(7):2126-2131

[37] Jonas A, Kézdy KE, Wald JH. Defined apolipoprotein A-I conformations in reconstituted high density lipoprotein discs. Journal of Biological Chemistry. 1989;**264**(9):4818-4824

[38] Jonas A et al. Reaction of discoidal complexes of apolipoprotein A-I and various phosphatidylcholines with lecithin cholesterol acyltransferase. Interfacial effects. Journal of Biological Chemistry. 1987;**262**(9):3969-3974

[39] Jonas A et al. Apolipoprotein A-I structure and lipid properties in homogeneous, reconstituted spherical and discoidal high density lipoproteins. Journal of Biological Chemistry. 1990;**265**(36):22123-22129

[40] Segrest JP et al. A detailed molecular belt model for apolipoprotein AI in discoidal high density lipoprotein. Journal of Biological Chemistry. 1999;**274**(45):31755-31758

[41] Koppaka V et al. The structure of human lipoprotein AI evidence for the "belt" model. Journal of Biological Chemistry. 1999;**274**(21):14541-14544

[42] Mishra VK et al. Association of a model class A (apolipoprotein) amphipathic α helical peptide with lipid high resolution NMR studies of peptide lipid discoidal complexes. Journal of Biological Chemistry. 2006;**281**(10):6511-6519

[43] Bhat S et al. Conformational adaptation of apolipoprotein AI to discretely sized phospholipid complexes. Biochemistry. 2007;**46**(26):7811-7821

[44] Martin DD et al. Apolipoprotein AI assumes a "looped belt" conformation on reconstituted high density lipoprotein. Journal of Biological Chemistry. 2006;**281**(29):20418-20426

[45] Wu Z et al. The refined structure of nascent HDL reveals a key functional domain for particle maturation and dysfunction. Nature Structural & Molecular Biology. 2007;**14**(9): 861-868

[46] Chetty PS et al. Comparison of apoA-I helical structure and stability in discoidal and spherical HDL particles by HX and mass spectrometry. Journal of Lipid Research. 2013; **54**(6):1589-1597

[47] Wu Z et al. Double superhelix model of high density lipoprotein. Journal of Biological Chemistry. 2009;**284**(52):36605-36619

[48] Jones MK et al. Assessment of the validity of the double superhelix model for reconstituted high density lipoproteins A combined computational-experimental approach. Journal of Biological Chemistry. 2010;**285**(52):41161-41171

[49] Zhang L et al. Morphology and structure of lipoproteins revealed by an optimized negative-staining protocol of electron microscopy. Journal of Lipid Research. 2011;**52**(1):175-184

[50] Murray SC et al. Direct measurement of the structure of reconstituted high-density lipoproteins by Cryo-EM. Biophysical Journal. 2016;**110**(4):810-816

[51] Bibow S et al. Solution structure of discoidal high-density lipoprotein particles with a shortened apolipoprotein AI. Nature Structural & Molecular Biology. 2017;**24**(2):187-193

[52] Segrest J et al. Surface density-induced pleating of a lipid monolayer drives nascent high-density lipoprotein assembly. Structure. 2015;**23**(7):1214-1226

[53] Silva RGD et al. Structure of apolipoprotein AI in spherical high density lipoproteins of different sizes. Proceedings of the National Academy of Sciences. 2008;**105**(34):12176-12181

[54] Gursky O. Crystal structure of Δ (185-243) apoA-I suggests a mechanistic framework for the protein adaptation to the changing lipid load in good cholesterol: From flatland to sphereland via double belt, belt buckle, double hairpin and trefoil/tetrafoil. Journal of Molecular Biology. 2013;**425**(1):1-16

[55] Wu Z et al. The low resolution structure of ApoA1 in spherical high density lipoprotein revealed by small angle neutron scattering. Journal of Biological Chemistry. 2011;**286**(14):12495-12508

[56] Huang R et al. Apolipoprotein AI structural organization in high-density lipoproteins isolated from human plasma. Nature Structural & Molecular Biology. 2011;**18**(4):416-422

[57] Segrest JP, Jones MK, Catte A. MD simulations suggest important surface differences between reconstituted and circulating spherical HDL. Journal of Lipid Research. 2013;**54**(10):2718-2732

[58] Goldstein JL, Brown MS. Low-density lipoprotein pathway and its relation to atherosclerosis. Annual Review of Biochemistry. 1977;**46**:897-930

[59] Vainio S, Ikonen E. Macrophage cholesterol transport: A critical player in foam cell formation. Annals of Medicine. 2003;**35**(3):146-155

[60] Born GV. New determinants of the uptake of atherogenic plasma proteins by arteries. Basic Research in Cardiology. 1994;**89**(Suppl 1(1)):103

[61] Proctor SD, Vine DF, Mamo JC. Arterial retention of apolipoprotein B48-and B100-containing lipoproteins in atherogenesis. Current Opinion in Lipidology. 2002;**13**(5):461-470

[62] Glass CK, Witztum JL. Atherosclerosis: The road ahead. Cell. 2001;**104**(4):503-516

[63] Kruth H. Macrophage foam cells and atherosclerosis. Frontiers in Bioscience: A Journal and Virtual Library. 2001;**6**:D429-D455

[64] Ross R. The pathogenesis of atherosclerosis (second of two parts). The New England Journal of Medicine. 1976;**295**:420-425

[65] Qiao J-H et al. Role of macrophage colony-stimulating factor in atherosclerosis: Studies of osteopetrotic mice. The American Journal of Pathology. 1997;**150**(5):1687

[66] Liu LK et al. Mulberry anthocyanin extracts inhibit LDL oxidation and macrophage-derived foam cell formation induced by oxidative LDL. Journal of Food Science. 2008;**73**(6)

[67] Prassl R, Laggner P. Molecular structure of low density lipoprotein: Current status and future challenges. European Biophysics Journal. 2008;**38**(2):145

[68] Chapman MJ, Guérin M, Bruckert E. Atherogenic, dense low-density lipoproteins. Pathophysiology and new therapeutic approaches. European Heart Journal. 1998;**19**:A24-A30

[69] Prassl R. Human low density lipoprotein: The mystery of core lipid packing. Journal of Lipid Research. 2011;**52**(2):187-188

[70] Galeano NF et al. Small dense low density lipoprotein has increased affinity for LDL receptor-independent cell surface binding sites: A potential mechanism for increased atherogenicity. Journal of Lipid Research. 1998;**39**(6):1263-1273

[71] Lundkatz S et al. Apolipoprotein B-100 conformation and particle surface charge in human LDL subspecies: Implication for LDL receptor interaction. Biochemistry. 1998;**37**(37):12867-12874

[72] Deckelbaum RJ et al. Thermal transitions in human plasma low density lipoproteins. Science. 1975;**190**(4212):392-394

[73] Pownall HJ et al. Effect of saturated and polyunsaturated fat diets on the composition and structure of human low density lipoproteins. Atherosclerosis. 1980;**36**(3):299-314

[74] Pregetter M et al. Microphase separation in low density lipoproteins. Journal of Biological Chemistry. 1999:**274**

[75] Baumstark MW et al. Structure of human low-density lipoprotein subfractions determined by X-ray small-angle scattering. Biochimica et Biophysica Acta. 1990;**1037**(1):48-57

[76] Spin JM, Atkinson D. Cryoelectron microscopy of low density lipoprotein in vitreous ice. Biophysical Journal. 1995;**68**(5):2115-2123

[77] Orlova EV et al. Three-dimensional structure of low density lipoproteins by electron cryomicroscopy. Proceedings of the National Academy of Sciences of the United States of America. 1999;**96**(15):8420-8425

[78] Sherman MB et al. Structure of triglyceride-rich human low-density lipoproteins according to cryoelectron microscopy. Biochemistry. 2003;**42**(50):14988-14993

[79] Segrest JP et al. Structure of apolipoprotein B-100 in low density lipoproteins. Journal of Lipid Research. 2001;**42**(9):1346

[80] Kumar V et al. Three-dimensional cryoEM reconstruction of native LDL particles to 16Å resolution at physiological body temperature. PLoS One. 2011;**6**(5):e18841

[81] Vauhkonen M, Somerharju P. Parinaroyl and pyrenyl phospholipids as probes for the lipid surface layer of human low density lipoproteins. Biochimica et Biophysica Acta. 1989;**984**(1):81-87

[82] Ren G et al. Model of human low-density lipoprotein and bound receptor based on CryoEM. Proceedings of the National Academy of Sciences of the United States of America. 2010;**107**(3):1059-1064

[83] Morehouse LA et al. Inhibition of CETP activity by torcetrapib reduces susceptibility to diet-induced atherosclerosis in New Zealand white rabbits. Journal of Lipid Research. 2007;**48**(6):1263-1272

[84] Rennings AJ, Stalenhoef A. JTT-705: Is there still future for a CETP inhibitor after torcetrapib? Expert Opinion on Investigational Drugs. 2008;**17**(10):1589

[85] Xie L et al. Drug discovery using chemical systems biology: Identification of the protein-ligand binding network to explain the side effects of CETP inhibitors. PLoS Computational Biology. 2009;**5**(5):e1000387

[86] Clark RW et al. Description of the torcetrapib series of cholesteryl ester transfer protein inhibitors, including mechanism of action. Journal of Lipid Research. 2006;**47**(3): 537-552

[87] Ranalletta M et al. Biochemical characterization of cholesteryl ester transfer protein inhibitors. Journal of Lipid Research. 2010;**51**(9):2739-2752

[88] Nicholls SJ et al. Assessment of the clinical effects of cholesteryl ester transfer protein inhibition with evacetrapib in patients at high-risk for vascular outcomes: Rationale and design of the ACCELERATE trial. American Heart Journal. 2015;**170**(6):1061-1069

[89] Zhang L et al. Structural basis of transfer between lipoproteins by cholesteryl ester transfer protein. Nature Chemical Biology. 2012;**8**(4):342-349

[90] Zhang L et al. An optimized negative-staining protocol of electron microscopy for apoE4 center dot POPC lipoprotein. Journal of Lipid Research. 2010;**51**(5):1228-1236

[91] Cilpakarhu G, Jauhiainen M, Riekkola ML. Atomistic MD simulation reveals the mechanism by which CETP penetrates into HDL enabling lipid transfer from HDL to CETP. Journal of Lipid Research. 2015;**56**(1):98-108

[92] Lei D et al. Structural features of cholesteryl ester transfer protein: A molecular dynamics simulation study. Proteins Structure Function & Bioinformatics. 2013;**81**(3):415-425

[93] Lei D et al. Insights into the tunnel mechanism of cholesteryl Ester transfer protein through all-atom molecular dynamics simulations. Journal of Biological Chemistry. 2016; **291**(27):14034-14044

[94] Lauer ME et al. Cholesteryl ester transfer between lipoproteins does not require a ternary tunnel complex with CETP. Journal of Structural Biology. 2016;**194**(2):191-198

[95] Zhang M et al. HDL surface lipids mediate CETP binding as revealed by electron microscopy and molecular dynamics simulation. Scientific Reports. 2015;**5**:8741

3

Cholesterol-Lowering Drugs and Therapies in Cardiovascular Disease

Zaid Almarzooq and Parmanand Singh

Abstract

Dyslipidemia is a major risk factor for cardiovascular disease (CVD). The relationship between low-density lipoprotein concentration and cardiovascular (CV) risk has been well established in numerous epidemiological studies. The benefit of cholesterol-lowering agents has been demonstrated in patients with known CVD. On the other hand, in patients without known CVD the decision to start therapy depends on their 10-year risk prediction of CV events. 3-Hydroxy-3-methylglutaryl-coenzyme A (HMG-CoA) reductase inhibitors ("statins"), a mainstay of cholesterol-lowering therapy, have been shown to reduce both CV events and all-cause mortality. Other lipid-lowering measures (both pharmacological and nonpharmacological) have also been demonstrated in clinical trials to reduce CV outcomes. In this chapter, we review contemporary therapies used to treat dyslipidemia and discuss future directions including novel agents on the horizon.

Keywords: cholesterol treatment, cardiovascular disease, dyslipidemia, cardiovascular risk stratification, hypercholesterolemia

1. Introduction

Atherosclerotic cardiovascular disease (CVD) affects more than 15 million Americans and is considered the leading cause of death in the United States (US) in both men and women (REF). Dyslipidemia is a major risk factor for atherosclerotic CVD [1]. We review current standard treatment of abnormal cholesterol levels and discuss future directions. Lipid-altering therapies favorably impact the lipid profile by lowering total cholesterol, low-density lipoprotein (LDL), and triglycerides (TGs), while beneficially increasing high-density lipoprotein (HDL; see **Table**

1) [2–4]. In addition, lipid-altering therapies cause a desirable shift toward less atherogenic cholesterol subparticles [5]. The benefit of lipid therapy has been borne out in studies evaluating their effects on coronary atherosclerosis regression (by angiography) and incidence of major adverse cardiovascular events (MACEs) [6–10]. The lipoprotein transport system mediates the movement of cholesterol and TG in plasma, in addition to numerous other important physiologic functions. These include transport of dietary fat absorbed in the intestines to the liver, transport of modified cholesterol to peripheral tissues for cell membrane and steroid hormone synthesis, and transport of free fatty acids that may be used for fuel [11]. Lipoproteins are typically classified by their size and density. The main lipoprotein carriers of cholesterol to peripheral tissues are LDL particles. They are internalized by LDL receptors, where they are then hydrolyzed. This is an important pathway in controlling plasma cholesterol levels, as evidenced in those with loss-of-function mutations of LDL receptors leading to an inherited hyperlipidemia [12]. Importantly, LDL particles vary in size. Those with fewer cholesteryl esters and more TGs are smaller, denser, and thus more atherogenic [11].

Drug class	LDL (%)	HDL (%)	TG (%)
Bile acid sequestrants	↓ 15–30	↑ 3–5	No change
Cholesterol absorption inhibitors (Ezetimibe)	↓ 17–22	↑ 2–5	↓ 4–11
Fibrates	↓ 5–20	↑ 10–20	↓ 20–50
Nicotinic acid (niacin)	↓ 5–25	↑ 15–35	↓ 20–50
PCSK9 inhibitors	↓ 61–62	↑ 5–7	↓ 13–17
HMG-CoA reductase inhibitors (Statins)	↓ 18–55	↑ 5–15	↓ 7–30

Abbreviations: LDL, low-density lipoprotein cholesterol; HDL, high-density lipoprotein; TC, total cholesterol; TG, triglycerides.

Table 1. Potencies of various lipid lowering agents.

Increased concentrations of LDL have been shown in epidemiological studies to be associated with an increased risk of MACE. This was demonstrated in The Lipid Research Clinics Prevalence Study, where after 10 years of follow-up in patients with known coronary heart disease (CHD), a higher death rate was evident in those with higher levels of plasma total cholesterol and LDL [13]. In addition, those with inherited hyperlipidemia have early athero-thrombosis [14]. Reducing LDL cholesterol is strongly linked to reductions in MACE, especially when using statins [10]. One-third of all middle-aged or older adults in the general population of the US and United Kingdom (UK) have an indication for statin therapy [15]. Notably decreased LDL and raising HDL levels have been associated with regression of atherosclerosis as evident in the Regression Growth Evaluation Statin Study (REGRESS) trial and several other trials [6–9].

Until recently, it was strongly recommended to treat to specific LDL targets [16]. These targets were based on post hoc analyses demonstrating greater reductions in MACE with LDL levels below certain levels. However, subsequent head-to-head statin trials compared different agents at different doses. These studies did not investigate the effects of different LDL target levels [17]. For such reasons, the most recent US guidelines advocate for using high-intensity statins for patients at high risk of cardiovascular events. By contrast, guidelines in Europe and Canada have maintained their recommendation on using LDL targets [18].

Statins are well known for pleotropic effects independent of cholesterol lowering, mainly anti-inflammatory properties [19]. In many statin trials, subjects with the largest reduction in high-sensitivity C-reactive protein (hsCRP) have decreased primary end points [20, 21]. In two statin trials, lower hsCRP and LDL levels were associated with a decrease in atheroma progression as assessed by serial intravascular ultrasound observation [22, 23]. Moreover, in the Justification for the Use of Statins in Prevention (JUPITER) trial, a decrease in MACE and all-cause mortality was seen in asymptomatic subjects with baseline elevated hsCRP levels and already low LDL level, which contemporary risk calculators would exclude from therapy. Notably, elevated LDL cholesterol is associated with MACE without the need for overt evidence of inflammation [24] .

1.1. Cardiovascular risk stratification: Who to treat?

In patients with known CVD, treatment with statins has been shown to reduce CV events and all-cause mortality, while other lipid-lowering agents have also been shown to reduce the incidence of CV events in patients not on statins [25–33]. However, in patients without known CVD, cholesterol-lowering agents have only been shown to be beneficial in those at a high risk of CV events. The absolute benefit of treatment is proportional to the underlying absolute CV risk. Therefore, it is important to target patients at a high risk of CV events rather than a specific LDL.

Various CV risk calculators have been used to identify patients at high risk. These calculators are modeled to a particular population; therefore, the choice of which risk calculator to use is important. Below, we will discuss the benefits and pitfalls of using risk calculators to guide decision to treat. The Framingham Risk score is a risk calculator based on a population from the northeastern US (https://www.framinghamheartstudy.org/risk-functions/cardiovascular-disease/10-year-risk.php#). The most current version includes major CV outcomes, stroke, and heart failure. Notably, statins have shown to reduce the incidence of major CV outcomes and stroke, but not heart failure [34]. The American Heart Association/American College of Cardiology (AHA/ACC) Pooled Cohort Equations Cardiovascular risk calculator (ASCVD) is based on a population of non-Hispanic whites and African Americans in the US (http://tools.acc.org/ASCVD-Risk-Estimator/). Compared to the Framingham risk calculator, it predicts major CV outcomes that are reduced by statins. Limitations of the ASCVD include its dichotomization of diabetes mellitus without considering its duration or type. It also does not take into account family history of premature CV disease, thus underestimating CV risk in those with significant family history of CV events [35].

The Joint British Societies (JBS-3) guidelines calculator is based on a population from the UK (http://www.jbs3risk.com/JBS3Risk.swf). In those with a low 10-year risk of CV events, the JBS-3 recommends using the QRISK® lifetime CV risk calculator [36]. Both the ASCVD and

JBS-3 predict both 10-year risk and lifetime risk of CV events. Without the data with long-term effects of statins, there is a limitation to use lifetime risk prediction for using cholesterol-lowering agents. Therefore, the use of the 10-year risk predictions has been recommended when making such decisions. In patient with diabetes, the UK Prospective Diabetes Study calculator incorporates factors important to those with diabetics that are not found in the ASCVD calculator such as diabetes duration and type [37].

Another factor used when making the decision to treat on a population-based approach is cost-effectiveness. The 2013 AHA/ACC guidelines have recommended the use of a 10-year risk of CV events threshold of 7.5% when deciding to use cholesterol-lowering agents. This was found to be more cost-effective when compared with ≥10% threshold [38].

In older patients, over age 65, the decision to treat is also influenced by the presence of other comorbidities not taken into account in the calculators above. For example, a patient with a concurrent illness with high mortality, such as metastatic pancreatic cancer, is unlikely to benefit from a cholesterol-lowering agent. Thus, clinical trials of cholesterol-lowering agents have typically excluded older patients. However, a healthy elderly patient may potentially benefit from these therapies, and in fact the absolute number to treat is much lower in a healthy elderly population, given the dramatic increase in absolute risk of CV disease in this cohort [39]. A barrier to using cholesterol-lowering agents in the elderly has been the notion that it takes years to see the benefit of cholesterol-lowering agents; however, many studies have shown that they can be beneficial in as early as 6 months, as seen in the 4S trial [40].

2. Pharmacological therapies

2.1. Statins

Statins have been shown to be beneficial in hypercholesterolemia for both primary and secondary prevention of CV events (see **Figure 1**) [41]. Their main mechanism of action involves competitive inhibition of an enzyme, 3-Hydroxy-3-methylglutaryl-coenzyme A (HMG-CoA) reductase, a rate-limiting step in cholesterol synthesis (see **Figure 2**) [42, 43]. This prevents substrate from binding to the enzymatic active site resulting in a decrease in intra-hepatic cholesterol synthesis [44]. The decrease in intrahepatic cholesterol leads to an increase in LDL receptors, and consequently an increase in LDL reuptake [45]. Other mechanisms described include alteration of hepatic Apolipoprotein B (Apo-B) secretion leading to a reduction in very low-density lipoprotein (VLDL) through decreased secretion and increased clearance. This consequently also contributes to the reduction in plasma TG [46]. Statins' effect on HDL has been attributed to their impact on hepatic microRNA33 (miR33) and consequent macrophage ATP-binding cassette transporter (ABCA)1-mediated efflux [47]. These additional mechanisms are thought to translate into clinical benefit through varied pathways including reversal of endothelial dysfunction, atheroma stabilization, and decreased thrombogenicity [48].

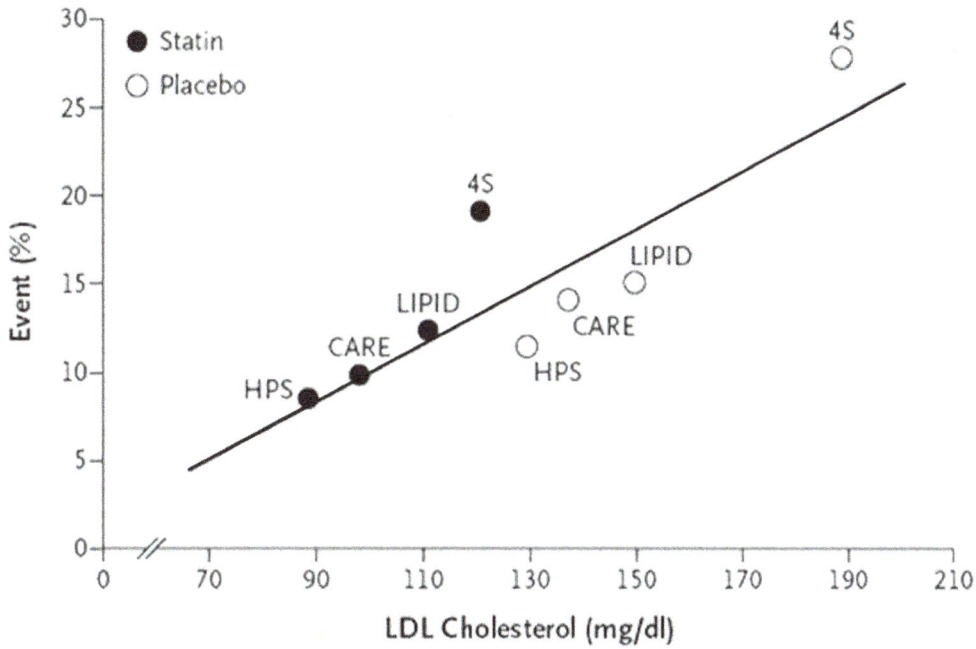

Figure 1. LDL, statins, and cardiovascular events. Reduction in cardiovascular event rates by lower low-density lipoprotein using statins in secondary prevention trials. *Abbreviations*: 4S, Scandinavian Simvastatin Survival Study; CARE, Cholesterol and Recurrent Events Trial; HPS, Heart Protection Study; LIPID, Long-term Intervention with Pravastatin in Ischemic Disease.

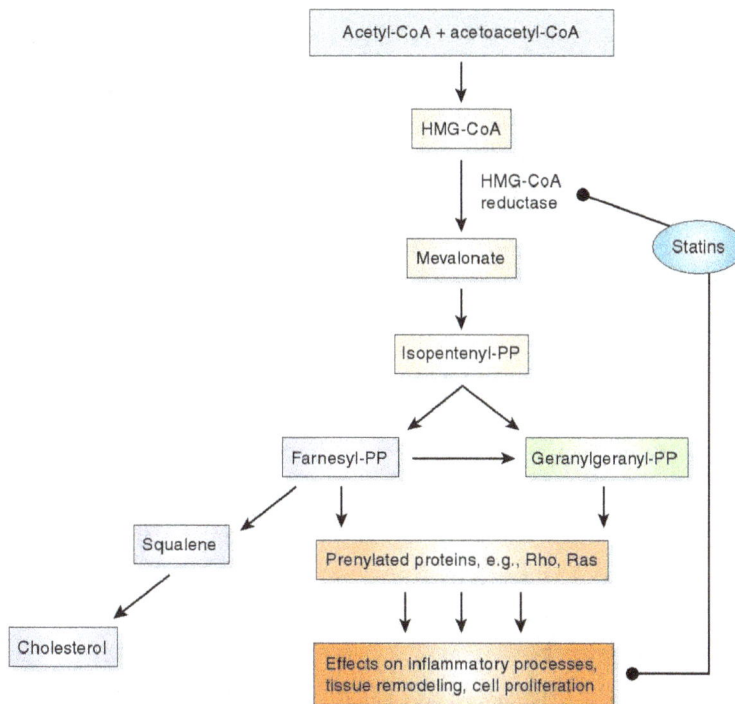

Figure 2. Mechanisms of HMG-CoA reductase inhibitors. Statins inhibit hepatic HMG-CoA reductase resulting in decreased downstream cholesterol production.

Statins are considered the most potent agents for lowering LDL cholesterol, and do so up to 63% [49]. They do have a predominant effect on small LDL particles leading to a shift in the LDL subfractions toward less atherogenic LDL [50]. Rosuvastatin has been shown to increase HDL by about 10%, appearing to be the most effective statins on HDL modification [51]. Regarding lowering TG, atorvastatin and rosuvastatin appear to be the most potent of the statins, with a dose-dependent decrease in TG of up to 33% [51].

Statins as a drug category demonstrate varying cholesterol-lowering potencies (see **Table 2**) [51–53]. Low-potency statins include simvastatin, lovastatin, pravastatin, and fluvastatin [51]. High-potency statins include atorvastatin and rosuvastatin [51]. Statins combined with a cholesterol absorption inhibitor (such as ezetimibe) or bile acid sequestrant show an additive cholesterol-lowering effect [54, 55].

Statin	TC (%)	LDL (%)	HDL (%)	TG (%)	Dose range (mg)
Atorvastatin	↓ 27–39	↓ 37–51	↑ 2–6	↓ 20–28	10–80
Rosuvastatin	↓ 33–40	↓ 46–55	↑ 8–10	↓ 20–26	10–40
Simvastatin	↓ 20–28	↓ 28–39	↑ 5–6	↓ 12–15	10–40
Pravastatin	↓ 15–22	↓ 20–30	↑ 3–6	↓ 8–13	10–40
Fluvastatin	↓ 13–19	↓ 17–23	↑ 1–3	↓ 5–13	20–80
Pitavastatin	↓ 22–31	↓ 31–44	↑ 1–4	↓ 13–22	1–4

Abbreviations: NNT, number needed to treat; WOSCOPS, West of Scotland Coronary Prevention Study; AFCAPS/ TEXCAPS, Air Force/Texas Coronary Atherosclerosis Prevention Study; ALLHAT-LLT, Antihypertensive and Lipid-Lowering Treatment to Prevent Heart Attack Trial; CARDS, Collaborative Atorvastatin Diabetes Study; MEGA, Management of Elevated Cholesterol in the Primary Prevention Group of Adult Japanese; JUPITER, Justification for the Use of statins in Prevention: an Intervention Trial Evaluating Rosuvastatin; 4S, Scandinavian Simvastatin Survival Study; CARE, Cholesterol and Recurrent Events trial; LIPID, Long-Term Intervention with Pravastatin in Ischemic Disease study;. HPS, Heart Protection Study; PROSPER, Prospective Study of Pravastatin in the Elderly at Risk; PROVE-IT, Pravastatin or Atorvastatin Evaluation and Infection Therapy; TNT, Treating to New Targets; IDEAL, Incremental Decrease in End Points through Aggressive Lipid Lowering.

Table 2. Potencies of different statins.

Numerous clinical trials have shown a trend toward improved CV outcomes, but not all have demonstrated statistical significance [56]. Statins have been shown to be effective in primary prevention of CHD (see **Table 3**) 21, 25–28, 32, 41, 57–63]. This was demonstrated in the Heart Protection Study [25], CARDS trial [26], and MEGA trial [27], where statins led to a significant reduction in MACE. Statins have also been shown to be effective in the secondary prevention of CHD as well (see **Table 3**). This benefit was evident in the Scandinavian Simvastatin Survival study (4S) [28], Lipid trial [29], and MIRACLE [30], where statin use resulted in a significant reduction in MACE. In a meta-analysis, which included 17,617 patients randomized to statins from the Cholesterol and Recurrent Events (CARE), Long-term Intervention with Pravastatin in Ischemic Disease (LIPID), and 4S trials, there was a significant reduction in MACE and all-cause mortality, but no effect on noncardiovascular mortality [31]. In addition, high-dose statin therapy was shown to have a significant reduction in MACE when compared to lower-dose therapy, as seen in the Treating to New Target (TNT) trial [41] and PROVE IT-TIMI 22 trial [32].

Study	Year	Patients	Statin and daily dose	Mean baseline LDL (mg/dL)	Mean LDL reduction (%)	Reduction in coronary events (%)	NNT
Primary prevention							
WOSCOPS	1995	6595	Pravastatin 40 mg	192	26	31 (P < 0.001)	42
AFCAPS/ TEXCAPS	1998	6605	Lovastatin 20–40 mg	150	25	37 (P < 0.001)	24
ALLHAT-LLT	2002	10,355	Pravastatin 40 mg	146	28	No significant reduction	
CARDS	2004	2838	Atorvastatin 10 mg	118	40	36 (P = 0.001)	32
MEGA	2006	7832	Pravastatin 10–20 mg	156	18	33 (P = 0.01)	119
JUPITER	2008	17,802	Rosuvastatin 20 mg	108	50	44 (P <0.001)	25
Secondary prevention							
4S	1994	4444	Simvastatin 20–40 mg	188	35	34 (P < 0.0001)	15
CARE	1998	4159	Pravastatin 40 mg	139	32	24 (P = 0.003)	33
LIPID	2002	9014	Pravastatin 40 mg	150	25	24 (P < 0.0001)	33
HPS	2002	20,536	Simvastatin 40 mg	3.4	1	24 (P <0.001)	20
PROSPER	2002	5804	Pravastatin 40 mg	147	34	14(P = 0.014)	47
PROVE-IT	2004	4162	Atorvastatin 80 mg versus Pravastatin 40 mg	106	41	16 (P = 0.005)	25
TNT	2005	10,003	Atorvastatin 80 mg versus Atorvastatin 10 mg	97	21	22 (P <0.001)	46
IDEAL	2005	8888	Atorvastatin 80 mg versus Simvastatin 20 mg	121	34	No significant reduction	

Table 3. Primary and secondary prevention statin trials.

The most important side effects associated with statins are hepatic injury and myopathy [64, 65]. The risk of liver injury with the use of statins appears to be dose dependent and is most likely to occur in the first 3 months. This risk was demonstrated in a meta-analysis of 35 randomized trials that showed an excess risk of 4.2 cases per 1000 patients associated with statin use [66]. Multiple mechanisms of liver injury have been demonstrated with statins including hepatocellular and cholestatic [67]. Among the different statins, the risk of liver injury appears to be similar, except with fluvastatin that has a higher risk [68]. Numerous studies have found no significant difference in elevated aminotransferases when statins were compared to placebo [25, 28, 57]. It was for this reason that the Food and Drug Administration

(FDA) revised the recommendation for liver function testing with regard to statin therapy in 2012 [69]. In the setting of rising aminotransferases three times the upper limit of normal, it is recommended to lower the statin dose or change medication.

Statin muscle injury remains the most concerning side effect, despite severe myopathy occurring in only 0.1–0.5% of patients [70, 71]. The degree of injury ranges from myalgia, myopathy, myositis, myonecrosis, to rhabdomyolysis [65]. Rhabdomyolysis, the most severe of the statin myopathy spectrum, was largely seen when statins were used with gemfibrozil or cyclosporine [72, 73]. This is thought to be related to the decrease in mevalonic acid associated with HMG-CoA reductase inhibition. Other mechanisms attributed to muscle injury include statins' effects on coenzyme Q10, also called ubiquinone, which is involved in muscle energy production [74]. Different statins possess varying risk to cause muscle injury, with fluvastatin exhibiting the lowest risk and simvastatin exhibiting a higher risk of muscle injury, especially at 80 mg/day dose, as shown in the SEARCH trial that was the basis of the FDA restriction of this dose of simvastatin [64, 70, 75]. The major predisposing factor for statin-induced myopathy injury includes hypothyroidism, obstructive liver disease, and renal failure; these contribute to both hypercholesterolemia and myopathy. Thus, it is important to test for thyroid-stimulating hormone (TSH) levels prior to starting statins [76].

Other notable side effects include proteinuria that has been reported to the Food and Drug Administration with rosuvastatin and simvastatin, but no increased risk of renal failure has been described [77–79]. In addition, there have been several meta-analyses of randomized trials that found a small, yet increased risk of diabetes with high-dose statin therapy when compared to lower-dose statin therapies, possibly related directly to its inhibition of HMG-CoA reductase [80]. However, given that statins have been shown to reduce CV events in diabetics, these studies have suggested that the beneficial effects of statins on CV events outweigh this risk [80, 81].

Despite physicians in practice witnessing the discontinuation of statins due to "intolerance," randomized control trials have failed to validate this finding. The difference between clinical practice and trials may relate to selection bias observed in clinical trials that limit their external validity [66, 82]. Intolerance is largely seen on the basis of muscle pain, leading to discontinuation of therapy. Another cause of intolerance is a rise in aminotransferases, which usually requires statins dose reduction, switch to another statin, or using an alternate drug. In patients, who are unable to tolerate statins, ezetimibe, fenofibrate, cholestyramine, and niacin have been recommended for those with known coronary heart disease (CHD) or at high-risk CV events (10-year risk >20%) [33]. Another option is the recently FDA-approved proprotein convertase subtilisin kexin type 9 (PCSK9) inhibitors.

2.2. PCSK9 inhibitors

PCSK9 is a serine protease that is mainly secreted by the liver in an inactive form, before undergoing catalytic changes in the endoplasmic reticulum. The mature PCSK9 is then released into the plasma where it has only one substrate, LDL receptors. Once in circulation, it regulates the LDL receptor recycling in the liver, intestines, pancreas, lungs, kidneys, and adipose tissue [83, 84]. PCSK9 binding to LDL receptors causes it to be internalized into endosomal or lysosomal compartments, where they are destroyed. This leads to a decrease in LDL receptors on the surface of the cell. It has therefore been shown that serum PCSK9 levels are inversely proportional to the number of LDL receptors (see **Figure 3**) [85, 86]. Blood levels of PCSK9 are influenced by the diurnal trend in secretion (peak levels at 4 am), gender (higher in females), and fasting states (lower levels) [87, 88]. A mutation in PCSK9 was first described in French families in 2003. It is the third gene implicated in the autosomal dominant familial hypercholesterolemia (FH); the other two genes encode LDL receptor and Apo-B, a component of the LDL particle [89]. It is usually a gain-of-function mutation in PCSK9 that results in a low level of LDL receptors leading to a high level of LDL and consequently increased risk of premature CV disease [90, 91]. On the other hand, loss-of-function PCSK9 mutations result in high level of LDL receptors, and a decrease in LDL and significant reduction in CV events. Of note, the reduction of CV events observed with PCSK9 mutation is higher than that associated with statins. This difference is attributed to the persistently low LDL levels caused by the underlying genetic predisposition. This was demonstrated in the ARIC study, Copenhagen Heart Study, and the Zimbabwe population study [92–94].

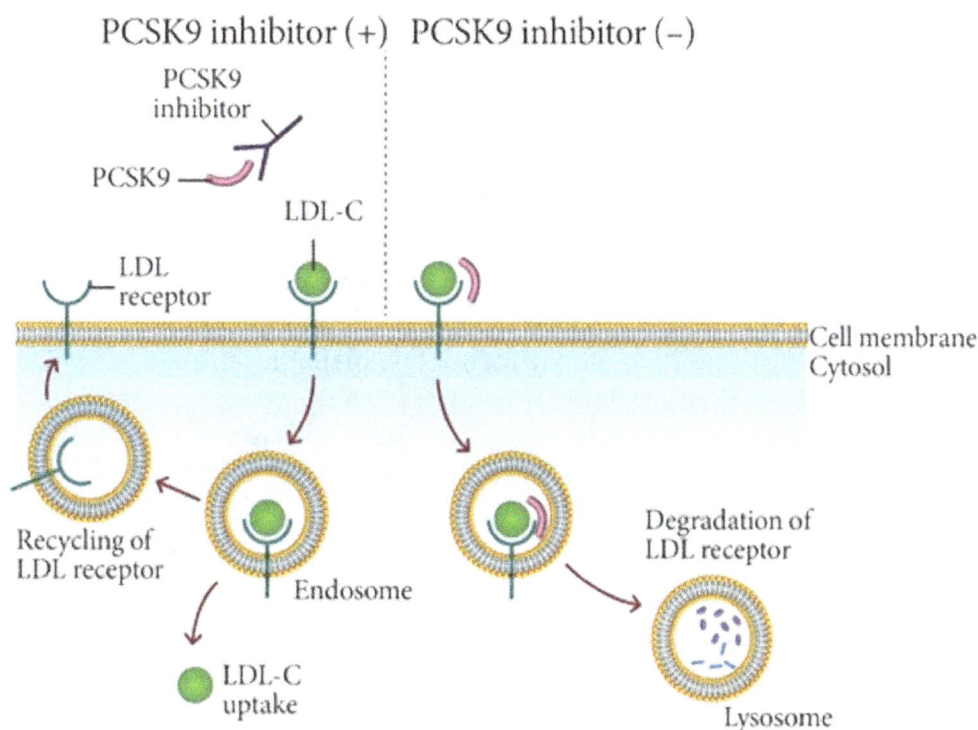

Figure 3. Mechanisms of PCSK9 inhibitors. Secreted PCSK9 binds to LDL receptors on the cell surface and forms an endosome that undergoes lysosomal degradation. In the presence of PCSK9 inhibitors, the interaction between PCSK9 and LDL receptors is disrupted, resulting in the recycling of LDL receptors and increased hepatic uptake of LDL from the bloodstream. *Abbreviations*: LDL, low-density lipoprotein cholesterol; PCSK9, proprotein convertase subtilisin kexin 9.

Statins have been described to increase the concentration of PCSK9 inhibitors by 14–47% in a dose- and time-dependent fashion. This is via a decrease in endogenous cholesterol synthesis caused by statin inhibition of HMG-CoA reductase with consequent up-regulation in LDL receptors. It has therefore been demonstrated that a PCSK9 mutation increases the response to statins [95–98]. Neutralizing antibodies to PCSK9 were first described in 2009, and in subsequent studies it was shown to decrease LDL levels by 30% in animal models [99].

Although statins are the most effective cholesterol-lowering agents for preventing CV events, there is a need for additional therapies in those patients who are (1) unable to take statins or (2) already on maximal statin doses with residual CV risk. The National Lipid Association in the US estimates that about 12% of patients discontinue statin therapy, of whom 62% experienced adverse effects [100]. These data signal the need for alternative effective agents, such as PCSK9 inhibitors, to be used with or instead of statins. As monotherapy, PCSK9 inhibitors lower LDL by up to approximately 66% [101]. In conjunction with statins, PCSK9 inhibitors reduce LDL by an additional 60% beyond statins [102]. Examples of monoclonal antibody PCSK9 inhibitors available in the market include evolocumab and alirocumab. Phase I, II, and III clinical trials have shown an additional decrease in LDL levels with the use of PCSK-9 inhibitors (monoclonal antibodies) in combination with statin therapy, as well as a significant decrease in CV events including mortality (hazard ratio (HR): 0.47–0.52) [2, 3]. Other PCSK9 inhibitors include the small interfering RNA (siRNA) molecules that block the synthesis of PCSK9 inhibitors and have been shown to decrease LDL by 40% in a phase I clinical trial when used at the highest dose compared to placebo [103].

Regarding their side effects, there were no significant differences in the incidence of adverse drug events between PCSK9 inhibitors (alirocumab, evolocumab) and placebo in the latest phase III trials, except for neurocognitive events, myalgia, injection site reactions, and ophthalmologic events [2, 3]. A major concern with PCSK9 inhibitors revolves around their cost and the very low LDL levels achieved (as low as 18 mg/dL compared to 44 mg/dL with rosuvastatin in the JUPITER study). Potential short- and long-term consequences of very low LDL levels include neurocognitive impairment, hemorrhagic stroke, hemolytic anemia, vitamin, and hormonal deficiencies [21, 104].

2.3. Ezetimibe

Ezetimibe inhibits the intestinal absorption of dietary and biliary cholesterol without affecting the absorption of fat-soluble vitamins or TG [105]. This possibly occurs by the inhibition of Niemann-Pick C1-like 1 (NPC1L1) protein function that is expressed in the intestines and liver [106]. The benefits of ezetimibe were demonstrated in the IMPROVE-IT trial where the addition of ezetimibe to statin therapy led to a decrease in CV events, excluding all-cause and CV mortality [54]. Ezetimibe is helpful in avoiding high doses of statin and the associated dose-dependent statin side effects, especially in patients who do not meet cholesterol targets. It has been well tolerated with the incidence of myopathy and serum transaminase elevations being similar when compared to placebo [54].

2.4. Bile acid sequestrants

Bile acid sequestrants, such as cholestyramine, colesevelam, and colestipol, lower cholesterol by binding to bile acids in the intestine preventing them from being reabsorbed [107]. The consequent decrease in intrahepatic cholesterol leads to an increase in LDL receptors that bind LDL from plasma with consequent small increase in HDL via increased intestinal synthesis of HDL [108]. They are relatively potent and exhibit a dose-dependent response achieving 10–25% reduction in LDL, exhibiting a synergistic effect when used with statins or niacin [55, 109, 110].

Major side effects have limited its overall use. Those described include abdominal discomfort with nausea, bloating, cramping, and rise in aminotransferases. Of the bile acid sequestrants, colesevelam is the better-tolerated drug. They also interact with common CV medications (warfarin and digoxin) by binding and inhibiting their absorption. This can be avoided by administering the other medications 1 h before or 4 h after ingestion of bile acid sequestrants [107].

2.5. Fibrates

Fibrates include gemfibrozil and fenofibrate [111]. The mechanism of action of fibrates is via activation of transcription factor, peroxisome proliferator-activated receptors (PPARs). It decreases TG via reduction in hepatic VLDL secretion, and stimulation of lipoprotein lipase that consequently leads to increased clearance of TG-rich lipoproteins. It also raises HDL by direct stimulation of HDL Apolipoprotein A-I/A-II synthesis and increased transfer of Apo A-I from HDL to VLDL [112].

This class of drugs lowers serum TG by 35–50%, and have also been shown to increase HDL by 5–20% directly proportional to the degree of hypertriglyceridemia [113–115]. Fibrates have not demonstrated any significant effect on cardiovascular outcomes, as seen in the FIELD trial [115], except in those with high TG (>200 mg/dL) or low HDL (<40 mg/dL) and metabolic syndrome, as was seen in the BIP trial [116].

The main side effect associated with fibrates is muscle injury. Muscle injury is often seen in patients who are already on a statin, and is thought to be mediated by fibrate-related inhibition of CYP3A4 with consequent decrease in statin metabolism [117]. Fibrates have also been shown to raise serum creatinine levels, but it remains unknown if there is direct parenchymal or tubular renal injury. Nevertheless, elevated creatinine has been found to be reversible on discontinuation of the medication, as was demonstrated in the FIELD trial [118]. Another noteworthy side effect is pancreatitis, which has been seen in patients with normal TG. However, the absolute risk remains low (number needed to harm over 5 years = 935) [119].

2.6. Nicotinic acid (niacin)

Nicotinic acid acts by inhibiting the hepatic production of VLDL and consequently decreasing LDL. It also increases HDL by reducing lipid transfer from HDL to VLDL, thus delaying HDL clearance [120]. This class of drugs has positive effects on HDL that occurs at relatively low dosages (1–1.5 g/day result in about 33% increase in HDL). Higher nicotinic acid doses are needed to lower LDL (3 g/day results in about 23% LDL decrease) [121, 122]. This class of drugs is also associated with a significant reduction of MACE in the HATS trial and ARBITER 6-HALTS trial when niacin was added to statin therapy [123, 124]. Contrary to these studies, the

AIM-HIGH, ARBITER-2, and HPS2-THRIVE trials found no significant benefit of adding niacin to statin therapy [125–127].

Unfortunately, its use is limited by poor tolerability. The most common side effect is flushing, which occurs in the majority (up to 80%) of patients at standard recommended doses. Other notable side effects include paresthesia, pruritis, and nausea, each of which occurs in 20% of patients at standard doses [120].

3. Lifestyle modification

All patients with an elevated LDL should be advised to attempt and undergo for therapeutic lifestyle changes. Therapeutic lifestyle changes involve weight loss (even in those who are only slightly overweight), exercise, and improvement in diet. Numerous studies have investigated and demonstrated the benefits of lifestyle modification. In the United Kingdom Lipid Clinics Program study, 2508 subjects who underwent diet modification experienced a 5–7% reduction in serum total and LDL cholesterol [128]. In the Lifestyle Heart Trial, 53 patients were randomized to either control diet (National Cholesterol Education Program-NCEP step 2 diet) or vegetarian therapy with exercise and relaxation therapy (intervention group). After 5 years of follow-up, the intervention group demonstrated a decrease in CV events (0.89 vs 2.25 events per patient) [129]. In the Lyon Diet Heart Study, 605 patients were randomized after a first myocardial infarction to either a Mediterranean diet or a control diet. After 4 years of follow-up, the Mediterranean diet group demonstrated lower rates of death and myocardial infarction [130].

4. Other potential therapy options

Statins are the preferred therapy for most patients with dyslipidemia, especially those with elevated total cholesterol and LDL cholesterol. However, in patients on maximal tolerated statin dose with a persistently elevated LDL, other therapies may be considered. These include niacin, bile acid sequestrants, and ezetimibe. Not uncommonly, these additional agents may not be sufficient to "normalize" abnormal cholesterol profiles, especially in patients with severe hypercholesterolemia and familial cholesterol diseases. Therapeutic options in this group of patients, who remain "at risk" for CV events, include LDL apheresis, lomitapide, surgical options, and gene therapy. Preferably, this cohort of patients should be managed by a specialist.

4.1. LDL apheresis

LDL apheresis is a procedure that involves extracorporeal removal of circulating Apo B-containing lipoprotein (e.g., LDL, VLDL, and lipoprotein-a). Regimens include weekly or biweekly depending on the rate LDL returns to baseline after therapy [131].

The National Lipid Associated Expert Panel on familial hypercholesterolemia recommended LDL apheresis in those with FH if LDL targets are not achieved with maximal tolerated medical therapy. These targets include LDL of ≥300 mg/dL in those with functional homozygous or heterozygous FH, LDL of ≥200 mg/dL in those with functional heterozygous FH, and ≥2 risk factors or high lipoprotein-a (≥50 mg/dL), or LDL of ≥160 mg/dL in those established CAD, CV disease, or diabetes [132]. In the absence of statin therapy, LDL apheresis lowers LDL by 50–75% acutely, by 30% after 6 months, and 38% after 18 months [133]. There are numerous studies showing benefit in outcomes such as myocardial infarction and reduction in arterial inflammation, but none have shown a survival benefit [134, 135]. Limitations to using LDL apheresis include patient burden, problems related to venous access, frequent long visits, and high costs [136].

4.2. Lomitapide

Lomitapide is a microsomal TG transfer protein inhibitor which inhibits the transfer of TG to Apo-B for the production of VLDL in the liver. However, lomitapide is metabolized by CYP3A4 and is also an inhibitor of CYP 3A4 and P-glycoprotein leading to numerous drug interactions. It was FDA approved in 2012 for use in patients with homozygous FH. It is used in addition to standard therapy, as well as other therapies such as LDL apheresis or liver transplantation. It has been shown to significantly decrease LDL (up to 50%) in a phase 3, open-label, non-randomized, dose-escalating study [137].

4.3. Mipomersen

Mipomersen is an injected antisense oligonucleotide that inhibits the production of Apo-B. Mipomersen binds to the Apo-B mRNA, affects Apo-B production, and consequently reduces the levels of LDL, VLDL, and intermediate dense lipoprotein. It has been approved by FDA in 2013 for use in homozygous FH patients; however, it is not approved in Europe. It has been shown that mipomersen can significantly decrease LDL in those patients with homozygous FH (up to 25%) [138]. Similar findings were found in studies involving other populations, including those with heterozygous FH and have CAD, statin intolerant, and at high risk of CV disease, and in those without FH who have or are at high risk of CVD [139–143].

4.4. Cholesteryl ester transfer protein inhibitors

Cholesteryl ester transfer protein (CETP) inhibitors, such as anacetrapib, have shown to significantly increase in HDL and lower LDL; however, there are no studies showing clinical benefit. In fact, in the REALIZE trial, despite a significant reduction in LDL in the intervention group compared to placebo, there was a significant increase in CV events, hence limiting its clinical use [144].

4.5. Anti-resistin antibodies

Anti-resistin antibodies inhibit resistin function, an adipokine (protein derived from adipose tissue) that is increased in obese individuals and positively correlated with atherosclerosis. In *in vitro* studies, resistin can decrease LDL receptor expression and increase PCSK9 expression.

By using anti-resistin antibodies, studies have shown an increase in LDL receptors in obese individuals [145].

4.6. Small molecule regulator of lipid metabolism

ETC-1002 is a small molecule regulator of carbohydrate and lipid metabolism. In a study of 177 subjects with LDL between 130 and 220 mg/dL not on statin therapy, patients were randomized to ETC-1002 (one of three different doses) or placebo. After 12 weeks of follow-up, treated subjects at the highest dose demonstrated a 27% decrease in LDL. There were no changes in TG or HDL. ETC-1002 also demonstrated a limited side effect profile [146, 147].

4.7. Recombinant Apo-A-I milano

Apo-A-I milano is a variant of the Apolipoprotein A-I (Apo-A-I). This variant leads to rapid mobilization of cholesterol with rapid regression of atherosclerosis. Subjects with Apo-A-I Milano have very low levels of HDL (10–30 mg/dL), longer survival, and reduced atherosclerosis compared to what is expected for their HDL levels [148]. Infusion of recombinant Apo-A-I milano (ETC-216) in an RCT was shown to lead to a significant regression of coronary atherosclerosis [149].

4.8. Lipoprotein-associated phospholipase A_2

Lipoprotein-associated phospholipase A_2 is also known as platelet-activating factor acetylhydrolase. It is a protein with pro-inflammatory properties that co-travels with circulating LDL particles and is found abundantly in atherosclerotic plaques [150]. Lipoprotein-associated phospholipase A_2 has been shown in a meta-analysis to significantly increase CHD and is an independent predictor of CHD and ischemic stroke [151]. However, in a large phase III randomized control trial (STABILITY trial), the lipoprotein-associated phospholipase A_2 inhibitor, darapladib, failed to show any CV benefit [152].

5. Conclusion

Over the last several years, the role of cholesterol-lowering agents in reducing cardiovascular disease and mortality has been further established. Statin therapy remains the cornerstone of lipid-lowering therapy; however, in patients already on maximal dose of statins or intolerant to statins with residual CV risk, other options are also available. As evidenced by the recent bench to bedside development of a new drug class (PCSK9), the emergence of drugs to specifically target a population, in this case, familial hypercholesterolemia, the national call for precision medicine is on the horizon. By continuing to scientifically probe biologic mechanisms in preclinical models related to cholesterol perturbation, drug development and translation to human clinical studies marks a bright and promising future.

Author details

Zaid Almarzooq and Parmanand Singh*

*Address all correspondence to: pas9062@med.cornell.edu

Weill Cornell Medical College, New York Presbyterian Hospital, New York, NY, USA

References

[1] Go AS, Mozaffarian D, Roger VL, Benjamin EJ, Berry JD, Borden WB, et al. Heart disease and stroke statistics—2013 update: a report from the American Heart Association. Circulation. 2013;127(1):e6.

[2] Sabatine MS, Giugliano RP, Wiviott SD, Raal FJ, Blom DJ, Robinson J, et al. Efficacy and safety of evolocumab in reducing lipids and cardiovascular events. N Engl J Med. 2015;372(16):1500–9.

[3] Robinson JG, Farnier M, Krempf M, Bergeron J, Luc G, Averna M, et al. Efficacy and safety of alirocumab in reducing lipids and cardiovascular events. N Engl J Med. 2015;372(16):1489–99.

[4] Expert Panel on Detection E. Executive summary of the Third Report of the National Cholesterol Education Program (NCEP) expert panel on detection, evaluation, and treatment of high blood cholesterol in adults (Adult Treatment Panel III). JAMA. 2001;285(19):2486.

[5] Salonen R, Nyyssönen K, Porkkala-Sarataho E, Salonen JT. The Kuopio Atherosclerosis Prevention Study (KAPS): effect of pravastatin treatment on lipids, oxidation resistance of lipoproteins, and atherosclerotic progression. Am J Cardiol. 1995;76(9):34C–9C.

[6] Jukema JW, Bruschke AV, van Boven AJ, Reiber JH, Bal ET, Zwinderman AH, et al. Effects of lipid lowering by pravastatin on progression and regression of coronary artery disease in symptomatic men with normal to moderately elevated serum cholesterol levels. The Regression Growth Evaluation Statin Study (REGRESS). Circulation. 1995;91(10):2528–40.

[7] Schartl M, Bocksch W, Koschyk DH, Voelker W, Karsch KR, Kreuzer J, et al. Use of intravascular ultrasound to compare effects of different strategies of lipid-lowering therapy on plaque volume and composition in patients with coronary artery disease. Circulation. 2001;104(4):387–92.

[8] Nissen SE, Tuzcu EM, Schoenhagen P, Brown BG, Ganz P, Vogel RA, et al. Effect of intensive compared with moderate lipid-lowering therapy on progression of coronary atherosclerosis: a randomized controlled trial. JAMA. 2004;291(9):1071–80.

[9] Lee JM, Robson MD, Yu LM, Shirodaria CC, Cunnington C, Kylintireas I, et al. Effects of high-dose modified-release nicotinic acid on atherosclerosis and vascular function: a randomized, placebo-controlled, magnetic resonance imaging study. J Am Coll Cardiol. 2009;54(19):1787–94.

[10] Mihaylova B, Emberson J, Blackwell L, Keech A, Simes J, Barnes EH, et al. The effects of lowering LDL cholesterol with statin therapy in people at low risk of vascular disease: meta-analysis of individual data from 27 randomised trials. Lancet. 2012;380(9841):581–90.

[11] Genest J. Lipoprotein disorders and cardiovascular risk. J Inherit Metab Dis. 2003;26(2–3):267–87.

[12] Goldstein JL, Brown MS. The LDL receptor. Arterioscler Thromb Vasc Biol. 2009;29(4):431–8.

[13] Pekkanen J, Linn S, Heiss G, Suchindran CM, Leon A, Rifkind BM, et al. Ten-year mortality from cardiovascular disease in relation to cholesterol level among men with and without preexisting cardiovascular disease. N Engl J Med. 1990;322(24):1700–7.

[14] Collaboration PS. Blood cholesterol and vascular mortality by age, sex, and blood pressure: a meta-analysis of individual data from 61 prospective studies with 55 000 vascular deaths. Lancet. 2007;370(9602):1829–39.

[15] Pencina MJ, Navar-Boggan AM, D'Agostino RB, Sr., Williams K, Neely B, Sniderman AD, et al. Application of new cholesterol guidelines to a population-based sample. N Engl J Med. 2014;370(15):1422–31.

[16] Panel NCEPNE. Third Report of the National Cholesterol Education Program (NCEP) Expert Panel on Detection, Evaluation, and Treatment of High Blood Cholesterol in Adults (Adult Treatment Panel III) final report. Circulation. 2002;106(25):3143.

[17] Hayward RA, Krumholz HM. Three reasons to abandon low-density lipoprotein targets: an open letter to the Adult Treatment Panel IV of the National Institutes of Health. Circ Cardiovasc Qual Outcomes. 2012;5(1):2–5.

[18] Ray KK, Kastelein JJ, Boekholdt SM, Nicholls SJ, Khaw KT, Ballantyne CM, et al. The ACC/AHA 2013 guideline on the treatment of blood cholesterol to reduce atherosclerotic cardiovascular disease risk in adults: the good the bad and the uncertain: a comparison with ESC/EAS guidelines for the management of dyslipidaemias 2011. Eur Heart J. 2014;35(15):960–8.

[19] Bu DX, Griffin G, Lichtman AH. Mechanisms for the anti-inflammatory effects of statins. Curr Opin Lipidol. 2011;22(3):165–70.

[20] Glynn RJ, Koenig W, Nordestgaard BG, Shepherd J, Ridker PM. Rosuvastatin for primary prevention in older persons with elevated C-reactive protein and low to average low-density lipoprotein cholesterol levels: exploratory analysis of a randomized trial. Ann Intern Med. 2010;152(8):488–96, W174.

[21] Hsia J, MacFadyen JG, Monyak J, Ridker PM. Cardiovascular event reduction and adverse events among subjects attaining low-density lipoprotein cholesterol< 50 mg/dl with rosuvastatin: the JUPITER trial (Justification for the Use of Statins in Prevention: an Intervention Trial Evaluating Rosuvastatin). J Am Coll Cardiol. 2011;57(16):1666–75.

[22] Nissen SE, Tuzcu EM, Schoenhagen P, Crowe T, Sasiela WJ, Tsai J, et al. Statin therapy, LDL cholesterol, C-reactive protein, and coronary artery disease. N Engl J Med. 2005;352(1):29–38.

[23] Puri R, Nissen SE, Libby P, Shao M, Ballantyne CM, Barter PJ, et al. C-reactive protein, but not low-density lipoprotein cholesterol levels, associate with coronary atheroma regression and cardiovascular events following maximally intensive statin therapy. Circulation. 2013:CIRCULATIONAHA. 113.004243.

[24] Varbo A, Benn M, Tybjaerg-Hansen A, Nordestgaard BG. Elevated remnant cholesterol causes both low-grade inflammation and ischemic heart disease, whereas elevated low-density lipoprotein cholesterol causes ischemic heart disease without inflammation. Circulation. 2013;128(12):1298–309.

[25] Collins R, Armitage J, Parish S, Sleight P, Peto R, Collaboration HPS. MRC/BHF Heart Protection Study of cholesterol lowering with simvastatin in 20 536 high-risk individuals: a randomised placebo controlled trial. Lancet. 2002;360(9326):7–22.

[26] Colhoun HM, Betteridge DJ, Durrington PN, Hitman GA, Neil HA, Livingstone SJ, et al. Primary prevention of cardiovascular disease with atorvastatin in type 2 diabetes in the Collaborative Atorvastatin Diabetes Study (CARDS): multicentre randomised placebo-controlled trial. Lancet. 2004;364(9435):685–96.

[27] Nakamura H, Arakawa K, Itakura H, Kitabatake A, Goto Y, Toyota T, et al. Primary prevention of cardiovascular disease with pravastatin in Japan (MEGA Study): a prospective randomised controlled trial. Lancet. 2006;368(9542):1155–63.

[28] Group SSSS. Randomised trial of cholesterol lowering in 4444 patients with coronary heart disease: the Scandinavian Simvastatin Survival Study (4S). Lancet. 1994;344(8934):1383–9.

[29] Marschner IC, Colquhoun D, Simes RJ, Glasziou P, Harris P, Singh BB, et al. Long-term risk stratification for survivors of acute coronary syndromes. Results from the Long-term Intervention with Pravastatin in Ischemic Disease (LIPID) Study. LIPID Study Investigators. J Am Coll Cardiol. 2001;38(1):56–63.

[30] Schwartz GG, Olsson AG, Ezekowitz MD, Ganz P, Oliver MF, Waters D, et al. Effects of atorvastatin on early recurrent ischemic events in acute coronary syndromes: the MIRACL study: a randomized controlled trial. JAMA. 2001;285(13):1711–8.

[31] LaRosa JC, He J, Vupputuri S. Effect of statins on risk of coronary disease: a meta-analysis of randomized controlled trials. JAMA. 1999;282(24):2340–6.

[32] Cannon CP, Braunwald E, McCabe CH, Rader DJ, Rouleau JL, Belder R, et al. Intensive versus moderate lipid lowering with statins after acute coronary syndromes. N Engl J Med. 2004;350(15):1495–504.

[33] Navarese EP, Kolodziejczak M, Schulze V, Gurbel PA, Tantry U, Lin Y, et al. Effects of proprotein convertase subtilisin/kexin type 9 antibodies in adults with hypercholesterolemia: a systematic review and meta-analysis. Ann Intern Med. 2015;163(1):40–51.

[34] D'Agostino RB, Vasan RS, Pencina MJ, Wolf PA, Cobain M, Massaro JM, et al. General cardiovascular risk profile for use in primary care the Framingham Heart Study. Circulation. 2008;117(6):743–53.

[35] Muntner P, Colantonio LD, Cushman M, Goff DC, Jr., Howard G, Howard VJ, et al. Validation of the atherosclerotic cardiovascular disease pooled cohort risk equations. JAMA. 2014;311(14):1406–15.

[36] Board JBS. Joint British Societies' consensus recommendations for the prevention of cardiovascular disease (JBS3). Heart. 2014;100(Suppl 2):ii1–67.

[37] Stevens RJ, Kothari V, Adler AI, Stratton IM, United Kingdom Prospective Diabetes Study G. The UKPDS risk engine: a model for the risk of coronary heart disease in type II diabetes (UKPDS 56). Clin Sci (Lond). 2001;101(6):671–9.

[38] Pandya A, Sy S, Cho S, Weinstein MC, Gaziano TA. Cost-effectiveness of 10-year risk thresholds for initiation of statin therapy for primary prevention of cardiovascular disease. JAMA. 2015;314(2):142–50.

[39] Grundy SM, Cleeman JI, Rifkind BM, Kuller LH. Cholesterol lowering in the elderly population. Coordinating Committee of the National Cholesterol Education Program. Arch Intern Med. 1999;159(15):1670–8.

[40] Miettinen TA, Pyorala K, Olsson AG, Musliner TA, Cook TJ, Faergeman O, et al. Cholesterol-lowering therapy in women and elderly patients with myocardial infarction or angina pectoris: findings from the Scandinavian Simvastatin Survival Study (4S). Circulation. 1997;96(12):4211–8.

[41] LaRosa JC, Grundy SM, Waters DD, Shear C, Barter P, Fruchart JC, et al. Intensive lipid lowering with atorvastatin in patients with stable coronary disease. N Engl J Med. 2005;352(14):1425–35.

[42] Istvan ES, Deisenhofer J. Structural mechanism for statin inhibition of HMG-CoA reductase. Science. 2001;292(5519):1160–4.

[43] Haslinger-Löffler B. Multiple effects of HMG-CoA reductase inhibitors (statins) besides their lipid-lowering function. Kidney Int. 2008;74(5):553–5.

[44] Ness GC, Zhao Z, Lopez D. Inhibitors of cholesterol biosynthesis increase hepatic low-density lipoprotein receptor protein degradation. Arch Biochem Biophys. 1996;325(2): 242–8.

[45] Ness GC, Chambers CM, Lopez D. Atorvastatin action involves diminished recovery of hepatic HMG-CoA reductase activity. J Lipid Res. 1998;39(1):75–84.

[46] Arad Y, Ramakrishnan R, Ginsberg HN. Lovastatin therapy reduces low density lipoprotein ApoB levels in subjects with combined hyperlipidemia by reducing the production of ApoB-containing lipoproteins: implications for the pathophysiology of ApoB production. J Lipid Res. 1990;31(4):567–82.

[47] Niesor EJ, Schwartz GG, Perez A, Stauffer A, Durrwell A, Bucklar-Suchankova G, et al. Statin-induced decrease in ATP-binding cassette transporter A1 expression via microRNA33 induction may counteract cholesterol efflux to high-density lipoprotein. Cardiovasc Drugs Ther. 2015;29(1):7–14.

[48] Davignon J, Ganz P. Role of endothelial dysfunction in atherosclerosis. Circulation. 2004;109(23 Suppl 1):III27–32.

[49] Rosenson RS, Otvos JD, Hsia J. Effects of rosuvastatin and atorvastatin on LDL and HDL particle concentrations in patients with metabolic syndrome: a randomized, double-blind, controlled study. Diabetes Care. 2009;32(6):1087–91.

[50] Otvos JD, Shalaurova I, Freedman DS, Rosenson RS. Effects of pravastatin treatment on lipoprotein subclass profiles and particle size in the PLAC-I trial. Atherosclerosis. 2002;160(1):41–8.

[51] Jones PH, Davidson MH, Stein EA, Bays HE, McKenney JM, Miller E, et al. Comparison of the efficacy and safety of rosuvastatin versus atorvastatin, simvastatin, and pravastatin across doses (STELLAR* Trial). Am J Cardiol. 2003;92(2):152–60.

[52] Jones P, Kafonek S, Laurora I, Hunninghake D. Comparative dose efficacy study of atorvastatin versus simvastatin, pravastatin, lovastatin, and fluvastatin in patients with hypercholesterolemia (the CURVES study). Am J Cardiol. 1998;81(5): 582–7.

[53] Stender S, Budinski D, Gosho M, Hounslow N. Pitavastatin shows greater lipid-lowering efficacy over 12 weeks than pravastatin in elderly patients with primary hypercholesterolaemia or combined (mixed) dyslipidaemia. Eur J Preventive Cardiol. 2013;20(1):40–53.

[54] Cannon CP, Blazing MA, Giugliano RP, McCagg A, White JA, Theroux P, et al. Ezetimibe added to statin therapy after acute coronary syndromes. N Engl J Med. 2015;372(25): 2387–97.

[55] Knopp RH, Brown WV, Corder CN, Dobs AS, Dujovne CA, Goldberg AC, et al. Comparative efficacy and safety of pravastatin and cholestyramine alone and combined in patients with hypercholesterolemia. Arch Int Med. 1993;153(11): 1321–9.

[56] Salonen R, Nyyssonen K, Porkkala E, Rummukainen J, Belder R, Park JS, et al. Kuopio Atherosclerosis Prevention Study (KAPS). A population-based primary preventive trial

of the effect of LDL lowering on atherosclerotic progression in carotid and femoral arteries. Circulation. 1995;92(7):1758–64.

[57] Downs JR, Clearfield M, Weis S, Whitney E, Shapiro DR, Beere PA, et al. Primary prevention of acute coronary events with lovastatin in men and women with average cholesterol levels: results of AFCAPS/TexCAPS. Air Force/Texas Coronary Atherosclerosis Prevention Study. JAMA. 1998;279(20):1615–22.

[58] Pedersen TR, Faergeman O, Kastelein JJ, Olsson AG, Tikkanen MJ, Holme I, et al. High-dose atorvastatin vs usual-dose simvastatin for secondary prevention after myocardial infarction: the IDEAL study: a randomized controlled trial. JAMA. 2005;294(19):2437–45.

[59] Shepherd J, Blauw GJ, Murphy MB, Bollen ELEM, Buckley BM, Cobbe SM, et al. Pravastatin in elderly individuals at risk of vascular disease (PROSPER): a randomised controlled trial. Lancet. 2002;360(9346):1623–30.

[60] Group WS. Baseline characteristics and screening experience in the West of Scotland Coronary Prevention Study. Am J Cardiol. 1995;76:485–91.

[61] Furberg CD, Wright JT, Davis BR, Cutler JA, Alderman M, Black H, et al. Major outcomes in moderately hypercholesterolemic, hypertensive patients randomized to pravastatin vs usual care—the antihypertensive and lipid-lowering treatment to prevent heart attack trial (ALLHAT-LLT). JAMA—J Am Med Assoc. 2002;288(23):2998–3007.

[62] Lewis SJ, Moye LA, Sacks FM, Johnstone DE, Timmis G, Mitchell J, et al. Effect of pravastatin on cardiovascular events in older patients with myocardial infarction and cholesterol levels in the average range. Results of the Cholesterol and Recurrent Events (CARE) trial. Ann Intern Med. 1998;129(9):681–9.

[63] Group LS. Long-term effectiveness and safety of pravastatin in 9014 patients with coronary heart disease and average cholesterol concentrations: the LIPID trial follow-up. The Lancet. 2002;359(9315):1379–87.

[64] Stroes ES, Thompson PD, Corsini A, Vladutiu GD, Raal FJ, Ray KK, et al. Statin-associated muscle symptoms: impact on statin therapy-European Atherosclerosis Society Consensus Panel Statement on Assessment, Aetiology and Management. Eur Heart J. 2015;36(17):1012–22.

[65] Rosenson RS, Baker SK, Jacobson TA, Kopecky SL, Parker BA, The National Lipid Association's Muscle Safety Expert P. An assessment by the Statin Muscle Safety Task Force: 2014 update. J Clin Lipidol. 2014;8(3 Suppl):S58–71.

[66] Kashani A, Phillips CO, Foody JM, Wang Y, Mangalmurti S, Ko DT, et al. Risks associated with statin therapy: a systematic overview of randomized clinical trials. Circulation. 2006;114(25):2788–97.

[67] Russo MW, Hoofnagle JH, Gu J, Fontana RJ, Barnhart H, Kleiner DE, et al. Spectrum of statin hepatotoxicity: experience of the drug-induced liver injury network. Hepatology. 2014;60(2):679–86.

[68] Hippisley-Cox J, Coupland C. Unintended effects of statins in men and women in England and Wales: population based cohort study using the QResearch database. BMJ. 2010;340:c2197.

[69] Marcum ZA, Vande Griend JP, Linnebur SA. FDA drug safety communications: a narrative review and clinical considerations for older adults. Am J Geriatr Pharmacother. 2012;10(4):264–71.

[70] Graham DJ, Staffa JA, Shatin D, Andrade SE, Schech SD, La Grenade L, et al. Incidence of hospitalized rhabdomyolysis in patients treated with lipid-lowering drugs. JAMA. 2004;292(21):2585–90.

[71] Dujovne CA, Chremos AN, Pool JL, Schnaper H, Bradford RH, Shear CL, et al. Expanded clinical evaluation of lovastatin (EXCEL) study results: IV. Additional perspectives on the tolerability of lovastatin. Am J Med. 1991;91(1B):25S–30S.

[72] Norman DJ, Illingworth DR, Munson J, Hosenpud J. Myolysis and acute renal failure in a heart-transplant recipient receiving lovastatin. N Engl J Med. 1988;318(1):46–7.

[73] Pierce LR, Wysowski DK, Gross TP. Myopathy and rhabdomyolysis associated with lovastatin-gemfibrozil combination therapy. JAMA. 1990;264(1):71–5.

[74] Rundek T, Naini A, Sacco R, Coates K, DiMauro S. Atorvastatin decreases the coenzyme Q10 level in the blood of patients at risk for cardiovascular disease and stroke. Arch Neurol. 2004;61(6):889–92.

[75] Armitage J, Bowman L, Wallendszus K, Bulbulia R, Rahimi K, Haynes R, et al. Intensive lowering of LDL cholesterol with 80 mg versus 20 mg simvastatin daily in 12 064 survivors of myocardial infarction: a double-blind randomised trial. Lancet. 2010;376(9753):1658–69.

[76] Bar SL, Holmes DT, Frohlich J. Asymptomatic hypothyroidism and statin-induced myopathy. Can Fam Phys. 2007;53(3):428–31.

[77] Howard W. The issue of statin safety: where do we stand? Grundy SM (University of Texas Southwestern Med Ctr, Dallas) Circulation 111:301 (6–9), 2005. Year Book Endocrinol. 2006 2006:126–7.

[78] Jacobson TA. Statin safety: lessons from new drug applications for marketed statins. Am J Cardiol. 2006;97(8A):44C–51C.

[79] Alsheikh-Ali AA, Ambrose MS, Kuvin JT, Karas RH. The safety of rosuvastatin as used in common clinical practice: a postmarketing analysis. Circulation. 2005;111(23):3051–7.

[80] Swerdlow DI, Preiss D, Kuchenbaecker KB, Holmes MV, Engmann JE, Shah T, et al. HMG-coenzyme A reductase inhibition, type 2 diabetes, and bodyweight: evidence from genetic analysis and randomised trials. Lancet. 2015;385(9965):351–61.

[81] Preiss D, Seshasai SR, Welsh P, Murphy SA, Ho JE, Waters DD, et al. Risk of incident diabetes with intensive-dose compared with moderate-dose statin therapy: a meta-analysis. JAMA. 2011;305(24):2556–64.

[82] Armitage J. The safety of statins in clinical practice. Lancet. 2007;370(9601):1781–90.

[83] Benjannet S, Rhainds D, Essalmani R, Mayne J, Wickham L, Jin W, et al. NARC-1/PCSK9 and its natural mutants: zymogen cleavage and effects on the low density lipoprotein (LDL) receptor and LDL cholesterol. J Biol Chem. 2004;279(47):48865–75.

[84] Seidah NG, Benjannet S, Wickham L, Marcinkiewicz J, Jasmin SB, Stifani S, et al. The secretory proprotein convertase neural apoptosis-regulated convertase 1 (NARC-1): liver regeneration and neuronal differentiation. Proc Natl Acad Sci USA. 2003;100(3): 928–33.

[85] Alborn WE, Cao G, Careskey HE, Qian YW, Subramaniam DR, Davies J, et al. Serum proprotein convertase subtilisin kexin type 9 is correlated directly with serum LDL cholesterol. Clin Chem. 2007;53(10):1814–9.

[86] Ahn CH, Choi SH. New drugs for treating dyslipidemia: beyond statins. Diabetes Metab J. 2015;39(2):87–94.

[87] Cui Q, Ju X, Yang T, Zhang M, Tang W, Chen Q, et al. Serum PCSK9 is associated with multiple metabolic factors in a large Han Chinese population. Atherosclerosis. 2010;213(2):632–6.

[88] Persson L, Cao G, Stahle L, Sjoberg BG, Troutt JS, Konrad RJ, et al. Circulating proprotein convertase subtilisin kexin type 9 has a diurnal rhythm synchronous with cholesterol synthesis and is reduced by fasting in humans. Arterioscler Thromb Vasc Biol. 2010;30(12):2666–72.

[89] Abifadel M, Varret M, Rabes JP, Allard D, Ouguerram K, Devillers M, et al. Mutations in PCSK9 cause autosomal dominant hypercholesterolemia. Nat Genet. 2003;34(2):154–6.

[90] Maxwell KN, Breslow JL. Proprotein convertase subtilisin kexin 9: the third locus implicated in autosomal dominant hypercholesterolemia. Curr Opin Lipidol. 2005;16(2):167–72.

[91] Humphries SE, Whittall RA, Hubbart CS, Maplebeck S, Cooper JA, Soutar AK, et al. Genetic causes of familial hypercholesterolaemia in patients in the UK: relation to plasma lipid levels and coronary heart disease risk. J Med Genet. 2006;43(12):943–9.

[92] Cohen JC, Boerwinkle E, Mosley TH, Jr., Hobbs HH. Sequence variations in PCSK9, low LDL, and protection against coronary heart disease. N Engl J Med. 2006;354(12):1264–72.

[93] Benn M, Nordestgaard BG, Grande P, Schnohr P, Tybjaerg-Hansen A. PCSK9 R46L, low-density lipoprotein cholesterol levels, and risk of ischemic heart disease: 3 independent studies and meta-analyses. J Am Coll Cardiol. 2010;55(25):2833–42.

[94] Hooper AJ, Marais AD, Tanyanyiwa DM, Burnett JR. The C679X mutation in PCSK9 is present and lowers blood cholesterol in a Southern African population. Atherosclerosis. 2007;193(2):445–8.

[95] Brown MS, Goldstein JL. A proteolytic pathway that controls the cholesterol content of membranes, cells, and blood. Proc Natl Acad Sci USA. 1999;96(20):11041–8.

[96] Dubuc G, Chamberland A, Wassef H, Davignon J, Seidah NG, Bernier L, et al. Statins upregulate PCSK9, the gene encoding the proprotein convertase neural apoptosis-regulated convertase-1 implicated in familial hypercholesterolemia. Arterioscler Thromb Vasc Biol. 2004;24(8):1454–9.

[97] Nohturfft A, DeBose-Boyd RA, Scheek S, Goldstein JL, Brown MS. Sterols regulate cycling of SREBP cleavage-activating protein (SCAP) between endoplasmic reticulum and Golgi. Proc Natl Acad Sci USA. 1999;96(20):11235–40.

[98] Berge KE, Ose L, Leren TP. Missense mutations in the PCSK9 gene are associated with hypocholesterolemia and possibly increased response to statin therapy. Arterioscler Thromb Vasc Biol. 2006;26(5):1094–100.

[99] Chan JC, Piper DE, Cao Q, Liu D, King C, Wang W, et al. A proprotein convertase subtilisin/kexin type 9 neutralizing antibody reduces serum cholesterol in mice and nonhuman primates. Proc Natl Acad Sci USA. 2009;106(24):9820–5.

[100] Toth PP, Harper CR, Jacobson TA. Clinical characterization and molecular mechanisms of statin myopathy. Expert Rev Cardiovasc Ther. 2008;6(7):955–69.

[101] Raal FJ, Stein EA, Dufour R, Turner T, Civeira F, Burgess L, et al. PCSK9 inhibition with evolocumab (AMG 145) in heterozygous familial hypercholesterolaemia (RUTHER-FORD-2): a randomised, double-blind, placebo-controlled trial. Lancet. 2015;385(9965): 331–40.

[102] Roth EM, McKenney JM, Hanotin C, Asset G, Stein EA. Atorvastatin with or without an antibody to PCSK9 in primary hypercholesterolemia. N Engl J Med. 2012;367(20): 1891–900.

[103] Fitzgerald K, Frank-Kamenetsky M, Shulga-Morskaya S, Liebow A, Bettencourt BR, Sutherland JE, et al. Effect of an RNA interference drug on the synthesis of proprotein convertase subtilisin/kexin type 9 (PCSK9) and the concentration of serum LDL cholesterol in healthy volunteers: a randomised, single-blind, placebo-controlled, phase 1 trial. Lancet. 2014;383(9911):60–8.

[104] LaRosa JC, Pedersen TR, Somaratne R, Wasserman SM. Safety and effect of very low levels of low-density lipoprotein cholesterol on cardiovascular events. Am J Cardiol. 2013;111(8):1221–9.

[105] Sudhop T, Lutjohann D, Kodal A, Igel M, Tribble DL, Shah S, et al. Inhibition of intestinal cholesterol absorption by ezetimibe in humans. Circulation. 2002;106(15):1943–8.

[106] Altmann SW, Davis HR, Jr., Zhu LJ, Yao X, Hoos LM, Tetzloff G, et al. Niemann-Pick C1 Like 1 protein is critical for intestinal cholesterol absorption. Science. 2004;303(5661): 1201–4.

[107] Davidson MH, Dillon MA, Gordon B, Jones P, Samuels J, Weiss S, et al. Colesevelam hydrochloride (cholestagel): a new, potent bile acid sequestrant associated with a low incidence of gastrointestinal side effects. Arch Intern Med. 1999;159(16):1893–900.

[108] Shepherd J, Packard CJ, Morgan HG, Third JL, Stewart JM, Lawrie TD. The effects of cholestyramine on high density lipoprotein metabolism. Atherosclerosis. 1979;33(4): 433–44.

[109] Insull W, Toth P, Mullican W, Hunninghake D, Burke S, Donovan JM, et al., editors. Effectiveness of colesevelam hydrochloride in decreasing LDL cholesterol in patients with primary hypercholesterolemia: a 24-week randomized controlled trial. Mayo Clinic Proceedings; 2001: Elsevier.

[110] Brown G, Albers JJ, Fisher LD, Schaefer SM, Lin JT, Kaplan C, et al. Regression of coronary artery disease as a result of intensive lipid-lowering therapy in men with high levels of Apolipoprotein B. N Engl J Med. 1990;323(19):1289–98.

[111] Oliver MF, Heady JA, Morris JN, Cooper MJ. Who cooperative trial on primary prevention of ischemic-heart-disease with clofibrate to lower serum-cholesterol—final mortality follow-up. Lancet. 1984;2(8403):600–4.

[112] Staels B, Dallongeville J, Auwerx J, Schoonjans K, Leitersdorf E, Fruchart JC. Mechanism of action of fibrates on lipid and lipoprotein metabolism. Circulation. 1998;98(19): 2088–93.

[113] Birjmohun RS, Hutten BA, Kastelein JJ, Stroes ES. Efficacy and safety of high-density lipoprotein cholesterol-increasing compounds: a meta-analysis of randomized controlled trials. J Am Coll Cardiol. 2005;45(2):185–97.

[114] Rubins HB, Robins SJ, Collins D, Fye CL, Anderson JW, Elam MB, et al. Gemfibrozil for the secondary prevention of coronary heart disease in men with low levels of high-density lipoprotein cholesterol. Veterans Affairs High-Density Lipoprotein Cholesterol Intervention Trial Study Group. N Engl J Med. 1999;341(6):410–8.

[115] Investigators FS. Effects of long-term fenofibrate therapy on cardiovascular events in 9795 people with type 2 diabetes mellitus (the FIELD study): randomised controlled trial. The Lancet. 2005;366(9500):1849–61.

[116] Group BS. Secondary prevention by raising HDL cholesterol and reducing triglycerides in patients with coronary artery disease the bezafibrate infarction prevention (BIP) study. Circulation. 2000;102(1):21–7.

[117] Athyros VG, Papageorgiou AA, Hatzikonstandinou HA, Didangelos TP, Carina MV, Kranitsas DF, et al. Safety and efficacy of long-term statin-fibrate combinations in patients with refractory familial combined hyperlipidemia. Am J Cardiol. 1997;80(5): 608–13.

[118] Davis TM, Ting R, Best JD, Donoghoe MW, Drury PL, Sullivan DR, et al. Effects of fenofibrate on renal function in patients with type 2 diabetes mellitus: the fenofibrate intervention and event lowering in diabetes (FIELD) study. Diabetologia. 2011;54(2): 280–90.

[119] Preiss D, Tikkanen MJ, Welsh P, Ford I, Lovato LC, Elam MB, et al. Lipid-modifying therapies and risk of pancreatitis: a meta-analysis. JAMA. 2012;308(8):804–11.

[120] Illingworth DR, Stein EA, Mitchel YB, Dujovne CA, Frost PH, Knopp RH, et al. Comparative effects of lovastatin and niacin in primary hypercholesterolemia. A prospective trial. Arch Intern Med. 1994;154(14):1586–95.

[121] Probstfield JL, Hunninghake DB. Nicotinic-acid as a lipoprotein-altering agent— therapy directed by the primary physician. Arch Int Med. 1994;154(14):1557–9.

[122] Grundy SM, Mok HY, Zech L, Berman M. Influence of nicotinic acid on metabolism of cholesterol and triglycerides in man. J Lipid Res. 1981;22(1):24–36.

[123] Zhao XQ, Morse JS, Dowdy AA, Heise N, DeAngelis D, Frohlich J, et al. Safety and tolerability of simvastatin plus niacin in patients with coronary artery disease and low high-density lipoprotein cholesterol (The HDL Atherosclerosis Treatment Study). Am J Cardiol. 2004;93(3):307–12.

[124] Villines TC, Stanek EJ, Devine PJ, Turco M, Miller M, Weissman NJ, et al. The ARBITER 6-HALTS Trial (arterial biology for the investigation of the treatment effects of reducing cholesterol 6-HDL and LDL treatment strategies in atherosclerosis): final results and the impact of medication adherence, dose, and treatment duration. J Am Coll Cardiol. 2010;55(24):2721–6.

[125] Investigators A-H, Boden WE, Probstfield JL, Anderson T, Chaitman BR, Desvignes-Nickens P, et al. Niacin in patients with low HDL cholesterol levels receiving intensive statin therapy. N Engl J Med. 2011;365(24):2255–67.

[126] Taylor AJ, Sullenberger LE, Lee HJ, Lee JK, Grace KA. Arterial biology for the investigation of the treatment effects of reducing cholesterol (ARBITER) 2: a double-blind, placebo-controlled study of extended-release niacin on atherosclerosis progression in secondary prevention patients treated with statins. Circulation. 2004;110(23):3512–7.

[127] Group H-TC. Effects of extended-release niacin with laropiprant in high-risk patients. N Engl J Med. 2014;371(3):203.

[128] Butowski PF, Winder AF. Usual care dietary practice, achievement and implications for medication in the management of hypercholesterolaemia. Data from the U.K. Lipid Clinics Programme. Eur Heart J. 1998;19(9):1328–33.

[129] Ornish D, Scherwitz LW, Billings JH, Brown SE, Gould KL, Merritt TA, et al. Intensive lifestyle changes for reversal of coronary heart disease. JAMA. 1998;280(23):2001–7.

[130] Michel de Lorgeril M, Salen P, Martin J-L, Monjaud I, Delaye J, Mamelle N. Mediterranean diet, traditional risk factors, and the rate of cardiovascular complications after myocardial infarction. Heart Failure. 1999;11(6): 779–785.

[131] Thompson GR, Catapano A, Saheb S, Atassi-Dumont M, Barbir M, Eriksson M, et al. Severe hypercholesterolaemia: therapeutic goals and eligibility criteria for LDL apheresis in Europe. Curr Opin Lipidol. 2010;21(6):492–8.

[132] Ito MK, McGowan MP, Moriarty PM, National Lipid Association Expert Panel on Familial H. Management of familial hypercholesterolemias in adult patients: recommendations from the National Lipid Association Expert Panel on familial hypercholesterolemia. J Clin Lipidol. 2011;5(3 Suppl):S38–45.

[133] Hemphill LC. Familial hypercholesterolemia: current treatment options and patient selection for low-density lipoprotein apheresis. J Clin Lipidol. 2010;4(5):346–9.

[134] Mabuchi H, Koizumi J, Shimizu M, Kajinami K, Miyamoto S, Ueda K, et al. Long-term efficacy of low-density lipoprotein apheresis on coronary heart disease in familial hypercholesterolemia. Hokuriku-FH-LDL-Apheresis Study Group. Am J Cardiol. 1998;82(12):1489–95.

[135] van Wijk DF, Sjouke B, Figueroa A, Emami H, van der Valk FM, MacNabb MH, et al. Nonpharmacological lipoprotein apheresis reduces arterial inflammation in familial hypercholesterolemia. J Am Coll Cardiol. 2014;64(14):1418–26.

[136] Stefanutti C, Vivenzio A, Di Giacomo S, Mazzarella B, Bosco G, Berni A. Aorta and coronary angiographic follow-up of children with severe hypercholesterolemia treated with low-density lipoprotein apheresis. Transfusion. 2009;49(7):1461–70.

[137] Cuchel M, Meagher EA, du Toit Theron H, Blom DJ, Marais AD, Hegele RA, et al. Efficacy and safety of a microsomal triglyceride transfer protein inhibitor in patients with homozygous familial hypercholesterolaemia: a single-arm, open-label, phase 3 study. Lancet. 2013;381(9860):40–6.

[138] Raal FJ, Santos RD, Blom DJ, Marais AD, Charng MJ, Cromwell WC, et al. Mipomersen, an Apolipoprotein B synthesis inhibitor, for lowering of LDL cholesterol concentrations in patients with homozygous familial hypercholesterolaemia: a randomised, double-blind, placebo-controlled trial. Lancet. 2010;375(9719):998–1006.

[139] Kastelein JJ, Wedel MK, Baker BF, Su J, Bradley JD, Yu RZ, et al. Potent reduction of Apolipoprotein B and low-density lipoprotein cholesterol by short-term administration of an antisense inhibitor of Apolipoprotein B. Circulation. 2006;114(16):1729–35.

[140] Akdim F, Stroes ES, Sijbrands EJ, Tribble DL, Trip MD, Jukema JW, et al. Efficacy and safety of mipomersen, an antisense inhibitor of Apolipoprotein B, in hypercholesterolemic subjects receiving stable statin therapy. J Am Coll Cardiol. 2010;55(15):1611–8.

[141] Stein EA, Dufour R, Gagne C, Gaudet D, East C, Donovan JM, et al. Apolipoprotein B synthesis inhibition with mipomersen in heterozygous familial hypercholesterolemia: results of a randomized, double-blind, placebo controlled trial to assess efficacy and safety as add-on therapy in patients with coronary artery disease. Circulation. 2012;126(19):2283–92. doi: 10.1161/CIRCULATIONAHA.112.104125.

[142] Visser ME, Wagener G, Baker BF, Geary RS, Donovan JM, Beuers UH, et al. Mipomersen, an Apolipoprotein B synthesis inhibitor, lowers low-density lipoprotein cholesterol in high-risk statin-intolerant patients: a randomized, double-blind, placebo-controlled trial. Eur Heart J. 2012;33(9):1142–9.

[143] Thomas GS, Cromwell WC, Ali S, Chin W, Flaim JD, Davidson M. Mipomersen, an Apolipoprotein B synthesis inhibitor, reduces atherogenic lipoproteins in patients with severe hypercholesterolemia at high cardiovascular risk: a randomized, double-blind, placebo-controlled trial. J Am Coll Cardiol. 2013;62(23):2178–84.

[144] Kastelein JJP, Besseling J, Shah S, Bergeron J, Langslet G, Hovingh GK, et al. Anacetrapib as lipid-modifying therapy in patients with heterozygous familial hypercholesterolaemia (REALIZE): a randomised, double-blind, placebo-controlled, phase 3 study. Lancet. 2015;385(9983):2153–61.

[145] Tavori H, Fan D, Blakemore JL, Yancey PG, Ding L, Linton MF, et al. Serum proprotein convertase subtilisin/kexin type 9 and cell surface low-density lipoprotein receptor: evidence for a reciprocal regulation. Circulation. 2013;127(24):2403–13.

[146] Pinkosky SL, Filippov S, Srivastava RA, Hanselman JC, Bradshaw CD, Hurley TR, et al. AMP-activated protein kinase and ATP-citrate lyase are two distinct molecular targets for ETC-1002, a novel small molecule regulator of lipid and carbohydrate metabolism. J Lipid Res. 2013;54(1):134–51.

[147] Ballantyne CM, Davidson MH, Macdougall DE, Bays HE, Dicarlo LA, Rosenberg NL, et al. Efficacy and safety of a novel dual modulator of adenosine triphosphate-citrate lyase and adenosine monophosphate-activated protein kinase in patients with hypercholesterolemia: results of a multicenter, randomized, double-blind, placebo-controlled, parallel-group trial. J Am Coll Cardiol. 2013;62'13':1154–62.

[148] Sirtori CR, Calabresi L, Franceschini G, Baldassarre D, Amato M, Johansson J, et al. Cardiovascular status of carriers of the Apolipoprotein A-I milano mutant. The Limone sul Garda Study. Circulation. 2001;103(15):1949–54.

[149] Nissen SE, Tsunoda T, Tuzcu EM, Schoenhagen P, Cooper CJ, Yasin M, et al. Effect of recombinant ApoA-I Milano on coronary atherosclerosis in patients with acute coronary syndromes: a randomized controlled trial. JAMA. 2003;290(17):2292–300.

[150] Karabina SA, Ninio E. Plasma PAF-acetylhydrolase: an unfulfilled promise? Biochim Biophys Acta. 2006;1761(11):1351–8.

[151] Collaboration L-PS. Thompson A, Gao P, Orfei L, Watson S, Di Angelantonio E, Kaptoge S, et al. Lipoprotein-associated phospholipase A2 and risk of coronary disease, stroke, and mortality: collaborative analysis of 32 prospective studies. Lancet. 2010;375(9725): 1536–44.

[152] Investigators S, White HD, Held C, Stewart R, Tarka E, Brown R, et al. Darapladib for preventing ischemic events in stable coronary heart disease. N Engl J Med. 2014;370(18): 1702–11.

4

Hormonal Regulation of Cholesterol Homeostasis

Zhuo Mao, Jinghui Li and Weizhen Zhang

Abstract

Cholesterol homeostasis is tightly regulated by a group of endocrine hormones under physiological conditions. Hormonal dysregulation is often associated with disturbed cholesterol homeostasis, resulting in many clinical disorders including atherosclerosis, fatty liver and metabolic syndrome. Circulating hormones regulate cholesterol metabolism by altering levels of relative genes either through their interactions with nuclear receptors or by interfering with bile acid signaling pathways. A better understanding of hormonal regulation of cholesterol metabolism would improve our likelihood of identifying effective and selective targets for the intervention of disturbed cholesterol. In this review, we discuss selected hormones critical for the cholesterol balance, including thyroid hormone, sex hormones, growth hormone, glucagon and irisin. We focus our discussion on the most recent advance in clinical epidemiology, animal mechanistic studies and the clinical application.

Keywords: cholesterol, thyroid hormone, sex hormones, growth hormone, glucagon and irisin

1. Introduction

Cholesterol is mainly composed of low-density lipoprotein (LDL), very-low-density lipoprotein (VLDL) and high-density lipoprotein (HDL). It plays a critical role in membrane biogenesis and steroid hormone biosynthesis. The disturbed plasma cholesterol is associated with many diseases, such as cardiovascular disease, diabetes and hepatic steatosis. Cholesterol is either uptaked exogenously from the diet or synthesized endogenously within cells. The liver is the major organ for cholesterol de novo synthesis which involves 19-step complex biochemical process. The rate-limiting enzyme is 3-hydroxy-3-methyl-glutaryl-CoA (HMG-CoA) reductase. Sterol regulatory element-binding protein 1c (SREBP-1c) is the master regulator of cholesterol by stimulating the transcription of LDL and HMG-CoA. LDL receptor (LDLr) is responsible for importing LDL from extracellular to intracellular environment for metabolism. Cholesterol is the primary source for biogenesis of steroid hormones. In turn, many hormones exert critical effects on cholesterol synthesis or metabolism. This occurs through the direct effect of these hormones on regulation of the expression or activity of HMG-CoA reductase, SREBP-1c or LDLr. In this chapter, we will discuss the regulatory role of several interesting hormones in cholesterol metabolism.

2. Thyroid hormone

2.1. Thyroid hormone and thyroid hormone receptors

Thyroid hormones (THs) include thyroxine (T4) and triiodothyronine (T3). They are synthesized and secreted by the thyroid gland. T4 is the major secreted hormone, while T3 has a higher affinity for TH receptors (TRs). T3 is considered as the active and more potent TH. T4 could be converted to T3 through a deiodination process catalyzed by deiodinases. TH regulates a number of biological functions including growth, development and metabolism in almost all tissues [1]. TH exerts these effects through binding to TRs which are expressed on different cells and tissues. TRs have two isoforms, TRα and TRβ, which are encoded by the THRA and THRB genes, respectively, in humans. Each TR isoform has several splice products, TRα1 (α2) and TRβ1 (β2). TRα1 and TRβ1 are ubiquitously expressed, while TRβ1 is the major TR existed in the liver. TRβ2 is expressed in the hypothalamus, the pituitary gland and the developing brain [2]. TRs are ligand-activated transcription factors, belonging to the family of nuclear receptors (NRs). It can bind to DNA sequences called TH-responsive elements (TREs) together with the retinoid X receptor alpha (RXR-α). In the absence of TH, TRs bind with corepressors, e.g., nuclear receptor corepressor and silencing mediator for retinoid and thyroid hormone receptor (NCOR2), suppressing the transcriptional activity. In the presence of TH, the binding induces a conformational change of TRs, releasing the corepressors and recruiting several co-activators to enhance the transcriptional activity. Since TRs associate with corepressors without ligand binding, it could decrease the transcriptional activity of the target genes. Therefore, it should be cautious to compare the data from animal models in which TRs are genetically deleted with the models with low levels of circulating THs, such as hypothyroidism or thyroidectomy [3].

2.2. Role of TH in cholesterol metabolism

There is substantial evidence linking TH status with cholesterol or lipid metabolism. Thyroid dysfunction exerts an important effect on the cholesterol level. Hypothyroidism patients typically have elevated plasma cholesterol and increased lipid accumulation in the liver. TH supplement can normalize this lipid dysregulation. THs promote cholesterol synthesis through inducing HMG-CoA reductase and farnesyl pyrophosphate gene expression [1]. THs markedly decrease the expression of apoB-100, the major protein of LDL, while increasing the expression of apo A-I, the major protein of HDL. In addition, THs increase LDLr gene expression. LDLr mediates the uptake of LDL from blood to the liver. Rat LDLr promoter contains two functional TREs. THs could directly bind to the TRE and upregulate the LDLr gene expression [4]. THs may also regulate the clearance of circulating remnant lipoproteins. Hepatic low-density lipoprotein receptor-related protein 1 (LRP1) is a receptor for remnant lipoproteins. Hepatic LRP1 protein expression and function are reduced in the hypothyroidism mouse model. T3 supplement partially normalizes its protein expression level [5]. THs also promote the cholesterol elimination by increasing conversion and secretion of cholesterol into bile acids. In this process, cholesterol 7α-hydroxylase (Cyp7A1), the enzyme in the cytochrome P450 family, is responsible for catalyzing the rate-limiting reaction in the degradation of cholesterol. Cyp7A1 is a direct TR target gene with TREs in its promoter region [6]. ATP-binding cassette (ABC) transporters G5 (ABCG5) and G8 (ABCG8) form a heterodimer that limits intestinal absorption and facilitates biliary secretion of cholesterol. Mice homozygous for disruption of Abcg5 demonstrate a significant reduction in basal biliary cholesterol secretion. T3 treatment does not increase the cholesterol secretion in Abcg5−/− mice as in the wild-type control mice. This observation suggests that THs induce secretion of cholesterol, largely dependent on the ABCG5/G8 transporter complex [7]. THs also modulate gene expression via micro-RNAs. In a human hepatic cell line, THs decrease sterol O-acyltransferase 2 (SOAT2 or ACAT2), the enzyme crucial for the hepatic secretion of cholesterol esters, via miR-181d [8].

T3 also upregulates LDLr gene expression by activating the expression of the sterol regulatory element-binding protein-2 (SREBP-2) and scavenger receptor class B1 (SR-B1) [9]. Cholesteryl ester transfer protein (CETP) mediates the exchange of cholesteryl esters from HDL to the VLDL and from total triglyceride (TG) to the opposite direction. THs could increase the activity of CETP to influence HDL metabolism [10]. In addition, THs stimulate the lipoprotein lipase (LPL) and hepatic lipase (HL) levels, catabolizing the TG-rich lipoproteins.

2.3. Interaction with other transcription factors

In addition to the direct action on the cholesterol-related genes, TRs also cross talk with many nuclear receptors to regulate their transcriptions. It shares the same DNA-binding site (direct repeat 4) with liver X receptor (LXR). Activation of TRβ1 by T3 upregulates mouse LXRα, but not LXRβ, mRNA expression in the liver at the transcriptional level [11]. TRβ1 is the major TR mediating the TH effects on plasma cholesterol. ATP-binding cassette transporter A1 (ABCA1) is important for HDL assembly and transporting cholesterol back to the liver for excretion. TR forms a heterodimer with retinoid X receptor (RXR) and binds to the DR-4 element of ABCA1 promoter, suppressing its transcription [12]. The apolipoprotein AV gene (APOA5) is a key determinant of the plasma triglyceride level. It affects the plasma TG level through promoting lipolysis of TG-rich lipoproteins and removal of their remnants [13]. TR-β mediates the effects of THs on the activation of APOA5 gene. Administration of TR-β-selective agonist increases apoAV and diminishes triglyceride levels [14]. In addition, TR-β may compete with LXR/RXR heterodimers for binding to the DR-4 element in the CYP7A1 promoter [15]. TR-β but not TR-α KO mice completely lost the induction effects of T3 on Cyp7a1 gene, confirming the critical role of TR-β in mediating the TH effect on cholesterol metabolism [16].

Taken together, TH regulates the serum cholesterol level in multiple crucial steps including stimulating its hepatic synthesis, serum uptake and the intrahepatic conversion to bile acids. The physiological level of TH is essential for maintaining the cholesterol homeostasis.

3. Sex hormones

It is well recognized that premenopausal females have better lipid profiles than males and are more protected from hypercholesterolemia-related diseases, such as cardiovascular diseases. Lipid screening has found that premenopausal women are associated with a lower level of LDL cholesterol and a higher level of HDL cholesterol. After menopause, the gender difference of lipid profiles disappears, and women even have higher-level LDL compared to age-matched men [17]. Estrogen replacement therapy would improve lipoprotein profiles in postmenopausal women [18]. Sex hormones, especially estrogen, account for the gender difference of cholesterol profiles.

3.1. Estrogen and estrogen receptors

The predominant and most important biologically relevant form of estrogen is 17β-estradiol (E2). Both women and men produce E2 through aromatization of androgen. In premenopausal women, estrogen is mainly synthesized in the ovaries. While in postmenopausal women and men, it is primarily converted from testosterone by aromatase (encoded by CYP19 gene) in extragonadal tissues such as adipose tissue, adrenal glands, bones, etc. [19]. There are at least three types of estrogen receptors, ER-α, ER-β and membrane-bound receptor G protein-coupled ER (GPER, also known as GPR 30). ER-α and ER-β are the classic estrogen receptors and are mainly expressed in the cytosol. Upon estrogen binding, ER-α and ER-β form homo- or heterodimers and bind to estrogen response element (ERE) in the downstream target genes, to initiate or suppress the transcriptional activity. The GPER and membrane-associated ER-α and ER-β variants are expressed in the plasma membrane. They mainly exert actions via non-genomic signaling. This membrane-initiated signaling involves protein kinase A (PKA), protein kinase C (PKC) and mitogen-activated protein kinase (MAPK)/extracellular signal-regulated protein kinase (ERK) signaling pathways [20–22].

3.2. Role of estrogens in cholesterol homeostasis

The influence and mechanism of estrogens on cholesterol metabolism have been investigated for a long time. Studies by Cypriani et al. in 1988 demonstrated that estrogens induced HMG-CoA reductase and subsequent cholesterol synthesis in breast cancer cell line [4]. Later, it was found that HMG-CoA reductase gene promoter contains an estrogen-responsive element-like sequence at position-93 (termed Red-ERE). And, estrogen induction of HMG-CoA reductase gene is dependent on the Red-ERE. The induction activity of estrogens occurs in the breast cancer cells but not in hepatic cells, indicating differential regulation of HMG-CoA reductase by estrogens in a tissue-specific manner [23]. Aromatase is an enzyme responsible for the key step in the biosynthesis of estrogens. Aromatase knockout (ArKO) mice display increased intra-abdominal adipose tissue and lipid droplet accumulation in the liver. Total cholesterol and LDL are also elevated in these transgenes [24]. Supplement of estrogens in both ArKO mice and rats with ovariectomy (OVX) normalizes LDL and total cholesterol levels, confirming the important role of estrogens in the lipid homeostasis in both males and females [25]. Hormone replacement therapy (HRT) increases the expression of leucocyte ABCA1 gene, which mediates the efflux of cholesterol to the HDL particles, leading to the subsequent increase in the HDL cholesterol level [26]. Estrogens thus play an important role in the modulation of the total cholesterol level by reducing LDL and concurrently increasing HDL.

The beneficial role of estrogens on cholesterol metabolism is mediated through nuclear and extra-nuclear ER-α and ER-β, as well as GPER. Genetic deletion of ER-α in mice results in upregulation of the genes involved in hepatic lipid biosynthesis and downregulation of the genes involved in lipid transport, indicating that estrogens act via ER-α to regulate lipid metabolism [27]. ER-α KO and ER-α/β double KO mice showed increased serum cholesterol and smaller LDL particles, but not in ER-β single KO mice [28]. Therefore, ER-α plays a more prominent role than ER-β. The roles of GPER in the regulation of metabolism are only beginning to emerge, which gains more attentions. GPER knockout mice exhibit impaired cholesterol homeostasis manifesting significantly a higher LDL level but a normal HDL level, suggesting that GPER mainly regulates LDL metabolism [29]. And, human individuals with a hypofunctional GPER P16L allele are associated with elevated plasma LDL. In vitro study shows that activation of GPER by the agonist upregulates hepatic LDLr expression [30]. The role of GPER signaling in cholesterol or metabolic control remains unclear and needs more further investigations [31]. In summary, estrogens protect against increases in the plasma cholesterol level mainly by activating ER-α and GPER.

3.3. Androgens

The human androgens include dehydroepiandrosterone, androstenedione, testosterone and dihydrotestosterone (DHT). Testosterone can be converted to DHT via 5α-reductase. Testosterones and DHT are active androgens, because they are the only androgens capable of binding to androgen receptors (ARs) to exert biological functions. AR is mainly expressed in the prostate, skeletal muscle, liver and central nervous system (CNS). Like ERs, AR is a member of the steroid and nuclear receptor superfamily. Ligand binding induces a conformation change of AR, leading to recruitment of cofactor proteins and transcriptional machinery and subsequent regulation of the target genes' transcription.

The effect of androgen on cholesterol is still not conclusive. Clinical studies show that androgen deficiency, such as in old men, is associated with increased risks of dyslipidemia, higher serum cholesterol and LDL levels [32]. Another study has found that AR antagonists might be useful in the treatment of obesity in men [33]. In the animal studies, dihydrotestosterone (DHT) treatment in castrated obese mice decreases LDL secretion and increases the expression of hepatic scavenger receptor class B member 1 (SR-1B) which is important in regulating cholesterol uptake from HDL. It also decreases the enzyme cholesterol 7α-hydroxylase which participates in bile formation and cholesterol removal. In another study using an orchidectomized Sprague–Dawley (SD) rat model, DHT treatment causes decreased lipid accumulation and cholesterol synthesis by increasing expression of carnitine palmitoyl transferase 1 and phosphorylation of HMG-CoA reductase via an AR-mediated pathway [34]. However, this finding in animals contradicts a clinical study showing that a single dose of testosterone injection increases the total cholesterol level by 15% through stimulating the hepatic expression of HMG-CoA reductase [35]. These contradictory results indicate a complex role of androgen on the cholesterol homeostasis in the liver.

4. Growth hormone

4.1. Growth hormone and growth hormone receptors

Growth hormone (GH) is secreted by the somatotroph cells of the anterior pituitary gland under neural, hormonal and metabolic control. GH regulates postnatal growth, as well as lipid, glucose and energy metabolism. The molecular mechanism of GH action is relatively complicated. It affects metabolism through direct or indirect action via insulin-like growth factor-1 (IGF-1) or antagonism of insulin action. GH receptor (GHR) is a member of the cytokine receptor superfamily. Upon binding to GH, GHR activates the cytoplasmic tyrosine kinase Janus kinase 2 (Jak2) and then recruits members of the signal transducer and activator of transcription (STAT) family of transcription factors. Phosphorylated STATs translocate into the nucleus and modulate the transcription of multiple target genes, including IGF-1, ALS and suppressor of cytokine signaling (SOCS) [36]. In addition to the Jak2/STAT signaling pathway, GHR can activate the Src tyrosine kinase signaling pathway and cross talk with insulin and IGF-1 signaling pathways.

4.2. Role of GH in cholesterol and lipid metabolism

There exists a negative relationship between obesity and GH. Enormous evidence supports that GH alters lipid metabolism. Clinical studies have shown a significant association between lower serum GH levels and non-alcoholic fatty liver disease (NAFLD). Hypopituitary patients with GH deficiency are more prone to NAFLD than control subjects [37–39]. GH supplementation has been shown to improve the NAFLD and the metabolic dysfunction [40, 41]. In rodent studies, high-fat diet feeding and obesity suppress pulsatile GH secretion [42]. In turn, chronic GH treatment ameliorates hepatic lipid peroxidation and improves lipid metabolism in high-fat diet-fed rats [43].

Hypophysectomy is a surgery process in which the pituitary gland (hypophysis) is removed, leading to an impairment of GH secretion. This model is used for investigating the GH function in animals under pathophysiology conditions. Increase of hepatic LDLr and hypocholesterolemia induced by estrogens is completely attenuated in hypophysectomized rats. Only GH supplementation is able to restore this effect of hypophysectomy. Further, GH treatment on the gallstone patients stimulates the expression of hepatic LDLr by twofold, leading to subsequent decrease in serum cholesterol by 25%. This study indicates that GH secretion is critical for the control of plasma LDL levels in humans [44]. GH is also important for the synthesis of bile acids by maintaining the normal activity of cholesterol 7α-hydroxylase. Hypophysectomized rats show significantly reduced activities of HMG-CoA reductase and cholesterol 7α-hydroxylase and hence an inhibition of cholesterol and bile acid biosynthesis. GH substitution restores the enzymatic activity of 7α-hydroxylase and increases the fecal excretion of bile acids [45]. Treatment of LDLr-deficient mice with GH reduces their elevated plasma cholesterol and triglyceride levels by stimulating the activities of HMG-CoA reductase and cholesterol 7α-hydroxylase [46]. GH thus regulates plasma lipoprotein levels and bile acid metabolism by altering hepatic LDLr expression and the enzymatic activity of cholesterol 7α-hydroxylase, respectively.

GHR is present in the liver and critical for the hepatic lipid metabolism. Laron dwarfism is a disorder characterized by an insensitivity to GH due to a genetic mutation of GHR. These male patients manifest NAFLD in adults [47]. Liver-specific deletion of GHR in mice leads to increased circulating free fatty acids and fatty liver as a result of increased synthesis and decreased efflux of triglyceride [48]. Binding of GH to GHR activates JAK2-STAT5 signaling pathway and modulates a number of target genes. Among these, altered expression of CD36, PPARγ and PGC1α/β, along with fatty acid synthase, lipoprotein lipase and very-low-density lipoprotein receptor (VLDLr) contributes to the hepatic lipid metabolism process [49, 50]. All these findings suggest that hepatic GH signaling is essential for the regulation of intrahepatic lipid and cholesterol metabolism.

5. Glucagon

Glucagon is a 29-aa peptide hormone secreted from the pancreatic islet alpha cells in response to low glucose. It is a well-known counter-regulatory hormone to insulin, mainly stimulating hepatic glucose production by increasing glycogenolysis and gluconeogenesis and concurrently inhibiting glycogen synthesis. Glucagon also affects hepatic cholesterol metabolism. The relationship between glucagon and cholesterol has been investigated since the 1950s [51]. The portacaval shunt surgery in a 6-year-old girl with the homozygous form of familial hypercholesterolemia disorder has been reported to significantly reduce LDL and cholesterol synthesis 5 months after surgery. This alteration is associated with a marked elevation of bile acids and the glucagon level, indicating that glucagon may improve hepatic lipid metabolism [52]. In the animal study, infusion of glucagon into the hyperlipidemic rat reduces circulating VLDL apoprotein and serum TG levels. It is due to the inhibition of incorporating amino acid into the apoprotein by glucagon [53]. Chronic glucagon administration in rats significantly reduces serum cholesterol and triglyceride levels but not in the liver. The internal secretion of cholesterol and cholesterol transformation into bile acids measured by an isotope balance method are strikingly increased, suggesting that glucagon stimulates cholesterol turnover rate [54]. Studies by Rudling et al. have found that injection of glucagon increases LDL binding to the LDLr in a dose-dependent manner and concomitantly decreases cholesterol and apoB/E in LDL and large HDL particles in rats. Moreover, the induction of LDLr by glucagon is not due to increased mRNA levels, indicating a novel posttranscriptional regulatory mechanism present in the liver [55]. In humans, glucagon administration represses cholesterol 7α-hydroxylase (CYP7A1) mRNA expression by increasing the PKA phosphorylation of HNF4a and reducing its ability to bind with the CYP7A1 gene, thus inhibiting bile acid synthesis [56].

Glucagon receptor, encoded by the GCGR gene, is a seven-transmembrane protein and belongs to the class II guanine nucleotide-binding protein (G protein)-coupled receptor superfamily. They are abundantly expressed in the liver and kidney. In the liver, glucagon receptors are mainly located in hepatocytes, with a small number expressed on the surface of Kupffer cells [57]. Mice with a null mutation of the glucagon receptor (Gcgr−/−) display low blood glucose and markedly elevated the plasma LDL level. Serum total cholesterol and HDL are not significantly changed in Gcgr−/− mice [58]. Gcgr−/− mice are more prone to develop hepatosteatosis following high-fat diet feeding [59]. Several glucagon receptor antagonists (GRA) have been developed to reduce hepatic glucose overproduction and improve the overall glycemic status. However, some GRAs including MK-0893 have been shown to dose-dependently increase LDL in T2DM patients. In the rodent preclinical trial, blockade of glucagon receptor using various GRAs elevates plasma LDL-c and total cholesterol. This is caused by increased cholesterol absorption instead of the change in cholesterol synthesis or secretion [60]. Taken together, these results suggest that glucagon plays a hypolipidemic effect through its glucagon receptors, making it an interesting and attractive pharmaceutical agent for the treatment of dyslipidemia and obesity.

6. Irisin

Irisin is a newly identified hormone encoded by the gene fibronectin type III domain-containing protein 5 (FNDC5). It is secreted into the circulation as a cleaved protein product and induced by exercise [61]. Irisin is proposed to mediate the metabolic benefits of exercising by promoting the browning of subcutaneous adipose tissue, reducing visceral obesity and improving glucose and cholesterol metabolism. Circulating the irisin level is negatively associated with fat mass, fasting glucose and dyslipidemia, as well as intrahepatic TG contents in humans [62, 63]. A higher baseline irisin level is associated with the metabolic benefits of diet-restricted treatment on human weight loss [64]. Lentivirus-mediated FNDC5 overexpression or subcutaneous perfusion of irisin promotes lipolysis and reduces hyperlipidemia in obese mice [65]. Irisin is negatively associated with HDL cholesterol and large HDL particles in adults with higher cardiovascular risk [66]. In addition, the serum irisin level is significantly higher in the NAFLD patients than in normal subjects [67]. Elevation of saliva irisin is positively related to total cholesterol [68]. Subcutaneous infusion of irisin decreases body weight, plasma total, VLDL, LDL, HDL cholesterol in diet-induced obese mice. The hepatic levels of total and esterified cholesterol are also reduced. These alterations are associated with significant reduction in the expression of the genes important for cholesterol synthesis, including *Srebp2*, HMG-CoA reductase (*Hmgcr*), the liver X receptor α (*Lxrα*, *Nr1h3*) and HMG CoA synthase (*Hmgcs*) in the liver and primary hepatocytes. Further experiments demonstrate that irisin inhibits cholesterol synthesis in hepatocytes through the activation of AMPK and SREBP2 [69]. As a novel hormone, evidence supporting the critical role of irisin in the regulation of cholesterol or lipid metabolism is still limited. More studies are needed to clarify the role of FNDC5/irisin in the lipid homeostasis under physiological and pathological conditions.

7. Conclusion

Cholesterol balance is regulated at multiple steps, including the biosynthesis, uptake, intracellular transport and conversion to bile acids for excretion. Hormones affect cholesterol biosynthesis and uptake by altering the transcription of genes critical for these biological processes (**Table 1**). Novel identified hormones are constantly added into the list implicated

	Origin	Biosynthesis	Uptake	Secretion	Conversion to bile acid
Thyroid hormone	Thyroid	↑	↑		↑
Sex hormone					
Estrogen	Ovary	↑		↑	
Androgen	Testis		↑	↑	↑
Growth hormone	Pituitary	↑	↑		↑
Glucagon	Islet α cells			↑	↓
Irisin	Skeletal muscle	↓			

Table 1. Effect of hormones on cholesterol metabolism.

in cholesterol balance process. Identification of hormonal receptor agonist/antagonist and understanding the hormonal regulatory mechanisms would help to identify potential effective and selective targets for the control of cholesterol dysfunction.

Acknowledgements

This work was supported by the National Natural Science Foundation of China (81500619), Natural Science Foundation of Guangdong Province (2016A030310040), Shenzhen Science and Technology Project (JCYJ20160422091658982, JCYJ20150324140036854), Shenzhen Peacock Plan (KQTD20140630100746562,827–000107) and Natural Science Foundation of SZU (201567).

Author details

Zhuo Mao, Jinghui Li and Weizhen Zhang*

*Address all correspondence to: weizhenzhang@bjmu.edu.cn

Department of Physiology, Center for Diabetes, Obesity and Metabolism, University Health Science Center, Shenzhen, Guangdong Province, China

References

[1] Sinha RA, Singh BK, Yen PM. Thyroid hormone regulation of hepatic lipid and carbohydrate metabolism. Trends in Endocrinology and Metabolism. 2014;**25**(10):538-545

[2] Schwartz HL et al. Quantitation of rat tissue thyroid hormone binding receptor isoforms by immunoprecipitation of nuclear triiodothyronine binding capacity. The Journal of Biological Chemistry. 1992;**267**:11794-11799

[3] Flamant F, Gauthier K. Thyroid hormone receptors: The challenge of elucidating iso-type-specific functions and cell-specific response. Biochimica et Biophysica Acta (BBA) – General Subjects. 2013;**1830**(7):3900-3907

[4] Cypriani B, Tabacik C, Descomps B. Effect of estradiol and antiestrogens on choles-terol biosynthesis in hormone-dependent and -independent breast cancer cell lines. Biochimica et Biophysica Acta. 1988;**972**(2):167-178

[5] Moon JH et al. Decreased expression of hepatic low-density lipoprotein receptor-related protein 1 in hypothyroidism: A novel mechanism of atherogenic dyslipidemia in hypo-thyroidism. Thyroid. 2013;**23**(9):1057-1065

[6] Lammel Lindemann JA et al. Thyroid hormone induction of human cholesterol 7 alpha-hydroxylase (Cyp7a1) in vitro. Molecular and Cellular Endocrinology. 2014; **388**(1-2):32-40

[7] Bonde Y et al. Stimulation of murine biliary cholesterol secretion by thyroid hormone is dependent on a functional ABCG5/G8 complex. Hepatology. 2012;**56**(5):1828-1837

[8] Yap CS et al. Thyroid hormone negatively regulates CDX2 and SOAT2 mRNA expression via induction of miRNA-181d in hepatic cells. Biochemical and Biophysical Research Communications. 2013;**440**(4):635-639

[9] Shin DJ, Osborne TF. Thyroid hormone regulation and cholesterol metabolism are con-nected through sterol regulatory element-binding protein-2 (SREBP-2). The Journal of Biological Chemistry. 2003;**278**(36):34114-34118

[10] Lagrost L. Regulation of cholesteryl ester transfer protein (CETP) activity: Review of in vitro and in vivo studies. Biochimica et Biophysica Acta. 1994;**1215**(3):209-236

[11] Hashimoto K et al. Liver X receptor-alpha gene expression is positively regulated by thyroid hormone. Endocrinology. 2007;**148**(10):4667-4675

[12] Huuskonen J et al. Regulation of ATP-binding cassette transporter A1 transcription by thyroid hormone receptor. Biochemistry. 2004;**43**(6):1626-1632

[13] Grosskopf I et al. Apolipoprotein A-V deficiency results in marked hypertriglyceridemia attributable to decreased lipolysis of triglyceride-rich lipoproteins and removal of their remnants. Arteriosclerosis, Thrombosis, and Vascular Biology. 2005;**25**(12):2573-2579

[14] Prieur X et al. Thyroid hormone regulates the hypotriglyceridemic gene APOA5. Journal of Biological Chemistry. 2005;**280**(30):27533-27543

[15] Hashimoto K et al. Cross-talk between thyroid hormone receptor and liver X receptor regulatory pathways is revealed in a thyroid hormone resistance mouse model. The Journal of Biological Chemistry. 2006;**281**(1):295-302

[16] Gullberg H et al. Thyroid hormone receptor beta-deficient mice show complete loss of the normal cholesterol 7alpha-hydroxylase (CYP7A) response to thyroid hormone but display enhanced resistance to dietary cholesterol. Molecular Endocrinology. 2000;**14**(11):1739-1749

[17] Atkins D et al. Lipid screening in women. Journal of the American Medical Women's Association. 2000;**55**:234-240

[18] Skafar DF et al. Female sex hormones and cardiovascular disease in Women1. The Journal of Clinical Endocrinology & Metabolism. 1997;**82**(12):3913-3918

[19] Simpson ER. Sources of estrogen and their importance. The Journal of Steroid Biochemistry and Molecular Biology. 2003;**86**(3-5):225-230

[20] Chambliss KL et al. Non-nuclear estrogen receptor alpha signaling promotes cardiovascular protection but not uterine or breast cancer growth in mice. The Journal of Clinical Investigation. 2010;**120**(7):2319-2330

[21] Kang L et al. Involvement of estrogen receptor variant ER-alpha36, not GPR30, in nongenomic estrogen signaling. Molecular endocrinology (Baltimore, Md.). 2010;**24**(4):709-721

[22] Nilsson B-O, Olde B, Leeb-Lundberg LMF. G protein-coupled oestrogen receptor 1 (GPER1)/GPR30: A new player in cardiovascular and metabolic oestrogenic signalling. British Journal of Pharmacology. 2011;**163**(6):1131-1139

[23] Di Croce L et al. The promoter of the rat 3-hydroxy-3-methylglutaryl coenzyme A reductase gene contains a tissue-specific estrogen-responsive region. Molecular Endocrinology. 1999;**13**(8):1225-1236

[24] Jones ME et al. Aromatase-deficient (ArKO) mice have a phenotype of increased adiposity. Proceedings of the National Academy of Sciences of the United States of America. 2000;**97**(23):12735-12740

[25] Hewitt KN et al. Estrogen replacement reverses the hepatic steatosis phenotype in the male aromatase knockout mouse. Endocrinology. 2004;**145**(4):1842-1848

[26] Darabi M et al. Increased leukocyte ABCA1 gene expression in post-menopausal women on hormone replacement therapy. Gynecological Endocrinology. 2011;**27**(9):701-705

[27] Bryzgalova G et al. Evidence that oestrogen receptor-alpha plays an important role in the regulation of glucose homeostasis in mice: Insulin sensitivity in the liver. Diabetologia. 2006;**49**(3):588-597

[28] Ohlsson C et al. Obesity and disturbed lipoprotein profile in estrogen receptor-alpha-deficient male mice. Biochemical and Biophysical Research Communications. 2000;**278**(3):640-645

[29] Sharma G et al. GPER deficiency in male mice results in insulin resistance, dyslipidemia, and a proinflammatory state. Endocrinology. 2013;**154**(11):4136-4145

[30] Hussain Y et al. G-protein estrogen receptor as a regulator of low-density lipoprotein cholesterol metabolism: Cellular and population genetic studies. Arteriosclerosis, Thrombosis, and Vascular Biology. 2015;**35**(1):213-221

[31] Sharma G, Mauvais-Jarvis F, Prossnitz ER. Roles of G protein-coupled estrogen receptor GPER in metabolic regulation. The Journal of Steroid Biochemistry and Molecular Biology. 2018;**176**:31-37

[32] Kelly DM, Jones TH. Testosterone: A metabolic hormone in health and disease. The Journal of Endocrinology. 2013;**217**(3):R25-R45

[33] Moverare-Skrtic S et al. Dihydrotestosterone treatment results in obesity and altered lipid metabolism in orchidectomized mice. Obesity (Silver Spring). 2006;**14**(4):662-672

[34] Zhang H et al. Differential effects of estrogen/androgen on the prevention of nonalcoholic fatty liver disease in the male rat. Journal of Lipid Research. 2013;**54**(2):345-357

[35] Garevik N et al. Single dose testosterone increases total cholesterol levels and induces the expression of HMG CoA reductase. Substance Abuse Treatment, Prevention, and Policy. 2012;**7**:12

[36] Vijayakumar A et al. Biological effects of growth hormone on carbohydrate and lipid metabolism. Growth Hormone & IGF Research. 2010;**20**(1):1-7

[37] Hong JW et al. Metabolic parameters and nonalcoholic fatty liver disease in hypopituitary men. Hormone and Metabolic Research. 2011;**43**(1):48-54

[38] Xu L et al. Association between serum growth hormone levels and nonalcoholic fatty liver disease: A cross-sectional study. PLoS One. 2012;**7**(8):e44136

[39] Nishizawa H et al. Nonalcoholic fatty liver disease in adult hypopituitary patients with GH deficiency and the impact of GH replacement therapy. European Journal of Endocrinology. 2012;**167**(1):67-74

[40] Chishima S et al. The relationship between the growth hormone/insulin-like growth factor system and the histological features of nonalcoholic fatty liver disease. Internal Medicine. 2017;**56**(5):473-480

[41] Pasarica M et al. Effect of growth hormone on body composition and visceral adiposity in middle-aged men with visceral obesity. The Journal of Clinical Endocrinology and Metabolism. 2007;**92**(11):4265-4270

[42] Steyn FJ et al. Increased adiposity and insulin correlates with the progressive suppression of pulsatile GH secretion during weight gain. The Journal of Endocrinology. 2013;**218**(2):233-244

[43] Qin Y, Tian YP. Preventive effects of chronic exogenous growth hormone levels on diet-induced hepatic steatosis in rats. Lipids in Health and Disease. 2010;**9**:78

[44] Rudling M et al. Importance of growth hormone for the induction of hepatic low density lipoprotein receptors. Proceedings of the National Academy of Sciences of the United States of America. 1992;**89**(15):6983-6987

[45] Rudling M, Parini P, Angelin B. Growth hormone and bile acid synthesis. Key role for the activity of hepatic microsomal cholesterol 7alpha-hydroxylase in the rat. The Journal of Clinical Investigation. 1997;**99**(9):2239-2245

[46] Rudling M, Angelin B. Growth hormone reduces plasma cholesterol in LDL receptor-deficient mice. The FASEB Journal. 2001;**15** 8 :1350-1356

[47] Laron Z, Ginsberg S, Webb M. Nonalcoholic fatty liver in patients with Laron syndrome and GH gene deletion–preliminary report. Growth Hormone & IGF Research. 2008;**18**(5):434-438

[48] Fan Y et al. Liver-specific deletion of the growth hormone receptor reveals essential role of growth hormone signaling in hepatic lipid metabolism. Journal of Biological Chemistry. 2009;**284**(30):19937-19944

[49] Barclay JL et al. GH-dependent STAT5 signaling plays an important role in hepatic lipid metabolism. Endocrinology. 2011;**152**(1):181-192

[50] Mueller KM et al. Impairment of hepatic growth hormone and glucocorticoid receptor signaling causes steatosis and hepatocellular carcinoma in mice. Hepatology. 2011;**54**(4):1398-1409

[51] Caren R, Carbo L. Pancreatic alpha-cell function in relation to cholesterol metabolism. The Journal of Clinical Endocrinology and Metabolism. 1956;**16**(4):507-516

[52] Bilheimer DW et al. Reduction in cholesterol and low density lipoprotein synthesis after portacaval shunt surgery in a patient with homozygous familial hypercholesterolemia. Journal of Clinical Investigation. 1975;**56**(6):1420-1430

[53] Eaton RP. Hypolipemic action of glucagon in experimental endogenous lipemia in the rat. Journal of Lipid Research. 1973;**14**(3):312-318

[54] Guettet C et al. Effects of chronic glucagon administration on cholesterol and bile acid metabolism. Biochimica et Biophysica Acta. 1988;**963**(2):215-223

[55] Rudling M, Angelin B. Stimulation of rat hepatic low density lipoprotein receptors by glucagon. Evidence of a novel regulatory mechanism in vivo. The Journal of Clinical Investigation. 1993;**91**(6):2796-2805

[56] Song KH, Chiang JYL. Glucagon and cAMP inhibit cholesterol 7 alpha-hydroxylase (CYP7A1) gene expression in human hepatocytes: Discordant regulation of bile acid synthesis and gluconeogenesis. Hepatology. 2006;**43**(1):117-125

[57] Watanabe J, Kanai K, Kanamura S. Glucagon receptors in endothelial and Kupffer cells of mouse liver. Journal of Histochemistry and Cytochemistry. 1988;**36**(9):1081-1089

[58] Gelling RW et al. Lower blood glucose, hyperglucagonemia, and pancreatic α cell hyperplasia in glucagon receptor knockout mice. Proceedings of the National Academy of Sciences of the United States of America. 2003;**100**(3):1438-1443

[59] Longuet C et al. The glucagon receptor is required for the adaptive metabolic response to fasting. Cell Metabolism. 2008;**8**(5):359-371

[60] Guan HP et al. Glucagon receptor antagonism induces increased cholesterol absorption. Journal of Lipid Research. 2015;**56**(11):2183-2195

[61] Bostrom P et al. A PGC1-alpha-dependent myokine that drives brown-fat-like development of white fat and thermogenesis. Nature. 2012;**481**(7382):463-468

[62] Ebert T et al. Association of metabolic parameters and rs726344 in FNDC5 with serum irisin concentrations. International Journal of Obesity. 2016;**40**(2):260-265

[63] Zhang HJ et al. Irisin is inversely associated with intrahepatic triglyceride contents in obese adults. Journal of Hepatology. 2013;**59**(3):557-562

[64] Lopez-Legarrea P et al. Higher baseline irisin concentrations are associated with greater reductions in glycemia and insulinemia after weight loss in obese subjects. Nutrition Diabetes. 2014;**4**:e110

[65] Xiong XQ et al. FNDC5 overexpression and irisin ameliorate glucose/lipid metabolic derangements and enhance lipolysis in obesity. Biochimica et Biophysica Acta. 2015;**1852**(9):1867-1875

[66] Panagiotou G et al. Circulating irisin, omentin-1, and lipoprotein subparticles in adults at higher cardiovascular risk. Metabolism. 2014;**63**(10):1265-1271

[67] Choi ES et al. Association between serum irisin levels and non-alcoholic fatty liver disease in health screen examinees. PLoS One. 2014;**9**(10):e110680

[68] Hirsch HJ et al. Irisin and the metabolic phenotype of adults with Prader-Willi syndrome. PLoS One. 2015;**10**(9):e0136864

[69] Tang H et al. Irisin inhibits hepatic cholesterol synthesis via AMPK-SREBP2 signaling. eBioMedicine. 2016;**6**(Supplement C):139-148

5

Natural Cholesterol Busters

Gamaleldin I. Harisa, Sabry M. Attia and

Gamil M. Abd Allah

Abstract

Hypercholesterolemia, a risk factor for cardiovascular and cerebrovascular diseases, is a silent health problem. It occurs due to buildup of large amount of cholesterol in blood vessels resulting in narrowed blood vessels or blockage of the flow of blood and causes cellular dysfunction. The predisposing factors for hypercholesterolemia are carbohydrates-enriched diet, unhealthy fats, and red meat. Moreover, family history, obesity, hypokinetic lifestyle, aging, and oxidative stress are associated with hypercholesterolemia. Therapeutic interventions of hypercholesterolemia involve cessation of bad habits, regular exercise, consumption of cholesterol buster diets, and cholesterol-lowering drugs. However, cholesterol-lowering drugs have low efficacy, and some patients cannot tolerate the adverse effects of hypocholesterolemic drugs. In light of this, there has been great interest to address natural cholesterol busters as first choice as cholesterol-lowering option. Healthy diet, regular exercise and natural cholesterol-lowering agents are documented to decrease blood cholesterol level. Natural cholesterol busters include dietary fibers, plant sterols, healthy fats, smart proteins, antinutrients, antioxidants, and L-arginine. These busters not only decrease cholesterol oxidation and absorption but also increase cholesterol catabolism and elimination. Most of these busters are found in cereals, oatmeal, fruits, vegetables, legumes, and fermented foods. The natural cholesterol busters are recommended strategies for treatment of hypercholesterolemia alone or in combination with cholesterol-lowering drugs.

Keywords: hypercholesterolemia, health diet, antioxidants, antinutrients, cardiovascular diseases, L-arginine

1. Introduction

Cholesterol is an important component in cell membrane that maintains the structure and function of the cells. Moreover, cholesterol is a precursor of sex hormones, corticosteroid, and vitamin D. This vitamin is involved in bone formation, modulates immune system, and regulates gene expression [1]. Cholesterol can be catabolized into bile acids that play an important role in digestion and absorption of fat diets and fat-soluble vitamins. The cells get its cholesterol through two pathways, endogenous source by means of biosynthesis in liver (80 %) and exogenous source from the diet (20%) [2]. Cholesterol is transported throughout the bloodstream by joining to specific proteins and lipids forming lipoproteins. There are four main types of lipoprotein acting as cholesterol carriers in circulation: chylomicrons, very low-density lipoproteins (VLDL), low-density lipoprotein (LDL) "bad cholesterol", and high-density lipoprotein (HDL) "good cholesterol" [1].

HDL elicits cardioprotective function by reverse cholesterol transport to the liver to be catabolized, moreover, HDL has antioxidant and anti-inflammatory effects as well as involved in nitric oxide (NO) homeostasis [3]. Under hypercholesterolemic conditions, HDL can be turned into a foe for vascular endothelium through production of free radicals that induced vascular cells and erythrocytes damage [3]. Moreover, cholesterol enrichment decreases membrane fluidity, disrupts cell signaling, induces toxic oxysterols, modulates gene expression, and induces apoptosis [4]. This results in disruption of redox balance and NO homeostasis, particularly in vascular cells and erythrocytes. Cholesterol-enriched erythrocyte membrane causes a reduction in the deformability of cells and impairment of the hemorheological behavior that can initiate cardiovascular disease [5]. Oxidative stress is one of the proposed mechanisms responsible for the changes in erythrocytes under hypercholesterolemic conditions; hence, erythrocytes lose their antioxidant power and become oxidized erythrocytes, which triggers foam cell formation by a mechanism similar to oxidized lipoproteins [5]. Therefore, oxidized erythrocytes are addressed as a new culprit in vascular diseases. **Figure 1** displays the double face of cholesterol.

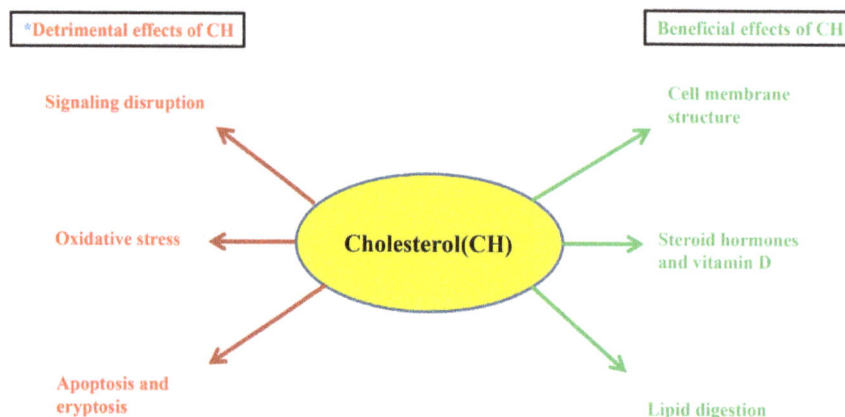

Figure 1. Beneficial and detrimental effects of cholesterol. Asterisk indicates hypercholesterolemic conditions.

Cholesterol-lowering drug therapies particularly with cholesterol biosynthesis inhibitors are associated with adverse effects such as myopathies, neuropathies, liver dysfunction, weakness, and depression [6]. However, intake of natural cholesterol busters reduces blood cholesterol level with minimal side effects [7–9]. Natural cholesterol busters include healthy diet — drinking excess cold water and avoidance of stress with regular exercise. Moreover, many nutraceuticals have cholesterol-lowering action; they include dietary fibers, plant sterols, healthy fats, smart proteins, antinutrients, antioxidants, and L-arginine [10]. These busters act by modulation biochemical pathways such as appetite suppression, inhibition of digestion, and absorption of dietary fats. In addition, they not only increase the metabolic rate and lipolysis but also decrease lipogenesis and inhibit adipocyte differentiation. **Figure 2** shows the possible mechanisms by which natural cholesterol-lowering agents decrease plasma cholesterol levels.

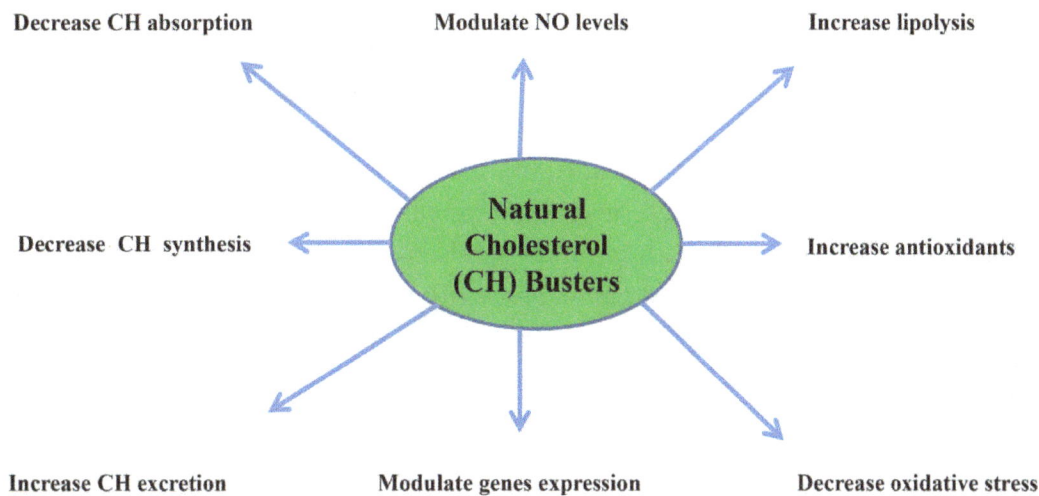

Decrease CH absorption   Modulate NO levels   Increase lipolysis

Decrease CH synthesis   **Natural Cholesterol (CH) Busters**   Increase antioxidants

Increase CH excretion   Modulate genes expression   Decrease oxidative stress

Figure 2. Beneficial effects of natural cholesterol busters.

On this basis, the selection of natural cholesterol-lowering agents with dual action such as lipid lowering and antioxidant activities with minimal side effects is very essential. Natural cholesterol busters can reduce blood cholesterol levels and risk of vascular diseases without adverse effects. This chapter highlights natural cholesterol busters as first line of cholesterol-lowering strategy.

2. Natural cholesterol busters

The first choice to decrease the blood cholesterol levels is lifestyle change including healthy diet — drinking excess of water, avoidance of stress and regular exercise. Moreover, there are a group of nutraceuticals that can be considered as cholesterol busters. Some of these nutraceuticals are plant sterols, healthy fats, dietary fibers, antinutrients, antioxidants, and L-arginine.

2.1. Healthy lifestyle as natural cholesterol busters

2.1.1. Health diet and exercise

Diet and lifestyle are major causes of dyslipidemia, diabetes, and cardiovascular diseases. Particularly, protein-enriched diet produces satiating effect and helps stave off hunger [10]. Consumption of plant-based foods lowers the rate of many chronic diseases; this is attributable to diets which contain smart proteins, trace elements, foliate, antioxidants, and antinutrients [10]. Additionally, low carbohydrate consumption modulates hormones release, increases lipolysis, and enhances fatty acids oxidation [10]. On the other hand, aerobic exercise decreases lipogenesis and activates lipoprotein lipase that increases lipolysis, resulted in enhancement of fat clearance and burning [11].

In these situations, depot fats and free fatty acids were utilized as fuel sources for muscle work [12]. Therefore, health diet with regular exercise (3h/week) at least for 5 days per week decreases subcutaneous fats, visceral fats as well as improve blood lipid levels [12]. Generally, the reduction of body fats is associated with a decrease of total cholesterol, triacylglycerol, LDL, while HDL levels were increased [10]. Furthermore, health diet and lifestyle modifications improve the availability of nitric oxide [10]. Therefore, healthy diets enriched with plant protein, low in carbohydrate and fat, devoid of trans fats (margarine, snack food, packaged baked food, and fried fast food), with regular exercise could be considered the best choice to treat hypercholesterolemia. Besides the aforementioned effects, caloric restrictions with exercise preserve antioxidant capacity as well as reduce reactive oxygen species formation and reduce apoptosis.

2.1.2. Cessation of bad habits

Cigarette smoking and alcohol drinking are most common bad habits worldwide. Combined use of both smoking and alcohol is more damaging to health than use of either alone. The most serious medical consequences of smoking and alcohol are vascular diseases and cancer [13]. This attribute of cigarette smoking enhances catecholamine release and inhibits lipoprotein lipase activity; this results in an increase in levels of chylomicrons, VLDL, and LDL with a decrease in HDL levels [14]. These resulted in alteration of lipid profile associated with decline of antioxidant power with an increase of lipid peroxidation, thrombosis, and vascular dysfunction [13]. Smoking cessation averts these deleterious effects on lipid abnormality, particularly HDL levels [14].

The liver plays a central role in the regulation of cholesterol homeostasis. Alcohol drinking causes fatty liver, besides this alcohol is metabolized into acetaldehyde and reactive oxygen radicals [15]. Acetaldehyde and reactive oxygen radicals can interact with proteins, lipids, and other biomolecules in the cell, resulting in adduct formation which is harmful to the liver. Moreover, acetaldehyde-protein adducts upregulate lipogenetic genes in the liver [15]. Several studies confirmed that chronic alcoholism induced abnormality in lipid metabolism with elevation of triacylglycerol and cholesterol-enriched lipoproteins in the blood [16].

2.2. Nutraceutical as natural cholesterol busters

2.2.1. Healthy fats

Dietary fatty acids are considered one of the main important dietary supplements that strongly determine the development of cardiovascular diseases. The dietary fatty acids include saturated fatty acids, monounsaturated fatty acids, and polyunsaturated fatty acids (PUFAs) [17]. Saturated fatty acid–rich diets are implicated in the promotion of cardiovascular diseases, while monounsaturated fatty acids and PUFAs have cardioprotective effects [17]. In particular, PUFAs are essential dietary elements for human body because human body lacks desaturating enzymes that are required for PUFAs' biosynthesis [18].

PUFAs are classified according to the position of first double bond from the methyl end (omega carbon) into omega-3 (ω3) PUFAs and omega-6 (ω6) PUFAs. Dietary intake of ω3-PUFAs with reduction in ω6-PUFAs consumption is beneficial for cardiac health [19], while higher consumption of ω6-PUFAs with lower ω3-PUFAs dietary contents is a risk for many diseases, particularly cardiovascular diseases. Inside the human body α-linolenic acid can be converted to eicosapentaenoic acid and docosahexaenoic acid by desaturase and elongase enzymes in a series of biochemical reactions [20]. The process of endogenous desaturation and elongation of α-linolenic acid into eicosapentaenoic acid and docosahexaenoic acid is usually inefficient. Therefore, intake of α-linolenic acid is essential for production of eicosapentaenoic and docosahexaenoic acids [21–24].

Omega-3 fatty acids are the precursors of biologically active mediators with health benefits with regard to their anti-inflammatory, antithrombotic, hypolipidemic, and cardioprotective effects [20]. However, ω6-PUFA produces pro-inflammatory, pro-thrombotic, and pro-atherogenic mediators [21–24]. Therefore, balanced ratio between ω3-PUFAs/ω6-PUFAs dietary intake is recommended for the decrease of cardiovascular risk. The reversal of this ratio has been considered responsible for the high prevalence of cardiovascular disease [21–24].

The ω3-PUFAs are involved in the formation of phospholipids that are involved in reverse cholesterol transport to the liver for catabolism [24]. Additionally, intake of ω3-PUFAs can reduce triacylglycerol levels through inhibition of hepatic lipogenesis and very low-density lipoproteins production by the liver and output into circulation. The ω3-PUFAs have been shown to increase plasma LDL with large particle size, which is much less atherogenic than LDL that cannot infiltrate blood vessels of vascular endothelium to start development of atherosclerosis [24]. Moreover, ω3-PUFAs downregulate sterol regulatory element-binding protein, resulting in suppression of gene expression of 3-hydroxy-3-methyl-glutaryl CoA reductase, a rate-limiting enzyme in cholesterol synthesis [25]. ω3-PUFAs also activate liver X receptors that upregulate expression of 7-α-hydroxylase, the main enzyme in conversion of cholesterol into bile acids [26].

Diet enriched with ω3-PUFAs is abundant in plant and marine sources, such as flaxseed, canola, salmon, mackerel, herring, and tuna. The fish oil is composed of higher percent of ω3-PUFAs; therefore, they are the best source of biologically active ω3-PUFAs mediators. The ω3-PUFAs have susceptibility to oxidative damage; therefore, antioxidants supplementation is recommended during ω3-PUFAs consumption. The ω3-PUFAs are promising therapeutic options for the prevention and treatment of hypercholesterolemia. The risk of antioxidants deficiency and mercury contamination during intake of fish oils must be considered.

2.2.2. Phytosterols

Phytosterols are plant source sterols; they are similar to animal sterol in the presence of steroid nucleus, whereas they differ in their side chain. Phytosterols have been incorporated in many dietary regimens to reduce plasma cholesterol levels and provide a cardioprotective action [27–28]. Phytosterols are classified according to their saturation into sterols and stanols; saturation of sterols produces stanols. The main physterols are sitosterol and campesterol, with their respective stanols, sitostanol and campestanol [27–28]. Phytosterols are relatively less absorbed than cholesterol, particularly stanols. Addition of phytosterols to the diet of hyper-cholesterolemic patients can effectively reduce blood cholesterol levels [29–30]. Phytostanols are preferred than sterols because the effect of sterols diminishes over time, while stanols' effect persists for a long time. Maximal reduction in cholesterol was reported with daily intake of 2.0 g of plant stanols. The effect of phytosterols is food dependent because the maximal bile secretion is with or directly after meals where stanols can target micelle formation to reduce the absorption of cholesterol and lipids [31–35]. Phytostanols esters showed greater effectiveness if taken on daily basis in sufficient amounts (0.8–2.0 g) with meals [31–35]. The beneficial effect of stanols over LDL reduction appears after 1–2 weeks of (2.0 g) daily consumption. Most importantly, this reduction in LDL persists as long as stanols being consumed [31–35].

Several mechanisms including interference with intestinal cholesterol solubility, inhibition of digestive enzymes, and decreasing cellular uptake of cholesterol have been proposed to explain the cholesterol-lowering effects of phytosterols [31–35]. Therefore, phytosterols reduce the absorption of both dietary and biliary cholesterol from the intestinal tract. Moreover, phytosterols induce the expression of ATP-binding cassette transporters, thus increasing the efflux of cholesterol from the intestinal cells [31–35]. In addition, phytosterols suppress the activity of acyl-cholesterol acyl transferase required for sterols absorption, consequently reducing intestinal cholesterol uptake. Phytosterols are partially inhibiting dietary and biliary cholesterol absorption by 30–50% through inhibition of cholesterol emulsification through disruption of the lipid micelles, reducing its solubility and availability for intestinal absorption [31–35]. Phytosterols are present naturally in many plants, such as corn, soybeans, and sunflower seeds. The risk of beta-sitosterolemia must be considered during intake of phytosterols as cholesterol-lowering therapy.

2.2.3. Dietary fibers

Dietary fibers including cellulose and its derivatives as well as lignin are considered as non-digestible parts of food. Diet rich in fiber has been reported to have an inverse relationship to cardiovascular risk. Therefore, fiber-enriched diets are recommended by many leading organizations to improve human health [36–37]. The chemical composition of dietary fibers is carbohydrate in nature; they are present in edible plants. Dietary fibers resist alimentary digestive enzymes, are non-absorbable and susceptible for partial fermentation by normal flora gastrointestinal tract [36–37]. Generally, dietary fibers are classified according to their solubility into soluble and insoluble fibers. Inulin, oligofructosides, pectin, mucilage, psyllium, gum, polysaccharides, and β-glucans are examples for soluble fibers, whereas lignin, cellulose, hemicellulose, and resistant starch are examples for insoluble fibers [38–41]. Chitosan can reduce the risk of cardiovascular diseases because it can lower triacylglycerol and cholesterol levels by increasing bile acid excretion [42].

Dietary fibers have hypolipidemic effect over both triacylglycerol and cholesterol-enriched lipoproteins [41]. The biochemical mechanisms underlying the hypolipidemic effect of dietary fibers may be due to different hypotheses. Dietary fibers form complexes with dietary fats, cholesterol, and bile acids. Therefore, fat digestion by pancreatic lipases is inhibited, while hepatic bile synthesis and cholesterol excretion are enhanced [41, 43]. In addition, dietary fibers can entrap water and water-soluble foodstuff, such as glucose, resulting in reduction in glucose absorption. Therefore, post-prandial plasma insulin declines with suppression of its stimulating action for 3-hydroxy-3-methylglutaryl-CoA reductase in cholesterol synthesis. This resulted in decrease of cholesterol biosynthesis with decrease in blood cholesterol levels [41, 43]. Fermentation of fibers by intestinal flora produces short chain fatty acids such as propionic and butyric acids. These acids can suppress hepatic cholesterol synthesis via competitive inhibition of 3-hydroxy-3-methyl-glutaryl CoA reductase and downregulate most of lipogenic enzymes [41, 43–45].

Dietary fibers promote growth of intestinal microflora such as *Lactobacillus acidophilus* [37]. Therefore, dietary fibers that selectively stimulate the growth and activity of beneficial microflora are known as "prebiotics"; "probiotics" in the gastrointestinal tract improve the intestinal microbial balance, thus improving human health. When probiotics and prebiotics are used in combination, they are known as "synbiotics" [46]. The use of synbiotics is to improve gut health and exert other health-promoting effects, such as modulation of the immune system, antihypertensive effects, prevention of cancer, antioxidant effects, reduction of dermatitis symptoms, facilitation of mineral absorption, and improvement of candidiasis [46]. Additionally, synbiotics has cholesterol-lowering properties through deconjugation of bile acids by bile-salt hydrolase, thus leading to coprecipitation of cholesterol with deconjugated bile [46]. Other explanations for cholesterol-lowering effects of probiotics include utilization of cholesterol in the cell membranes during growth of probiotics, conversion of cholesterol into coprostanol and production of short-chain fatty acids upon prebiotics fermentation by probiotics [46].

Dietary fibers are present in nuts, beans, lentil, lupin, blueberries, cucumber, green leafy vegetables, green beans, carrot, celery, yoghurt, and fermented foods.

2.2.4. Antioxidants

Antioxidants can minimize cellular damage by inactivating free radicals, which could attack other cellular molecules. Enzymatic antioxidants that could provide a protection against free radicals are superoxide dismutase, catalase, and glutathione peroxidases [47]. Non-enzymatic antioxidants with similar function are present widely in the biological system and able to quench many types of free radicals. They include glutathione, vitamin E, vitamin C, β-carotene, retinols, selenium, copper, zinc, manganese, and others [47]. Hypercholesterolemia upregulates the activity of free radical–generating enzymes; however, it downregulates the activity of antioxidant enzymes that trigger the production of reactive oxygen metabolites [48]. These reactive metabolites provoke lipoproteins oxidation, protein glycation, and glucose auto-oxidation. Therefore, hypercholesterolemia has been implicated as pathogenesis of pancreatitis, hepatitis, renal injury, stroke, atherosclerosis, and metabolic syndrome by oxidative damage-dependent mechanism [49].

There are scientific evidences of the protective effects of naturally occurring antioxidants in biological systems. Consequently, the identification of natural antioxidants with cholesterol-lowering effect in diet consumed by human is very important. Antioxidants are attractive alternative therapy to treat hypercholesterolemic patients [50]. The antioxidants with cholesterol-lowering capability include antioxidant vitamins, coenzymeQ-10, resveratrol, grape seed, cherry seed, and spices. Moreover, flavonoids, such as silymarin, rutin, quercetin, naringin, and hesperidin, were used for the same purpose [7–9]. Chrysin is a natural flavonoid that is able to decrease plasma lipid concentration and has an antioxidant property [51]. Moreover, rice bran oil is involved in lipid metabolism and oxidation; therefore, it has significant health benefits by the modulation of lipid profiles and preservation of normal redox balance in hypercholesterolemic conditions [52]. Antioxidants are exerting their beneficial effects as free radical scavengers and as chelators of pro-oxidant metals. Furthermore, administration of antioxidants augments endogenous antioxidant power as well as inhibits free radicals generating enzymes [54]. Antioxidants inhibit the oxidation of lipoproteins, protect the oxidative damage of erythrocytes and preserve the availability of nitric oxide in the body [53]. Consequently, antioxidants prevent hypercholesterolemia-induced vascular cells damage. Vegetables and fruits are good source of antioxidants; they include reddish, lettuce, carrot, tomato, cucumber, red cabbage, and low caloric fruits such as apple, grape fruits and orange.

2.2.5. Antinutrients

Antinutrients are plant secondary metabolites such as saponins, flavonoids, alkaloids, tannins, oxalates, phytates, protease inhibitors, amylase inhibitors, lipase inhibitors, and lectins. They are secreted by the plant as a part of the defense mechanism [54, 55]. Human beings use these agents for many beneficial purposes. Some of the antinutrients are used in modulation of gastrointestinal function. Lectins have high binding capacity to the intestinal brush border membrane. This stimulates the release of anorectic neuropeptides that produce satiety and decrease food intake [55]. However, lectins can cause severe intestinal damage with disrupting digestion provoking food allergies and other immune responses [55]. Saponins are amphipathic antinutrients which can reduce cholesterol absorption by disruption of cholesterol micelle formation and downregulate the activity of lipogenic enzymes [54, 55]. Furthermore, saponins also reduce the uptake of glucose from the gut through intraluminal physicochemical interaction [54, 55].

Tannins are present in most cereals and are able to inhibit the activities of protease, amylase and lipase [54–56]. Chlorogenic acid is a member of antinutrients present in green coffee.

Soybeans, fenugreek, bean, and ginseng are good sources of antinutrients. Antinutrients have immune-potentiating action, anticancer effect, and antioxidant power, which could prevent cardiovascular diseases. However, the risk of hemolysis, pancreatic hypertrophy, minerals deficiency, vitamins deficiency, and other malabsorption syndrome must be considered during intake of antinutrients for treatment of hypercholesterolemia [54–56]. **Table 1** annotated the common dietary sources, the main mechanisms of action, and the probable side effects of natural cholesterol lowering agents.

Cholesterol buster	Dietary source	Main mechanism of action	Probable side effects
Healthy fats	Salmon, flaxseed, and canola oils	Decrease cholesterol synthesis and increase its catabolism	Depletion of antioxidant
Phytosterols	Corn, soybeans, and sunflower seeds	Induce expression of ATP-binding cassette transporters	Beta-Sitosterolemia
Dietary fibers	Legumes, beans, and vegetables	Form complexes with dietary cholesterol and bile acids	Abdominal discomfort
Antinutrients	Beans, fenugreek, and ginseng	Produce satiety and decrease cholesterol micelles formation	Hemolysis and malabsorption syndrome
Antioxidants	Fruits, vegetables, and rice bran oil	Decrease free radicals formation and lipoprotein oxidation	-
L-arginine	Poultry, seafood, and lupine	Antioxidants and restores nitric oxide bioavailability	Hypotension

Table 1. The common dietary sources, the main mechanisms of action, and the probable side effects of natural cholesterol busters.

2.2.6. L-Arginine

Nitric oxide is an important vasodilator and has many biological functions. Several cells including endothelial cells and erythrocytes can produce nitric oxide which uses L-arginine as a substrate and tetrahydrobiopterin and flavoproteins as cofactors [57, 58]. Hypercholesterolemia is associated with the increased oxidative stress that reduces the nitric oxide bioavailability through disruption of L-arginine transport into cells, inactivation of nitric oxide synthase, and activation of arginase [9, 58, 59]. Furthermore, high blood cholesterol levels increase endogenous L-arginine analogues that are able to inhibit nitric oxide synthesis. In particular, asymmetric dimethylarginine competes with L-arginine at the catalytic site of nitric oxide synthase, and symmetric dimethylarginine blocks the transport of L-arginine into the cells via the transporter for cationic amino acids [9, 58, 59]. In hypercholesterolemia, erythrocytes and endothelial cells float in cholesterol-enriched media. This results in a decrease of nitric oxide production and endothelial dysfunction [9, 58, 59]. On the contrary, L-arginine supplementation restores nitric oxide levels and reduces vascular oxidative damage in hypercholesterolemic conditions [57]. It has been reported that L-arginine–enriched foods lower LDL levels; this indicates positive health benefits associated with L-arginine on cardiovascular system [60]. Moreover, dietary supplementation with L-arginine stimulates nitric oxide biosynthetic pathway. In addition, polyphenolic compound mediates L-arginine transport into cells and enhances nitric oxide production [60, 61]. L-arginine–enriched foods include dairy products, poultry, seafood, wheat germ, lupine, granola, oatmeal, peanuts, nuts, pumpkin seed, and chickpeas. The risk of hypotension must be considered during intake of L-arginine as a cholesterol-lowering agent. **Figure 3** shows role of cholesterol busters in prevention hypercholesterolemia induced endothelial dysfunction.

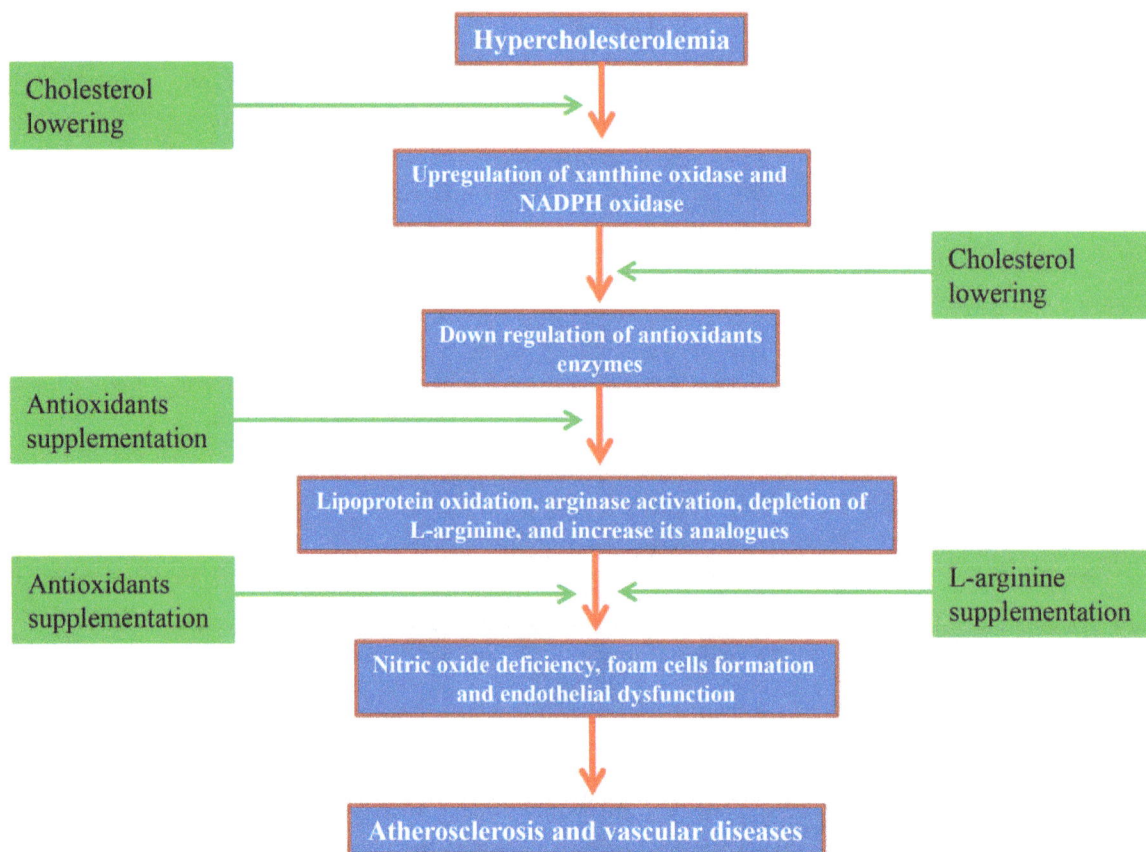

Figure 3. Mechanisms of action of cholesterol busters in prevention hypercholesterolemia induced endothelial dysfunction. Green color indicates the site of action of therapeutic agent.

3. Suggestion and recommendations

Based on the current data in this chapter, the following recommendations aid in maintaining a healthy life.

- Eat three to five healthy diet daily containing different foods. Healthy diets contain fruits, vegetables, and legumes with less fat and carbohydrate.

- Reduce the intake of salt, flour, and sugar; use more fibers and reduce the amount of food in your plate.

- Consume cold water and sugar-free gum during a feeling of false or emotional hunger.

- Motivate regularly such as walking, riding a bike, and other activities (30–45 min), at least 5 days weekly to burn off the excess calories.

- Prohibit bad habits such smoking and alcohol drinking as conceivable.

- Avoid overcrowding, noise, and contaminant exposure as possible.

- Check your body weight weekly.

- Examine your blood sugar level and plasma lipids profile for every 6 months.

4. Summary

Healthy diet and exercise can successfully manage blood cholesterol levels, besides supplementation of natural cholesterol busters. Natural cholesterol busters not only decrease cholesterol absorption, but also increase cholesterol metabolism and elimination. The intervention of natural cholesterol busters is the safest strategy in the prevention and treatment of hypercholesterolemia. The hypocholesterolemic properties of natural cholesterol busters have been proved; however, further studies are required to address general recommendations considering human variability in response to dietary regimen. The natural cholesterol busters are found in cereals, oatmeal, fruits, vegetables, and legumes. In case of failure of natural cholesterol busters as first choice cholesterol-lowering option, the cholesterol-lowering drugs are recommended with natural cholesterol busters. Take care that high intake of antinutrients may be associated with serious health problems due to the presence of phytate, oxalate, cyanogenic glycoside, and other toxic antinutrients.

Acknowledgements

The authors extend their appreciation to Kayyali Chair for Pharmaceutical Industry, Department of Pharmaceutics, College of Pharmacy, King Saud University for funding this work through the research project Number (G-2016-1).

Author details

Gamaleldin I. Harisa[1,3*], Sabry M. Attia[2] and Gamil M. Abd Allah[3]

*Address all correspondence to: harisa@ksu.edu.sa

1 Kayyali Chair for Pharmaceutical Industry, College of Pharmacy, King Saud University, Riyadh, Saudi Arabia

2 Department of Pharmacology and Toxicology, College of Pharmacy, King Saud University, Riyadh, Saudi Arabia

3 Department of Biochemistry, College of Pharmacy, Al-Azhar University (Boys), Nasr City, Cairo, Egypt

References

[1] Widmaier E, Raff H, Strang K. Vander's human physiology: the mechanisms of body function. 13th ed. New York, NY: McGraw-Hill Science/Engineering/Math; 2013.

[2] Ikonen E. Cellular cholesterol trafficking and compartmentalization. Nat Rev Mol Cell Biol. 2008; 9(2):125–38.

[3] Xu S, Liu Z, Liu P. HDL cholesterol in cardiovascular diseases: the good, the bad, and the ugly? Int J Cardiol. 2013; 168(4):3157–9.

[4] Tabas I. Consequences of cellular cholesterol accumulation: basic concepts and physiological implications. J Clin Invest. 2002; 110(7):905–11.

[5] Harisa GI, Badran M, Alanazi F, Attia S, Shazly G. Influence of pravastatin chitosan nanoparticles on erythrocytes cholesterol and redox homeostasis: an in vitro study. Arab J Chem. 2015; http://dx.doi.org/10.1016/j.arabjc.2015.10.016. In press.

[6] Petyaev IM. Improvement of hepatic bioavailability as a new step for the future of statin. Arch Med Sci. 2015; 11(2):406–10.

[7] Franiak-Pietryga I, Koter-Michalak M, Broncel M, Duchnowicz P, Chojnowska-Jezierska J. Anti-inflammatory and hypolipemic effects in vitro of simvastatin comparing to epicatechin in patients with type-2 hypercholesterolemia. Food Chem Toxicol. 2009; 47(2):393–7.

[8] Duchnowicz P, Bors M, Podsędek A, Koter-Michalak M, Broncel M. Effect of polyphenols extracts from Brassica vegetables on erythrocyte membranes (in vitro study). Environ Toxicol Pharmacol. 2012; 34(3):783–90.

[9]   Csonka C, Sárközy M, Pipicz M, Dux L, Csont T. Modulation of hypercho-
      lesterolemia-induced oxidative/nitrative stress in the heart. Oxid Med Cell
      Longev. 2016;3863726.

[10] Harisa GI, Alanazi FK. The beneficial roles of Lupineus luteus and lifestyle
      changes in management of metabolic syndrome: a case study. Saudi Pharm J.
      2015; 23(6):712–5.

[11] Plaisance EP, Fisher G. Exercise and dietary-mediated reductions in postprandial
      lipemia. J Nutr Metab. 2014;902065.

[12] Togashi K, Masuda H, Iguchi K. Effect of diet and exercise treatment for obese Japanese
      children on abdominal fat distribution. Res Sports Med. 2010; 18(1):62–70.

[13] McCullough ML, Patel AV, Kushi LH, Patel R, Willett WC, Doyle C, Thun MJ, Gapstur
      SM. Following cancer prevention guidelines reduces risk of cancer, cardiovascular
      disease, and all-cause mortality. Cancer Epidemiol. Biomarkers Prev. 2011; 20(6):1089–
      97.

[14] Chelland Campbell S, Moffatt RJ, Stamford BA. Smoking and smoking cessation the
      relationship between cardiovascular disease and lipoprotein metabolism: a review.
      Atherosclerosis. 2008; 201(2):225–35.

[15] Oliva J, French SW, Li J, Bardag-Gorce F. Proteasome inhibitor treatment reduced fatty
      acid, triacylglycerol and cholesterol synthesis. Exp Mol Pathol. 2012; 93(1):26–34.

[16] Wang Z, Yao T, Song Z. Chronic alcohol consumption disrupted cholesterol
      homeostasis in rats: down-regulation of low-density lipoprotein receptor and
      enhancement of cholesterol biosynthesis pathway in the liver. Alcohol Clin Exp
      Res. 2010; 34(3):471–8.

[17] Gillingham LG, Harris-Janz S, Jones PJ. Dietary monounsaturated fatty acids are
      protective against metabolic syndrome and cardiovascular disease risk factors. Lipids.
      2011; 46:209–28.

[18] Engler MM, Engler MB. Omega-3 fatty acids: role in cardiovascular health and disease.
      J Cardiovasc Nurs. 2006; 21:17–24; quiz 25–6.

[19] Grenon SM, Hughes-Fulford M, Rapp J, Conte MS. Polyunsaturated fatty acids and
      peripheral artery disease. Vasc Med. 2012; 17:51–63.

[20] Seo T, Blaner WS, Deckelbaum RJ. Omega-3 fatty acids: molecular approaches to
      optimal biological outcomes. Curr Opin Lipidol. 2005; 16:11–8.

[21] Brenna JT. Efficiency of conversion of alpha-linolenic acid to long chain n–3 fatty acids
      in man. Curr Opin Clin Nutr Metab Care. 2002; 5:127–32.

[22] Adkins Y, Kelley DS. Mechanisms underlying the cardioprotective effects of omega-3
      polyunsaturated fatty acids. J NutrBiochem. 2010; 21:781–92.

[23] Gomez Candela C, Bermejo Lopez LM, Loria Kohen V. Importance of a balanced omega 6/omega 3 ratio for the maintenance of health: nutritional recommendations. Nutr Hosp. 2011; 26:323–9.

[24] Balogun K, & Cheema S. Cardioprotective role of omega-3 polyunsaturated fatty acids through the regulation of lipid metabolism. Ch. 27 in: Jagadeesh J, et al. (editors). Pathophysiology and pharmacotherapy cardiovascular disease. 1st ed. 2015. Aids (an imprint of Springer), Germany.

[25] Le Jossic-Corcos C, Gonthier C, Zaghini I, Logette E, Shechter I, Bournot P. Hepatic farnesyl diphosphate synthase expression is suppressed by polyunsaturated fatty acids. Biochem J. 2005; 385:787–94.

[26] Davidson MH. Mechanisms for the hypotriglyceridemic effect of marine omega-3 fatty acids. Am J Cardiol. 2006; 98:27i–33.

[27] Genser B, Silbernagel G, De Backer G, Bruckert E, Carmena R, Chapman MJ et al. Plant sterols and cardiovascular disease: a systematic review and meta-analysis. Eur Heart J. 2012; 33(4):444–51.

[28] Thompson GR, Grundy SM. History and development of plant sterol and stanol esters for cholesterol-lowering purposes. Am J Cardiol. 2005; 96(Suppl):3D–9D.

[29] O'Neill FH, Sanders TA, Thompson GR. Comparison of efficacy of plant stanol ester and sterol ester: short-term and longer-term studies. Am J Cardiol. 2005; 96(1A):29D–36D.

[30] Miettinen TA, Gylling H. Effect of statins on noncholesterol sterol levels: implications for use of plant stanols and sterols. Am J Cardiol. 2005; 96(1A):40D–6D.

[31] Cater NB, Garcia-Garcia AB, Vega GL, Grundy SM. Responsiveness of plasma lipids and lipoproteins to plant stanol esters. Am J Cardiol 2005; 96(Suppl): 23D–8D.

[32] Assmann G, Seedorf U. Phytosterols, plasma lipids and CVD risk. Ch. 29 in: Mancini M, et al. (editors). Nutritional and metabolic bases of cardiovascular disease. 1st ed. 2011. Blackwell Publishing Limited, USA.

[33] Rosin S, Ojansivu I, Kopu A, Keto-Tokoi M, Gylling H. Optimal use of plant stanol ester in the management of hypercholesterolemia. Cholesterol. 2015; 2015:706970.

[34] King ED. Dietary fiber, inflammation, and cardiovascular disease. Mol Nutr Food Res. 2005; 49(6):594–600.

[35] Mudagil D, Barak S. Composition, properties and health benefits of indigestible carbohydrate polymers as dietary fiber: a review. Int J Biol Macromol. 2013; 61:1–6.

[36] Papathanasopoulos A, Camilleri M. Dietary fiber supplements: effects in obesity and metabolic syndrome and relationship to gastrointestinal functions. Gastroenterology. 2010; 138:65–72.

[37]   Slavin JL. Carbohydrates, dietary fiber, and resistant starch in white vegetables: links to health outcomes. Adv Nutr. 2013; 4:351S–15S.

[38]   Cani PD, Possemiers S, Van de Wiele T, et al. Changes in gut microbiota control inflammation in obese mice through a mechanism involving GLP-2-driven improvement of gut permeability. Gut. 2009; 58(8):1091–103.

[39]   Urías-Silvas JE, Cani PD, Delmée E, Neyrinck A, López MG, Delzenne NM. Physiological effects of dietary fructans extracted from Agave tequilanaGto and Dasylirion spp. Br J Nutr. 2008; 99(2):254–61.

[40]   Retelny VS, Neuendorf A, Roth JL. Nutrition protocols for the prevention of cardiovascular disease. Nutr Clin Pract. 2008; 23(5):468–76.

[41]   Theuwissen E, Mensink RP. Water-soluble dietary fibers and cardiovascular disease. Physiol Behav. 2008; 94(2):285–92.

[42]   Xia, W. Liu P, Zhang J, Chen J. Biological activities of chitosan and chitooligosaccharides. Food Hydrocoll. 2011; 25:170–9.

[43]   Giovane A, Napoli C. Protective effects of food on cardiovascular disease. Ch. 24 in: Sauer H, et al. (editors). Studies on cardiovascular disorders. 2010. Humana Press (an imprint of Springer), USA.

[44]   Artiss JD, Brogan K, Brucal M, Moghaddam M, Jen KL. The effects of a new soluble dietary fiber on weight gain and selected blood parameters in rats. Metabolism. 2006; 55(2):195–202.

[45]   Delzenne NM, Williams CM. Prebiotics and lipid metabolism. Curr Opin Lipidol. 2002; 13(1):61–67.

[46]   Ooi LG, Liong MT. Cholesterol-lowering effects of probiotics and prebiotics: a review of in vivo and in vitro findings. Int J Mol Sci. 2010; 11(6):2499–522.

[47]   Chitra KP, KS Pillai. Antioxidants in health. Ind J Physiol Pharmacol. 2002; 46(1):1–5.

[48]   Costa LG1, Giordano G, Furlong CE. Pharmacological and dietary modulators of paraoxonase 1 (PON1) activity and expression: the hunt goes on. Biochem Pharmacol. 2011; 81(3):337–44.

[49]   Olorunnisola OS, Bradley G, Afolayan AJ. Protective effect of T. violacea rhizome extract against hypercholesterolemia-induced oxidative stress in Wistar rats. Molecules. 2012; 17(5):6033–45.

[50]   Deng R. Food and food supplements with hypocholesterolemic effects. Recent Pat Food Nutr Agric. 2009; 1(1):15–24.

[51]   Zarzecki, MS, Araujo SM, Bortolotto VC, de Paula MT. Hypolipidemic action of chrysin on Triton WR-1339-induced hyperlipidemia in female C57BL/6 mice. Toxicol Rep. 2014; 1:200–8.

[52] Minhajuddin M1, Beg ZH, Iqbal J. Hypolipidemic and antioxidant properties of tocotrienol rich fraction isolated from rice bran oil in experimentally induced hyperlipidemic rats. Food Chem Toxicol. 2005; 43(5):747–53.

[53] Vogiatzi G, Tousoulis D, Stefanadis C. The role of oxidative stress in atherosclerosis. Hell J Cardiol. 2009; 50(5):402–9.

[54] Soetan KO. Pharmacological and other beneficial effects of antinutritional factors in plants: a review. Afr J Biotechnol 2008; 7(25):4713–21.

[55] Ramírez-Jiménez AK, Reynoso-Camacho R, Elizabeth Tejero M, León-Galván F, Loarca-Piña G. Potential role of bioactive compounds of *Phaseolus vulgaris L.* on lipid-lowering mechanisms. Food Res Int 2015; 7692–104.

[56] Meng S, Cao J, Feng Q, Peng J, Hu Y. Roles of chlorogenic acid on regulating glucose and lipids metabolism: a review. Evid Based Complement Alternat Med. 2013; 2013:801457.

[57] Ramírez-Zamora S, Méndez-Rodríguez ML, Olguín-Martínez M, Sánchez-Sevilla L, Quintana-Quintana M, García-García N, Hernández-Muñoz R. Increased erythrocytes by-products of arginine catabolism are associated with hyperglycemia and could be involved in the pathogenesis of type 2 diabetes mellitus. PLoS One. 2013; 8(6):e66823.

[58] Harisa GI. L-Arginine ameliorates arylesterase/ paraoxonase activity of paraoxonase-1 in hypercholesterolemic rats. Asian J Biochem. 2011; 6(3):263–72.

[59] Eligini S, Porro B, Lualdi A, Squellerio I, Veglia F, Chiorino E, Crisci M, Garlaschè A, Giovannardi M, Werba JP, Tremoli E, Cavalca V. Nitric oxide synthetic pathway in red blood cells is impaired in coronary artery disease. PLoS One. 2013; 8(8):e66945.

[60] Palloshi A, Fragasso G, Piatti P, Monti LD, Setola E, Valsecchi G, Galuccio E, Chierchia SL & Margonato A. Effect of oral L -arginine on blood pressure and endothelial function in patients and symptoms with systemic hypertension, Positive exercise tests, and normal coronary arteries. Am J Cardiol. 2004; 93:933–5.

[61] Harisa GI, Mariee AD, Abo-Salem OM, Attia SM. Erythrocyte nitric oxide synthase as a surrogate marker for mercury-induced vascular damage: the modulatory effects of naringin. Environ Toxicol. 2014; 29(11):1314–22.

Treatment of Homozygous Familial Hypercholesterolemia: Challenges and Latest Development

Min-Ji Charng

Abstract

Familial hypercholesterolemia (FH) is an autosomal codominant genetic disorder of lipoprotein metabolism. Patients can be heterozygous (HeFH) with one mutated allele, homozygous (HoFH) with two identical mutations, or compound heterozygous with different mutations in each allele. HoFH is the more severe form of the disease and is associated with extremely elevated levels of total cholesterol and low-density lipoprotein cholesterol (LDL-C). These lipid abnormalities are associated with accelerated atherosclerosis and cardiovascular disease (CVD) and an increased risk of cardiac events and early death. The prevalence of HoFH has been estimated to be 1 in 1 million; however, this is likely an underestimation as the disease is substantially underdiagnosed and undertreated. Early diagnosis and treatment are important to reduce CVD events. Aggressive therapy with conventional agents such as statins and ezetimibe produce substantial reductions in LDL-C, but patients rarely reach target goals. Apheresis should be considered in all patients with HoFH, although LDL-C levels rapidly rebound to baseline levels. Three recently introduced novel agents (mipomersen, lomitapide, and evolocumab)—each with a unique mechanism of action—have increased therapeutic options in this difficult-to-treat population. When added to standard therapy, these agents produce significant additional LDL-C lowering and can potentially improve clinical outcomes.

Keywords: evolocumab, familial hypercholesterolemia, lomitapide, mipomersen, treatment

1. Introduction

Familial hypercholesterolemia (FH) is an autosomal codominant genetic disorder of lipoprotein metabolism, usually caused by mutations in the low-density lipoprotein (LDL) receptor (*LDLR*) gene or other genes that affect LDLR function. Patients can be heterozygous (HeFH) with one mutated allele, homozygous (HoFH) with two identical mutations, or compound heterozygous with different mutations in each allele [1]. Patients with HoFH have either a complete absence or marked impairment (i.e., 2–30% activity) in LDLR function [1]. There are a number of defects in lipid metabolism among patients with FH that include reduced LDLR-mediated catabolism of LDL, impairment of apolipoprotein B (apo B)-mediated clearance of LDL, and increased proprotein convertase subtilisin/kexin type 9 (PCSK9) levels, which mediates posttranslational destruction of LDLRs [2, 3].

Since the reduction of LDLRs in HoFH is more pronounced than that seen with HeFH, hypercholesterolemia is usually more severe in HoFH than in HeFH and is characterized by very high serum levels of total cholesterol and LDL-cholesterol (LDL-C). Levels of LDL-C are typically above 500 mg/dL and total cholesterol levels range from 650 to 1000 mg/dL when HoFH is untreated, whereas LDL-C levels are typically greater than 300 mg/dL when treated [2–5]. High-density lipoprotein cholesterol (HDL-C) is often decreased and triglyceride levels are generally normal [4].

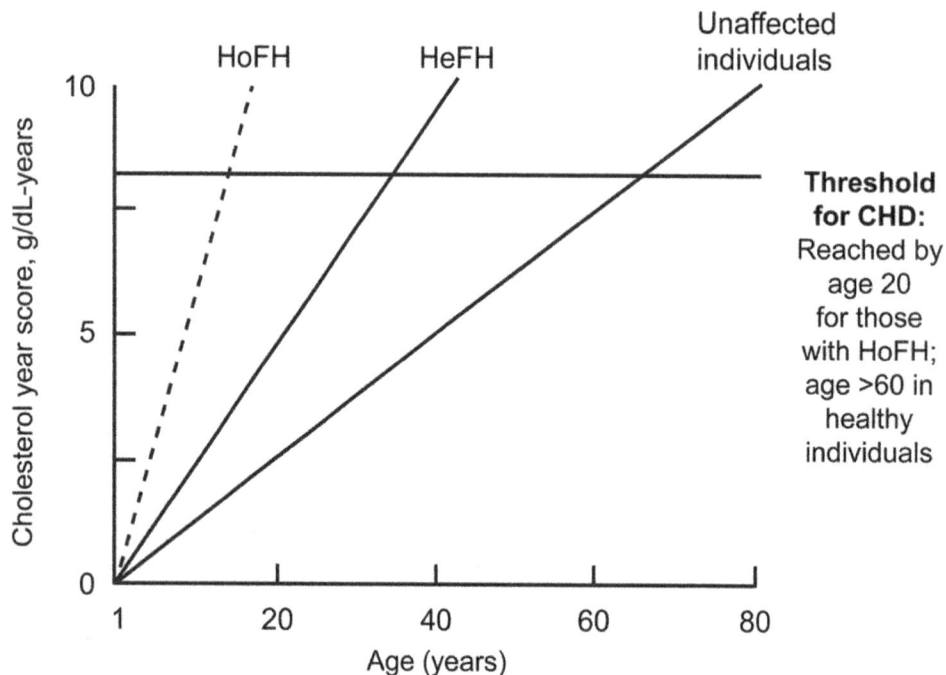

Figure 1. Cumulative LDL exposure in patients with FH [8, 9]. Modified from Horton et al. 2009 [9].

The severe lipid abnormalities associated with HoFH result in accelerated atherosclerosis, accelerated cardiovascular disease (CVD), and an increased risk of cardiac events and early death. It is estimated that CVD risk is increased by up to 20-fold in untreated patients and still elevated approximately 10-fold in patients receiving statins [5–7]. The lifelong exposure of highly elevated lipid levels means that signs/symptoms of CVD occur at an early age— typically prior to 20 years of age and as early as preteen years with the highest risk in males [5, 8]. Females develop CVD about 10 years later than males [6]. Young patients often have severe and widespread atherosclerosis in all major arterial beds, including the carotid, coronary, femoral, and iliac, and there have been instances of acute myocardial infarction and sudden death in patients as young as 4 years of age [8]. The CVD risk is related to cumulative LDL-C exposure. As seen in **Figure 1**, patients with HoFH exceed the theoretical threshold of LDL-C exposure in early childhood compared with early middle age for patients with HeFH and after age 60 years for normal healthy individuals [8, 9]. Although, as with all individuals, the risk of developing CVD is also related to the presence of other genetic or environmental risk factors, the effect of each risk factor is amplified in the setting of dramatically elevated cholesterol levels [4].

The physical signs and symptoms of HoFH are characterized by accelerated atherosclerosis and the deposition of cholesterol. Atherosclerotic manifestations include vascular endothelial damage that produces premature coronary artery disease (CAD), peripheral artery disease, and valvular disease (e.g., aortic stenosis) [4]. Deposition of cholesterol results in the development of cutaneous or tendinous xanthomas and corneal arcus [8]. Xanthomas typically occur around the eyelids and tendons of the feet, hands, and elbows [5].

HoFH is substantially underdiagnosed and undertreated [7]. For example, it is estimated that less than 1% of patients with FH are diagnosed in most countries and that only 48% of patients with FH were receiving statin therapy in one Danish study [7]. Most patients with FH are not identified because of inconsistent screening and general unawareness [6]. Indeed, the disease is often not recognized until the initial cardiovascular (CV) event [6].

2. Epidemiology

The exact prevalence rate of HoFH is unknown. Although the prevalence is historically estimated to be approximately 1 in 1 million [7], this likely underestimates true prevalence rates. More recent estimates, based on surveys of unselected general populations that found a prevalence of HeFH of 1 in ~200 or 1 in 244, suggest a prevalence of 1 in 160,000 to 1 in 300,000 for HoFH [10]. Founder mutations that reduce genetic variation can influence the prevalence in certain racial groups or geographic locations, resulting in increased prevalence in certain groups (e.g., French Canadian, the Netherlands, Lebanese, Hokuriku district of Japan, South African Afrikaners) [11–15]. National programs that include patient registries and cascade screening have been useful for identifying patients and facilitating treatments.

3. Genetics

True HoFH is caused by two identical mutations that are inherited in an autosomal dominant pattern [16]. Two mutant alleles of the *LDLR* gene (*MIM 606945*) cause the majority (85–95%)

of cases [7, 10, 17]. Mutations in this gene cause a reduction in LDLR activity and are associated with decreased clearance of LDL particles and increased LDL-C levels.

Secondary genes associated with HoFH include *APOB* (*MIM107730*), *PCSK9* (*MIM 607786*), and *LDLR-adaptor protein 1* (*LDLRAP1*; *MIM 605747*) [8, 10, 17]. In addition to "true" HoFH, patients with HoFH can have compound heterozygous mutations (different mutations in each allele of the same gene) or double heterozygous mutations (mutations in two different genes affecting LDLR function) [7, 10]. The severity of the HoFH depends on residual LDLR activity. Irrespective of the underlying genetic defect, patients with HoFH are classified as either receptor negative (i.e., <2% residual activity) or receptor defective (i.e., 2–25% residual activity) [10]. The effect on LDL-C concentrations is also related to genotype. Homozygous *LDLR*-defective mutations are generally associated with the highest LDL-C levels, followed by compound heterozygous *LDLR*-defective + *LDLR*-negative mutations, homozygous *LDLRAP1* or *LDLR*-defective mutations, homozygous *APOB* or *PCKS9* gain-of-function mutation, and double heterozygous mutation [5, 10]. Metabolic defects include impaired LDL uptake (the most common functional defect), hepatic oversecretion of apo B, decreased catabolism of triglyceride-rich lipoproteins, increased plasma levels of lipoprotein(a) (Lp(a)), and low levels of HDL-C [10].

4. Diagnosis

Since CV risk is related to the cumulative exposure to elevated lipids, early diagnosis is important for earlier treatment of HoFH to reduce CV risk. Although genetic testing can confirm FH, it is not well defined since genetic confirmation can be difficult to verify in some patients [10]. Indeed, genetic testing is generally not needed as the disease is primarily diagnosed via clinical and biochemical features [6–8, 10, 18]. A number of diagnostic criteria have been proposed [8], but they are typically based on family history (i.e., HeFH in both parents and/or premature CAD), the presence of physical manifestations (i.e., tendon xanthomas, corneal arcus) at an early age, severely increased LDL-C, and molecular diagnosis. Patients with HoFH generally have untreated LDL-C levels >500 mg/dL (>13 mmol/L) or treated levels ≥300 mg/dL (≥7.76 mmol/L) [8]. However, not all patients (especially children) with HoFH have significantly elevated LDL-C, with more than one-half of Dutch children with HoFH having LDL-C levels between 217 and 379 mg/dL (5.6–9.8 mmol/L) [10]. Patients with a suspected diagnosis of HoFH should typically be referred to a specialized center for proper comprehensive management [6, 10].

Since early detection of patients with HoFH is crucial for the prevention of CVD, targeted and cascade (i.e., identifying family members at risk) screening is recommended for the identification of new cases in adults [6, 7, 16, 19, 20]. Targeted screening to identify index cases is recommended for patients with hypercholesterolemia and at least one of the following features: personal/family history of xanthomas or premature CVD or family history of significant hypercholesterolemia or sudden premature cardiac death [6, 7]. Specific criteria in Europe (i.e., European Atherosclerosis Society [EAS]) are similar, but somewhat different than those of the National Lipid Association in the United States (US), with slightly different cholesterol cut-points for screening [21]. Such testing is important because most patients identified via screening were not aware of the diagnosis and were therefore not receiving therapy [17]. The index subject should be referred for genetic screening and a family pedigree should be created to identify potential cases, followed by cascade screening with LDL-C measurements [7]. Targeted screening is also recommended in children and adolescents with CV risk factors [6, 16]. Prenatal diagnosis is possible, and it is recommended that the partners of known cases of HeFH should be tested to exclude the disease [22]. Economic modeling has shown that comprehensive screening using cholesterol and DNA testing is cost-effective [19].

5. Treatment options

Given the severity of hypercholesterolemia with increased CV risk, HoFH requires intensive therapy. However, HoFH is often unresponsive to traditional treatment [20]. A number of societies and associations in the United States (American College of Cardiology/American Heart Association; National Lipid Association) [20, 23, 24], Europe (EAS; National Institute for Health and Care Excellence) [10, 25], and Canada (Canadian Cardiovascular Society) [6] have published guidelines on the treatment of HoFH. The primary target of treatment in these guidelines is the reduction of LDL-C via a combination of lifestyle, antihyperlipidemic pharmacotherapy, and apheresis [6, 10, 20, 23, 26]. Since lipid-lowering therapy is associated with a delayed onset of CVD and prolonged survival, early and aggressive therapy should be initiated as soon as possible [6, 10]. The EAS has recommended LDL-C targets of <100 mg/dL (<2.5 mmol/L) in children and <70 mg/dL (<1.8 mmol/L) in adults [10].

Statins, the first line of pharmacotherapy to lowering cholesterol level, effectively lower LDL-C 10% to 25% in patients with HoFH [10, 26], and even more (approximately 50% reduction of LDL-C) in those with HeFH [26]. The combination with ezetimibe (acholesterol absorption inhibitor) leads to additive 15–20% LDL-C reductions [6, 10]. Other agents such as bile acid sequestrants, niacin, fibrates, and probucol can be considered. A clinical study of HoFH patients from South Africa found that statin use was associated with a 51% reduction in the risk of major CV events and a 66% reduction in the risk of death although the mean LDL-C levels in the patients were only reduced 26% [27].

Because of very high LDL-C levels in HoFH, its target level is extremely difficult to achieve though cholesterol has been reduced [10]. The inability of standard lipid-lowering therapies to produce the necessary effect is further exacerbated by the fact that these agents work by increasing expression of LDLRs. Thus, lipoprotein apheresis should be considered in all patients with HoFH and should be initiated early. For example, the EAS guidelines recommend that apheresis should ideally be initiated by age 5 and not later than age 8 in children with HoFH [10]. Canadian guidelines recommend apheresis in adults with HoFH with LDL-C >329 mg/dL (>8.5 mmol/L) and in children (weighing >15 kg or >7 years of age) with an LDL-C >193 mg/dL (>5 mmol/L) [6]. LDL apheresis selectively removes LDL-C without affecting immu-noglobulins or other proteins with reductions of approximately 60% [18]. However, a rapid rebound in LDL-C is seen with levels returning to baseline within 2 to 4 weeks [18, 20]. Although there are no randomized trials evaluating the effect of apheresis on clinical outcomes, there is clinical evidence that apheresis can contribute to regression and/or stabilization of atherosclerotic plaque [10]. Limitations to the use of apheresis include lack of availability in some locations, high cost, long procedure duration, and the need to maintain vascular access [4]. It is recommended that patients on apheresis undergo routine monitoring to assess carotid atherosclerosis (carotid ultrasound), progression of aortic valve/root disease (echocardiography), and progression of coronary atherosclerosis (stress exercise test) [6].

6. New pharmacologic therapies

Recently, three novel agents have become available—mipomersen, lomitapide, and evolocumab—each with a unique mechanism of action. Two of these agents (mipomersen and lomitapide) target very low-density lipoprotein (VLDL) production, while the other (evolocumab) causes increased catabolism of LDL-C via LDLR recycling (**Figure 2**) [10].

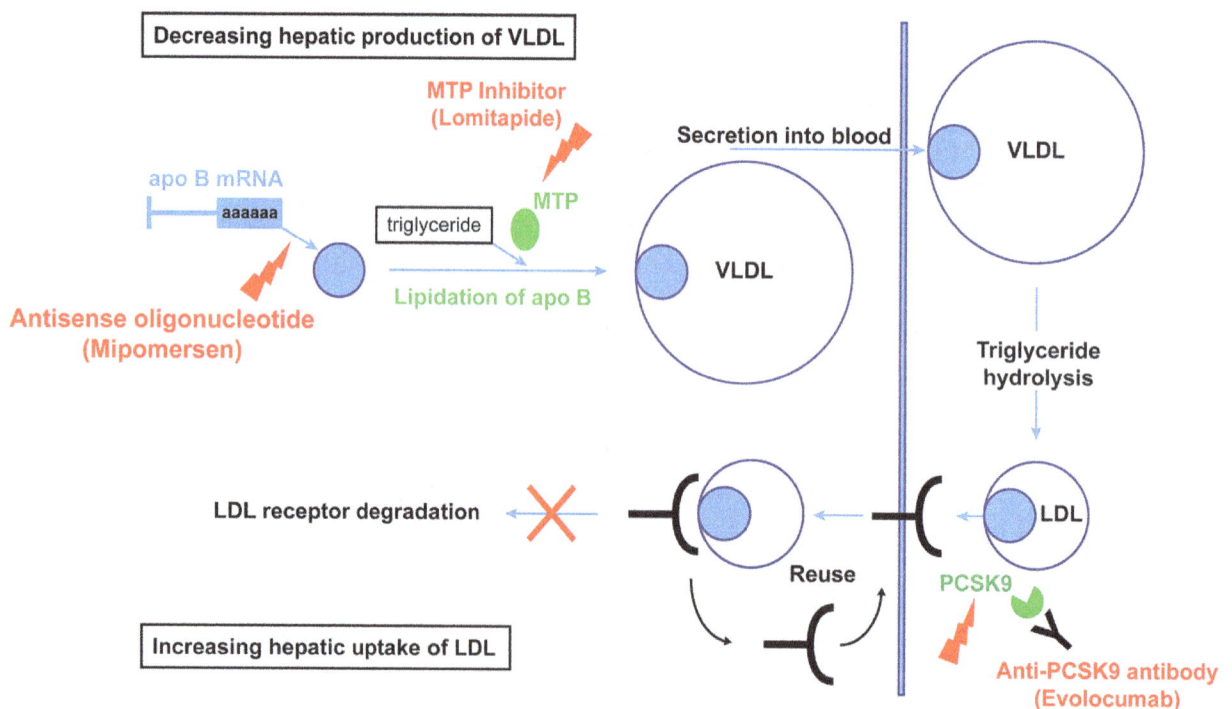

Figure 2. Mechanisms of action of mipomersen, lomitapide, and evolocumab. Modified from Cuchel et al. 2014 [10].

Properties of these agents are summarized in **Table 1** [28–32] and are discussed in detail in the following sections. These agents produce additive LDL-C lowering when combined with other lipid-lowering therapies such as statins, ezetimibe, and apheresis [10] and represent promising approaches to the treatment of HoFH for those patients who cannot achieve LDL-C targets with conventional therapy.

Agent	MOA	Indication	Dosage and administration	LDL-C lowering	Adverse events
Mipomersen[29]	Oligonucleotide inhibitor of apolipoprotein B-100 synthesis	Adjunctive therapy in HoFH	**HoFH:** 200 mg SC once weekly	25%	Increased transaminases Hepatic steatosis Injection-site reactions
Lomitapide [28,30,31]	Microsomal triglyceride transfer protein inhibitor	Adjunctive therapy in HoFH	**HoFH:** Initiate at 5 mg/day, titrating to max of 60 mg/day	46%	Increased transaminases Hepatic steatosis
Evolocumab[32]	PCSK9 inhibitor	Adjunctive therapy in HeFH and HoFH	**HeFH:** 140 mg SC every 2 weeks or 420 mg SC once monthly[b] **HoFH:** 420 mg SC once monthly	23%	Nasopharyngitis, upper respiratory tract infection, influenza, back pain, and injection-site reactions

[a]Based on phase III trials in HoFH;

[b]Administered as three injections consecutively within 30 minutes.

HeFH, heterozygous familial hypercholesterolemia; HoFH, homozygous familial hypercholesterolemia; LDL-C, low-density lipoprotein cholesterol; MOA, mechanisms of action; PCSK9, proprotein convertase subtilisin/kexin type 9; SC, subcutaneous.

Table 1. Novel agents for the treatment of HoFH.

6.1. Mipomersen

6.1.1. Pharmacodynamics

Apo B is the primary protein of VLDL, intermediate density lipoprotein, and LDL and is essential for the production and catabolism of VLDL and LDL [33, 34]. Apo B is involved in the packaging and distribution of both dietary and endogenously produced cholesterol and triglycerides by lipoproteins [35]. The atherosclerotic potential of apo B is evidenced by the observation that apo B concentrations are highly predictive for atherosclerotic disease, including patients with FH [8, 33].

Mipomersen is an antisense oligonucleotide against the mRNA of apo B-100, the primary ligand for the LDLR [33, 34]. The drug reduces apo B mRNA translation, and thereby the synthesis of apo B by ribosomes, resulting in a reduction in the secretion of VLDL. Thus, mipomersen targets the production of LDL rather than its clearance (**Figure 2**) [34]. In animal models, species-specific inhibition of antisense apo B leads to reductions in apo B-100, LDL-C, and total cholesterol in a dose- and time-dependent manner [29, 35].

Mipomersen is readily absorbed after subcutaneous administration with the highest drug concentrations in the liver and kidney. Bioavailability ranges from 54% to 78% over a dose range of 50 to 400 mg [29]. Elimination is primarily via metabolism by endonucleases and renal excretion (as parent drug and metabolites) and the half-life ranges from 1 to 2 months [29, 35]. In the United States, mipomersen is indicated as an adjunct to lipid-lowering medications and diet to reduce LDL-C, apo B, total cholesterol, and non-HDL-C in patients with HoFH [36]. The drug is administered once weekly by subcutaneous injection [29].

6.1.2. Efficacy

Based on its mechanism of action and its demonstrated activity in patients with hypercholesterolemia as either monotherapy or in combinations, it is reasonable that mipomersen would be effective in the treatment of HoFH [35]. In a phase II, open-label, study, mipomersen was administered in a dose-escalation fashion (50, 100, 200, and 300 mg) to nine patients with HoFH. Patients received five doses over 2 weeks followed by weekly dosing through week 6 ($n = 5$) or week 13 ($n = 4$). At week 6, LDL-C reductions ranged from 0.5% to 36%. By week 13, the reductions ranged from 9.0% to 51.1%[29].

The phase III trial of mipomersen in patients with HoFH included 51 patients with clinical diagnosis or genetically confirmed HoFH [37]. Mean baseline LDL-C was 402 mg/dL (10.4 mmol/L). Patients who received maximally tolerated doses of lipid-lowering drug were randomized to receive mipomersen 200 mg subcutaneously ($n = 34$) or placebo ($n = 17$) once weekly for 26 weeks [37]. The primary endpoint was the percent change in LDL-C concentration from baseline. Secondary endpoints were changes from baseline in apo B, total cholesterol, and non-HDL-C concentrations. At 26 weeks, mipomersen-treated patients achieved significant reductions in all primary and secondary endpoints versus placebo: LDL-C (–24.7%), apo B (–26.8%), total cholesterol (–21.2%), and non-HDLC (–24.5%). By comparison, reductions for those in the placebo group were: LDL-C (–3.3%), apo B (–2.5%), total cholesterol (–2.0%), and non-HDL-C (–2.9%). In addition, mipomersen was also associated with substantial reductions in Lp(a) (–31.1%), triglycerides (–17.4%), and VLDL (–17.4%), and a significant increase in HDL-C (+15.1%). Notably, there was substantial variability in the reduction of LDL-C concentrations among HoFH patients receiving mipomersen with values ranging from +2% to –82%. The magnitude of treatment effect was independent of baseline LDL-C, age, race, or sex in multivariate analysis [37].

6.1.3. Safety/tolerability

In the phase III HoFH trial, the most common adverse events among patients with HoFH were injection-site reactions (76%), flu-like symptoms (29%), nausea (18%), headache (15%), and chest pain (12%). Injection-site reactions included erythema (56%), hematoma (35%), pain (35%), pruritus (29%), discoloration (29%), macule (15%), papule (12%), and swelling (12%). Similar rates of injection-site reactions were observed in pooled data from other clinical trials with rates of 84% and 33%, respectively, for those in the mipomersen and placebo groups [29]. Most reactions were of mild to moderate severity with only 5% discontinuing treatment because of an injection-site reaction. In pooled phase III trials that included all patients with hypercholesterolemia, 30% of patients experienced flu-like symptoms (e.g., pyrexia, chills, myalgia, arthralgia, malaise, fatigue) compared with 16% of those receiving placebo [29].

Laboratory abnormalities in the phase III HoFH trial were primarily characterized by elevated liver transaminases. Alanine aminotransferase (ALT) increases of ≥1 but ≤3 times the upper limit of normal (ULN) were observed in 50% of patients in the mipomersen groups but was similar to that seen with placebo (53%). However, increased ALT of ≥3 × ULN was seen in 12% of mipomersen-treated patients but none of the placebo-treated patients [37]. In the pooled phase III trials, 8.4% of patients receiving mipomersen experienced an elevated ALT >3 × ULN on two consecutive occasions at least 7 days apart compared to 0.0% of placebo-treated patients [29]. These ALT changes were generally associated with lesser elevations of aspartate aminotransferase (AST). Mipomersen was also associated with an increase in hepatic fat in 9.6% of patients compared with 0.02% of placebo-treated patients. However, this increase was not accompanied by changes in patient weight, plasma glucose, or HbA1c, suggesting that there is no associated increased risk of metabolic syndrome. It is suggested that the hepatic steatosis and elevated transaminase concentrations are inherent consequences of attenuating apo B production. Nevertheless, mipomersen carries a black box warning for the risk of hepatotoxicity (i.e., increased transaminases and hepatic steatosis) and the drug is only available in the United States via a Risk Evaluation and Mitigation Strategy program [29].

6.2. Lomitapide

6.2.1. Pharmacodynamics

The microsomal triglyceride transfer protein (MTP) is an intracellular lipid-transfer protein located in the lumen of the endoplasmic reticulum. It is responsible for binding and moving individual lipid molecules between membranes. MTP is a major mediator of the assembly and secretion of apo B-containing lipoproteins such as VLDL from the liver, which is converted into LDL-C, and chylomicrons, which contain dietary cholesterol and triglycerides, from the intestine [30, 31, 38]. The rare genetic condition abetalipoproteinemia provides insight into the importance of MTP in lipid handling and transport. Abetalipoproteinemia is characterized by loss-of-function mutations in the gene encoding MTP (i.e., *MTTP*) and is associated with marked hypocholesterolemia and an absence of apo B-containing lipoproteins in the plasma [35]. Lack of functional MTP in abetalipoproteinemia results in the inability to load apo B with lipoproteins and the targeted proteasomal degradation of apo B. This leads to a loss of intestinal secretion of chylomicrons and liver secretion of VLDL and a consequent lack of LDL-C in the plasma [35]. Thus, inhibition of MTP is a potentially powerful therapeutic target to reduce the production of apo B-containing lipoproteins, particularly VLDL (the precursor of LDL-C) [30].

Lomitapide is a small molecule that inhibits MTP action. By binding directly to MTP, lomitapide inhibits the synthesis of triglyceride-rich chylomicrons in the intestine and VLDL in the liver, with a resulting reduction in plasma LDL-C [39]. The mechanism of action of lomitapide in inhibiting MTP is illustrated in **Figure 2**.

Oral absorption of lomitapide is poor with an absolute bioavailability of 7%, thought to be due to a first-pass effect. Lomitapide pharmacokinetics is approximately dose proportional after single oral doses of 10–100 mg. The drug is extensively metabolized in the liver and has a terminal half-life of 39.7 hours [28, 30]. Lomitapide is indicated in the United States and the European Union as an adjunct to a low-fat diet and other lipid-lowering treatments, including LDL apheresis where available, to reduce LDL-C, total cholesterol, apo B, and non-HDL-C in patients with HoFH [28, 39].

6.2.2. Efficacy

An initial study in 18 patients with HoFH evaluated the addition of lomitapide to usual lipid-lowering therapy, including apheresis [40]. The dose of lomitapide was gradually titrated during the first 14–18 weeks to a target dose of 60 mg/day (80 mg/day if LDL and safety criteria were met). The mean overall LDL-C reduction was 44% at 6 months compared with baseline but the individual values ranged from an increase in LDL-C of 19% to a reduction of 93%, indicating a wide variability of effect. Four patients achieved an LDL-C <100 mg/dL (<2.6 mmol/L) and another two achieved levels <170 mg/dL (<4.4 mmol/L) [40].

The pivotal phase III open-label trial included 29 patients with HoFH based on clinical criteria or documented genetic mutations [41]. Upon enrollment, patients were required to enter a 6-week run-in phase in which patients were initiated on concomitant lipid-lowering therapy (including apheresis), vitamin E, essential fatty acids, and a low-fat diet. Patients then entered a 26-week efficacy phase where lomitapide was initiated at 5 mg/day and titrated (at 4-week intervals) up to a maximum of 60 mg/day. Following the efficacy phase, patients continued lomitapide therapy in a 52-week safety phase. Mean baseline total cholesterol and LDL-C levels were 429 mg/dL (11.1 mmol/L) and 336 mg/dL (8.7 mmol/L), respectively [41]. Twenty-three of 29 patients completed both the efficacy phase (26 weeks) and safety phase (52 weeks). At the end of 26 weeks, patients achieved statistically significant mean reductions from baseline in total cholesterol (–46%; $P < 0.0001$) and LDL-C (–50%; $P < 0.0001$) [41]. The large majority of patients ($n = 19/23$ [83%]) achieved LDL-C reductions >25% and one-half ($n = 12/23$) had a >50% reduction [41]. Furthermore, 8 patients achieved LDL-C concentrations <100 mg/dL (<2.6 mmol/L). Based on these LDL-C reductions, three patients permanently discontinued apheresis and three permanently increased the time interval between apheresis treatments. Significant reductions from baseline were also seen for VLDL cholesterol (–45%), non-HDL-C (–50%), triglycerides (–45%), and apo B (–49%). Lipid lowering was independent of the use of apheresis, suggesting that apheresis does not affect the lipid-lowering efficacy of lomitapide [42]. These reductions were maintained throughout the 52-week safety phase with reductions of 35% and 38%, respectively, for total cholesterol and LDL-C despite changes in concomitant lipid-lowering therapy [41]. Nineteen of the 23 patients who competed the efficacy and safety phases entered a long-term extension study [43, 44]. As of 2015, the median duration of treatment was 5.1 years [43]. At 126 weeks, mean LDL-C levels were reduced by 46%. Similar reductions were also observed in apo B (–54%), non-HDL-C (–47%), VLDL cholesterol (–37%), and triglycerides (–38%) [43, 44].

Additional evidence of the efficacy of lomitapide in HoFH comes from a Japanese trial [45] and the Lomitapide Observational Worldwide Evaluation Registry (LOWER) [45, 46]. The Japanese trial included nine patients with a mean baseline LDL-C of 199 mg/dL (5.2 mmol/L), which was reduced to 118 mg/dL (3.1 mmol/L) at week 26 (–42%) [45]. Significant reductions were also seen for total cholesterol (–32%), non-HDL-C (–40%), VLDL (–42%), apo B (–45%), and triglycerides (–42%) [45]. LOWER is a noninterventional registry open to lomitapide-treated patients that is designed to evaluate the long-term safety and efficacy of lomitapide in clinical practice and is eventually expected to enroll at least 300 patients and follow them for at least 10 years [47]. As of March 2015, 84 patients had enrolled in LOWER, with all but one from the United States [46]. Titration of lomitapide occurred slower than in the pivotal phase III trial, with a mean dose of 10 mg reached only after 12 months. The mean reduction in LDL-C at month 4 was 42%, with 38% of patients achieving a reduction of at least 50% at 6 months [46, 47].

6.2.3. Safety/tolerability

Oral lomitapide was generally well tolerated in patients with HoFH. Although the majority of patients experienced an adverse event in the phase III trial ($n = 27/29$ [93%] in the efficacy phase; $n = 21/23$ [91%] in the safety phase), most events were mild to moderate in intensity [41]. The most common adverse events were gastrointestinal in nature, with 27/29 patients in the efficacy phase and 21/23 patients in the safety phase experiencing a gastrointestinal event [41]. The most common events in the phase III trial were gastrointestinal in nature (27 patients during the efficacy phase and 17 during the safety phase), most commonly manifested as diarrhea, nausea, dyspepsia, and vomiting [41, 43]. Three patients discontinued treatment due to a gastrointestinal event [41]. The incidence of gastrointestinal events decreased during the extension phase: diarrhea (42%), nausea (32%), vomiting (26%), and dyspepsia (11%) [43].

Ten patients in the phase III trial had elevated levels of ALT, AST, or both >3 × ULN at least once during the trial, and four patients had elevations at least 5 × ULN [41]. No patient discontinued treatment permanently because of these elevations and all were managed by either dose reduction or temporary interruption of lomitapide [41, 43]. In the LOWER registry, elevated transaminase levels ≥3 × ULN were observed in only 16 patients (19%) [46].

Among the 20 patients from the phase III trials with evaluable nuclear magnetic resonance spectroscopy data, hepatic fat increased from 1% at baseline to 8.6% at the end of week 26 and 8.3% at week 78 [41]. Hepatic fat continued to increase through the extension trial [43], although the accumulation of fat appears to be reversible after discontinuation of lomitapide [39]. Whether this fat accumulation is a risk factor for the development of steatohepatitis and cirrhosis is currently unknown. No cases of cirrhosis or late-stage liver disease have been identified in the long-term extension studies [43].

6.3. Evolocumab

6.3.1. Pharmacodynamics

PCSK9 is a key regulator of LDLR function. When PCSK9 binds to the LDLR, LDLR degradation is enhanced in the liver, thereby increasing LDL-C plasma concentrations [4].Although some patients with HoFH have no LDLR function, up to 75% have residual activity (between 2% and 25%) [2]. Patients with HoFH also have increased PCSK9 function. Among patients with residual LDLR function, PCSK9 inhibition may be useful for lowering LDL-C [2]. Evolocumab is a human immunoglobulin G2 monoclonal antibody directed against human PCSK9. By binding to PCSK9, evolocumab inhibits circulating PCSK9 from binding to the LDLR, preventing PCSK9-mediated LDLR degradation and permitting LDLR to recycle back to the liver cell surface. This increases the number of LDLRs available to clear LDL from the blood, thereby lowering LDL-C level (**Figure 2**) [32, 48, 49].

6.3.2. Efficacy

The addition of evolocumab to stable lipid-lowering therapy was evaluated in an open-label pilot trial in eight patients with LDLR-negative or LDLR-defective HoFH [32]. Patients received subcutaneous evolocumab 420 mg every 4 weeks for 12 weeks, maintained for an additional 12 weeks at 4-week intervals, and then 420 mg of evolocumab every 2 weeks for an additional 12 weeks [32]. All eight patients had LDLR mutations, with six patients having defective receptor status (i.e., residual LDLR function) and two having negative LDLR function. Mean baseline LDL-C was 441 mg/dL (11.4 mmol/L) [32]. After 12 weeks of every 4-week dosing, mean LDL-C decreased by a mean of 17% (range, +5% to −44%). The two patients with negative LDLR activity did not achieve reductions in LDL-C [32]. After 12 weeks of every 2-week dosing, mean LDL-C was reduced by 14%, again with no reductions in the two patients that were LDLR-negative. Apo B was reduced by 14.9% and 12.5% by the 4-week and 2-week dosing schedules and Lp(a) was reduced by 11.7% and 18.6%, respectively, by the two schedules. However, there was little change in triglycerides, HDL-C, or apolipoprotein A1 with either schedule [32].

The pivotal randomized, phase III, double-blind, placebo-controlled trial included 49 patients with HoFH on stable lipid-lowering therapy (but not apheresis) for at least 4 weeks. Patients were randomized in a 2:1 ratio to receive evolocumab 420 mg or placebo every 4 weeks [48]. LDLR mutations in both alleles were present in 45 of 48 patients (94%), with 22 of these having the same mutation in both alleles (true HoFH) and 23 having different mutations in each LDLR allele (i.e., compound heterozygous FH) [48]. One patient receiving evolocumab had LDLR receptor-negative mutations in both alleles and another had autosomal recessive hypercholesterolemia. The mean decrease in ultracentrifugation LDL-C was 23.1% for those receiving evolocumab compared with a 7.9% increase for the placebo group (primary endpoint) [48]. Evolocumab was also associated with a 19.2% reduction in apo B at week 12, although changes in Lp(a), HDL-C, and triglycerides were not significantly different relative to placebo [48]. Response to evolocumab correlated with the underlying genetic cause of HoFH, with a greater reduction in LDL-C among those with two LDLR-defective mutations than in those with even a single LDLR-negative mutation. However, among the 20 patients receiving evolocumab who had defects in either one or both alleles, a 29.5% reduction in ultracentrifugation LDL-C was achieved [48]. The patient with LDLR-negative mutations in both alleles and the one with autosomal recessive hypercholesterolemia did not respond to evolocumab (LDL-C levels increased by 3–10%) [48].

The efficacy of evolocumab in combination with apheresis is under evaluation in the Trial Assessing Long Term Use of PCSK9 Inhibition in Subjects with Genetic LDL Disorders (TAUSSIG) in patients with severe FH not controlled with current lipid therapy [50]. Patients received evolocumab 420 mg and apheresis every 2 weeks. An interim analysis found that evolocumab was associated with a mean reduction of 17% in LDL-C at week 12 ($n = 24$) and 20% at week 24 ($n = 12$) [50]. Four patients were able to stop or decrease the frequency of apheresis. The three patients with LDLR-negative mutations in both alleles did not respond to evolocumab. Evolocumab is indicated in the United States and EU as an adjunct to diet and other LDL-lowering therapies for the treatment of patients with HoFH who require additional lowering of LDL-C.

6.3.3. Safety/tolerability

In the phase III trial in patients with HoFH, the most common adverse events among those receiving evolocumab were upper respiratory tract infection (9%), influenza (9%), gastroenteritis (6%), nasopharyngitis (6%), and increased ALT or AST $\geq 3 \times$ ULN [48]. There were no adverse event-related treatment discontinuations. These rates of adverse events are generally consistent with those seen in other large randomized trials evaluating evolocumab in the treatment of hypercholesterolemia [49]. Immunogenicity appears to be uncommon, with only 0.1% of patients in pooled clinical trials testing positive for binding antibody development. There was no evidence of neutralizing antibodies and no evidence that the presence of antidrug antibodies impacted the pharmacokinetic profile, clinical response, or safety of evolocumab [49].

7. Conclusions

HoFH is a rare disease that is underdiagnosed and undertreated and is associated with substantial morbidity and mortality. Early diagnosis and aggressive therapy are the cornerstones of the management of HoFH. Until recently, therapeutic options were limited and insufficient to get patients to their treatment goals. The availability of novel pharmacologic agents provides clinicians with additional treatment options in this difficult-to-treat population. **Figure 3** summarizes the suggested treatment algorithm of the EAS for patients with HoFH [10].

This algorithm highlights the novel treatment options that will allow greater reductions in lipid levels in HoFH patients and let them achieve their target goals. It is hoped and expected that these expanded options will ultimately translate into improvements in clinical outcomes including a decrease in CV events and CVD-related mortality.

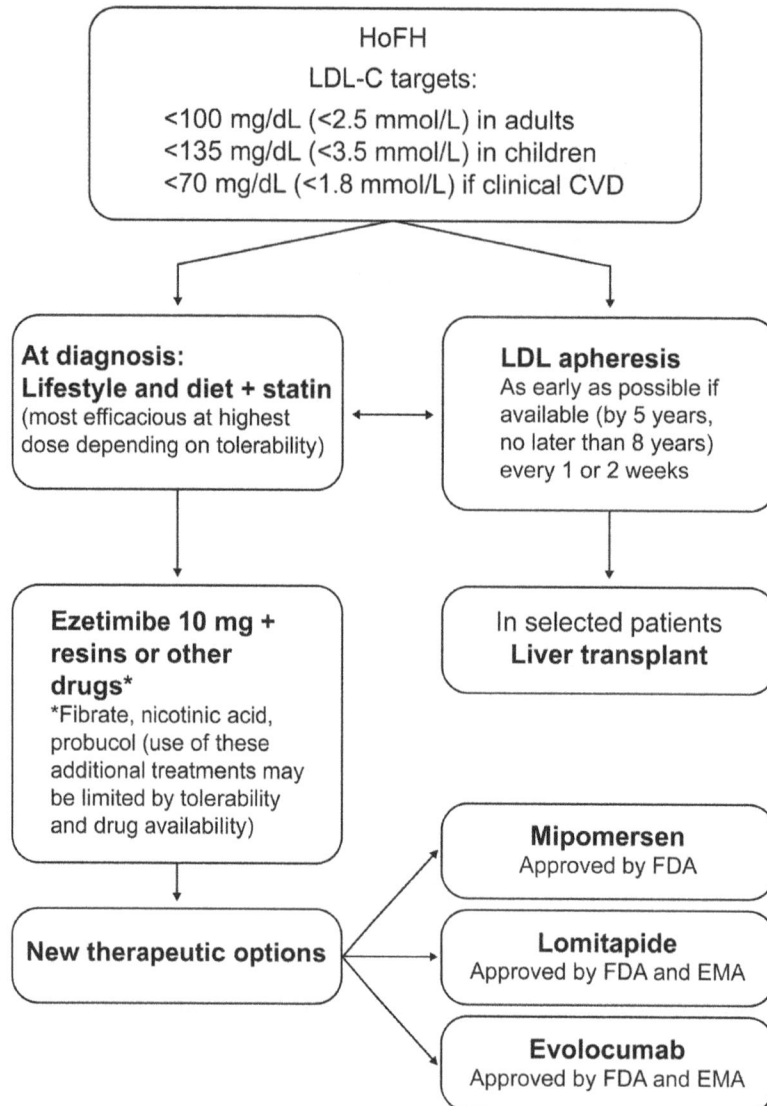

Figure 3. European Atherosclerosis Society treatment algorithm for the management of HoFH. Modified from Cuchel et al. 2014 [10].

Author details

Min-Ji Charng

Address all correspondence to: mjcharng@vghtpe.gov.tw

Division of Cardiology, Taipei Veterans General Hospital and National Yang-Ming University, Taipei, Taiwan, R.O.C.

References

[1] Sniderman AD, Tsimikas S, Fazio S. The severe hypercholesterolemia phenotype: clinical diagnosis, management, and emerging therapies. J Am Coll Cardiol. 2014;63:1935–1947.

[2] Chiou KR, Charng MJ. Genetic diagnosis of familial hypercholesterolemia in Han J Clin Lipidol. 2016;10:490–496.

[3] Marais AD, Blom DJ. Recent advances in the treatment of homozygous familial hypercholesterolaemia. Curr Opin Lipidol. 2013;24:288–294.

[4] Farnier M, Bruckert E. Severe familial hypercholesterolaemia: current and future management. Arch Cardiovasc Dis. 2012;105:656–665.

[5] Singh S, Bittner V. Familial hypercholesterolemia—epidemiology, diagnosis, and screening. Curr Atheroscler Rep. 2015;17:482–485.

[6] Genest J, Hegele RA, Bergeron J, Brophy J, Carpentier A, Couture P, et al. Canadian Cardiovascular Society position statement on familial hypercholesterolemia. Can J Cardiol. 2014;30:1471–1481.

[7] Nordestgaard BG, Chapman MJ, Humphries SE, Ginsberg HN, Masana L, Descamps OS, et al. Familial hypercholesterolaemia is underdiagnosed and undertreated in the general population: guidance for clinicians to prevent coronary heart disease: consensus statement of the European Atherosclerosis Society. Eur Heart J. 2013;34:3478–3490.

[8] Raal FJ, Santos RD. Homozygous familial hypercholesterolemia: current perspectives on diagnosis and treatment. Atherosclerosis. 2012;223:262–268.

[9] Horton JD, Cohen JC, Hobbs HH. PCSK9: a convertase that coordinates LDL catabolism. J Lipid Res. 2009;50(Suppl):S172–S177.

[10] Cuchel M, Bruckert E, Ginsberg HN, Raal FJ, Santos RD, Hegele RA, et al. Homozygous familial hypercholesterolaemia: new insights and guidance for clinicians to improve detection and clinical management. A position paper from the Consensus Panel on Familial Hypercholesterolaemia of the European Atherosclerosis Society. Eur Heart J. 2014;35:2146–2157.

[11] Fahed AC, Safa RM, Haddad FF, Bitar FF, Andary RR, Arabi MT, et al. Homozygous familial hypercholesterolemia in Lebanon: a genotype/phenotype correlation. Mol Genet Metab. 2011;102:181–188.

[12] Kusters DM, Huijgen R, Defesche JC, Vissers MN, Kindt I, Hutten BA, et al. Founder mutations in the Netherlands: geographical distribution of the most prevalent mutations in the low-density lipoprotein receptor and apolipoprotein B genes. Neth Heart ˇ. 2011;19:175–182.

[13] Mabuchi H, Nohara A, Noguchi T, Kobayashi J, Kawashiri MA, Tada H, et al. Molecular genetic epidemiology of homozygous familial hypercholesterolemia in the Hokuriku district of Japan. Atherosclerosis. 2011;214:404–407.

[14] Moorjani S, Roy M, Gagne C, Davignon J, Brun D, Toussaint M, et al. Homozygous familial hypercholesterolemia among French Canadians in Quebec Province. Arteriosclerosis. 1989;9:211–216.

[15] Seftel HC, Baker SG, Sandler MP, Forman MB, Joffe BI, Mendelsohn D, et al. A host of hypercholesterolaemic homozygotes in South Africa. Br Med J. 1980;281:633–636.

[16] Feldman DI, Blaha MJ, Santos RD, Jones SR, Blumenthal RS, Toth PP, et al. Recommendations for the management of patients with familial hypercholesterolemia. Curr Atheroscler Rep. 2015;17:473. DOI: 10.1007/s11883-014-0473-6

[17] Alonso R, Mata P, Zambon D, Mata N, Fuentes-Jimenez F. Early diagnosis and treatment of familial hypercholesterolemia: improving patient outcomes. Expert Rev Cardiovasc Ther. 2013;11:327–342. DOI: 10.1586/erc.13.7

[18] Mombelli G, Pavanello C. Novel therapeutic strategies for the homozygous familial hypercholesterolemia. Recent Pat Cardiovasc Drug Discov. 2013;8:143–150. DOI: 10.2174/15748901112079990001

[19] Minhas R, Humphries SE, Qureshi N, Neil HA. Controversies in familial hypercholesterolaemia: recommendations of the NICE Guideline Development Group for the identification and management of familial hypercholesterolaemia. Heart. 2009;95:584–587. DOI: 10.1136/hrt.2008.162909

[20] Robinson JG. Management of familial hypercholesterolemia: a review of the recommendations from the National Lipid Association Expert Panel on Familial Hypercholesterolemia. J Manag Care Pharm. 2013;19:139–149.

[21] Gouni-Berthold I, Berthold HK. Familial hypercholesterolemia: etiology, diagnosis and new treatment options. Curr Pharm Des. 2014;20:6220–6229.

[22] Reiner Z, Catapano AL, De Backer G, Graham I, Taskinen MR, Wiklund O, et al. ESC/EAS Guidelines for the management of dyslipidaemias: the Task Force for the management of dyslipidaemias of the European Society of Cardiology (ESC) and the European Atherosclerosis Society (EAS). Eur Heart J. 2011;32:1769–1818. DOI: 10.1093/eurheartj/ehr158

[23] Ray KK, Kastelein JJ, Boekholdt SM, Nicholls SJ, Khaw KT, Ballantyne CM, et al. The ACC/AHA 2013 guideline on the treatment of blood cholesterol to reduce atherosclerotic cardiovascular disease risk in adults: the good the bad and the uncertain: a comparison with ESC/EAS guidelines for the management of dyslipidaemias 2011. Eur Heart J. 2014;35:960–968. DOI: 10.1093/eurheartj/ehu107

[24] Stone NJ, Robinson JG, Lichtenstein AH, Bairey Merz CN, Blum CB, Eckel RH, et al. 2013 ACC/AHA guideline on the treatment of blood cholesterol to reduce atheroscler-

otic cardiovascular risk in adults: a report of the American College of Cardiology/ American Heart Association Task Force on Practice Guidelines. Circulation. 2014;129:S1–S45. DOI: 10.1161/01.cir.0000437738.63853.7a

[25] National Institute on Clinical Care and Excellence (NICE). Familial hypercholesterolaemia: identifification and management.2008. Available from: http://www.nice.org.uk/guidance/cg71. [Accessed Nov 23, 2015]

[26] Bruckert E. Recommendations for the management of patients with homozygous familial hypercholesterolaemia: overview of a new European Atherosclerosis Society consensus statement. Atheroscler Suppl. 2014;15:26–32.

[27] Raal FJ, Pilcher GJ, Panz VR, van Deventer HE, Brice BC, Blom DJ, et al. Reduction in mortality in subjects with homozygous familial hypercholesterolemia associated with advances in lipid-lowering therapy. Circulation. 2011;124:2202–2207.

[28] JUXTAPID (lomitapide): package insert. Cambridge, MA: Aegerion Pharmaceuticals, Inc.; 2015.

[29] McGowan MP, Moriarty PM, Backes JM. The effects of mipomersen, a second-generation antisense oligonucleotide, on atherogenic (apoB-containing) lipoproteins in the treatment of homozygous familial hypercholesterolemia. Clin Lipidol. 2014;9:487–503.

[30] Perry CM. Lomitapide: a review of its use in adults with homozygous familial hypercholesterolemia. Am J Cardiovasc Drugs. 2013;13:285–296.

[31] Raal FJ. Lomitapide for homozygous familial hypercholesterolaemia. Lancet. 2013;381:7–8.

[32] Stein EA, Honarpour N, Wasserman SM, Xu F, Scott R, Raal FJ. Effect of the proprotein convertase subtilisin/kexin 9 monoclonal antibody, AMG 145, in homozygous familial hypercholesterolemia. Circulation. 2013;128:2113–2120.

[33] Parhofer KG. Mipomersen: evidence-based review of its potential in the treatment of homozygous and severe heterozygous familial hypercholesterolemia. Core Evid. 2012;7:29–38.

[34] Patel N, Hegele RA. Mipomersen as a potential adjunctive therapy for hypercholesterolemia. Expert Opin Pharmacother. 2010;11:2569–2572.

[35] Rader DJ, Kastelein JJ. Lomitapide and mipomersen: two first-in-class drugs for reducing low-density lipoprotein cholesterol in patients with homozygous familial hypercholesterolemia. Circulation. 2014;129:1022–1032.

[36] KYNAMRO (mipomersen sodium): package insert. Cambridge, MA: Genzyme Corporation; 2015.

[37] Raal FJ, Santos RD, Blom DJ, Marais AD, Charng MJ, Cromwell WC, et al. Mipomersen, an apolipoprotein B synthesis inhibitor, for lowering of LDL cholesterol concentrations

in patients with homozygous familial hypercholesterolaemia: a randomised, double-blind, placebo-controlled trial. Lancet. 2010;375:998–1006.

[38] Liao W, Hui TY, Young SG, Davis RA. Blocking microsomal triglyceride transfer protein interferes with apoB secretion without causing retention or stress in the ER. J Lipid Res. 2003;44:978–985.

[39] Lyseng-Willliamson KA, Perry CM. Lomitapide: a guide to its use in adults with homozygous familial hypercholesterolaemia in the EU. Drugs Ther Perspect. 2013;29:373–378.

[40] Cuchel M, Meagher E, Marais AD, Blom DJ, Theron HD, Baer AL, et al. Abstract 1077: a phase III study of microsomal triglyceride transfer protein inhibitor lomitapide (AEGR-733) in patients with homozygous familial hypercholesterolemia: interim results at 6 months [Abstract]. Circulation. 2009;120:S441.

[41] Cuchel M, Meagher EA, du Toit Theron H, Blom DJ, Marais AD, Hegele RA, et al. Efficacy and safety of a microsomal triglyceride transfer protein inhibitor in patients with homozygous familial hypercholesterolaemia: a single-arm, open-label, phase 3 study. Lancet. 2013;381:40–46.

[42] Averna M, Cuchel M, Meagher E, Du H, Theron T, Blom DJ, et al. Apheresis treatment does not affect the lipid-lowering efficacy of lomitapide, a microsomal triglyceride transfer protein inhibitor, in patients with homozygous familial hypercholesterolemia (HoFH). In: Deutschen Atherosklerosekongress 2012; 7–8 December 2012; Munich, Germany. Perfusion. 2012.

[43] Blom DJ, Averna M, Meagher E, Theron H, Sirtori C, Hegele RA, et al. Long-term efficacy and safety of lomitapide for the treatment of homozygous familial hypercholesterolemia: results of the phase 3 extension trial. In: American Heart Association; 7–11 November 2015; Orlando, FL.

[44] Cuchel M, Blom DJ, Averna MR, Meagher EA, Theron HD, Sirtori CR, et al. Sustained LDL-C lowering and stable hepatic fat levels in patients with homozygous familial hypercholesterolemia treated with the microsomal triglyceride transfer protein inhibitor, lomitapide: results of an ongoing long-term extension study [Abstract]. Circulation. 2013;128:A16516.

[45] Harada-Shiba M, Ikewaki K, Nohara A, Yanagi K, Otsubo Y, Foulds P, et al. Efficacy and safety of lomitapide in Japanese patients with homozygous familial hypercholesterolemia on cucurrent lipid-lowering therapy [Abstract]. Circulation. 2015;132:A12468.

[46] Blom DJ, Kastelein JJ, Larrey D, Makris L, Schwamiein C, Phillips H, et al. Lomitapide Observational Worldwide Evaluation Registry (LOWER): one-year data [Abstract]. Circulation. 2015;132:A10818.

[47] Blom DJ, Fayad ZA, Kastelein JJP, Larrey D, Makris L, Schwamiein C, et al. LOWER, a

registry of lomitapide-treated patients with homozygous familial hypercholesterole-mia: rationale and design. J Clin Lipidol. 2015;10:273–282.

[48] Raal FJ, Honarpour N, Blom DJ, Hovingh GK, Xu F, Scott R, et al. Inhibition of PCSK9 with evolocumab in homozygous familial hypercholesterolaemia (TESLA Part B): a randomised, double-blind, placebo-controlled trial. Lancet. 2015;385:341–350.

[49] REPATHA (evolocumab): package insert. Thousand Oaks, CA: Amgen, Inc.; 2015.

[50] Bruckert E, Blaha V, Stein EA, Raal FJ, Kurtz CE, Honarpour N, et al. Trial assessing long-term use of PCSK9 inhibition in patients with genetic LDL disorders (TAUSSIG): efficacy and safety in patients with homozygous familial hypercholesterolemia receiving lipid apheresis [Abstract]. Circulation. 2014;130:A17016.

7

Vascular Inflammation and Genetic Predisposition as Risk Factors for Cardiovascular Diseases

Zeynep Banu Gungor

Abstract

Atherosclerosis previously defined as an obstructive disease leads to fatty deposits in the arterial wall. Nowadays, according to the best of our knowledge, specific cells, molecular mechanisms, and genes play crucial roles in the pathogenesis of the disease. Inflammatory reaction contributes to atherosclerotic lesion formation, since fatty streak leads to a plaque erosion or rupture. Experimental and clinical studies have shown that besides well-known risk factors, such as smoking, hypertension, diabetes, and dyslipidemia, genetic variations in certain locuses affect the disease burden. A common genetic variability at the apoE locus has been shown to be associated with a risk for cardiovascular disease. In many studies, a higher cardiovascular risk has been associated with the presence of the apo ε4 allele, whereas the apo ε2 allele has been protective. Recent studies stated that pro-inflammatory cytokines increase the binding of low-density lipoprotein (LDL) to endothelium and smooth muscle cells, so inflammatory response solely increases lipoprotein accumulation within the vessel wall. As a conclusion, cholesterol accumulation leads to atherosclerotic plaque via several mechanisms. Genetic predisposition and inflammatory process may affect disease severity.

Keywords: vascular inflammation, apoE, Lp-PLA2, LDL subtypes, endothelial dysfunction

1. Introduction

Cholesterol is one of the important molecules of the organism due to its strong relationship with cardiovascular disease. In clinical practice, the term of lipids is mainly used instead of lipoprotein metabolism because of its association with atherosclerosis. Certain lipoprotein fractions lead to the deposition and retention of cholesterol in the vessel wall causing atherosclerosis. Different guidelines recommend that lowering plasma cholesterol level by diet or drugs results in the reduction in cardiovascular disease.

Cholesterol is a hydrophobic macromolecule, transported in the circulation by lipoproteins such as chylomicrons, very low-density lipoprotein (VLDL), and high-density lipoprotein (HDL). Low-density lipoprotein (LDL) and intermediate-density lipoprotein (IDL) are synthesized from VLDL. Cholesterol, which is taken from the diet, is absorbed from the intestine and transported via chylomicrons to the liver. In the liver, endogen lipids with cholesterol are packaged into VLDL and secreted to bloodstream. LDL is responsible for peripheral cholesterol transport. Lipoproteins contain different proportions of lipids and proteins and have different physical and chemical properties. Apolipoproteins (apo) are the protein components of lipoproteins. Each lipoprotein class differs by its apoprotein content and proportions. ApoB100 is the main apoprotein of LDL and VLDL. ApoA-I and ApoA-II are the main apoproteins of HDL. ApoC-I, apoC-II, apoC-III, and apoE are present in all lipoproteins in different proportions. These apoproteins have various functions and help in the metabolic pathways of lipoprotein metabolism such as the activation of specific enzymes and the stabilization of the lipoprotein structure and recognized by cell surface of specific cells/ tissues. Among different types of apolipoproteins, ApoE has a crucial importance due to its link with cardiovascular diseases.

1.1. ApoE and its relationship with cholesterol metabolism

Apolipoprotein (apo) E is synthesized mainly by the liver, and less is produced by other cell types such as macrophages. It has a great biological and biomedical importance in lipid metabolism such as cholesterol transportation, triglyceride metabolism, and lipoprotein metabolism. It is a structural component of plasma chylomicrons, very low-density lipoproteins (VLDL) and high-density lipoproteins (HDL), and a ligand for apo B/E (LDL) receptor and LDL receptor-related protein (LRP) [1]. It also facilitates the interlocation of lipoproteins with proteoglycans. ApoE consists of 299 amino acid residue and has three common isoforms apoE2, apoE3, and apoE4 which differ structurally by two amino acid substitutions at residues 112 and 158: ApoE2 (Cys112, Cys158), ApoE3 (Cys112, Arg158), and ApoE4 (Arg112, Arg158) [2]. Each isoform is encoded by three different apoE alleles (ε2, ε3, and ε4), resulting in six different genotypes (E2/2, E3/2, E4/2, E3/3, E4/3, and E4/4) [3] (**Figure 1**).

ApoE consists of two functional domains joined by a flexible hinge region: an amino-terminal domain that contains a highly positively charged receptor-binding region composed mainly of arginine and lysine residues, and a carboxyl-terminal domain which includes a lipid-binding region. Substitutions of two amino acid residues in the three ApoE isoforms significantly alter their receptor-binding and lipid-binding affinities and lead to differences in lipid metabolism [4]. ApoE2 has a lower-binding affinity for low-density lipoprotein (LDL) receptors compared to ApoE3 and ApoE4. ApoE3 and ApoE4 bind similarly to the LDLR; however, compared to apoE3, apoE4 reduces plasma cholesterol less in humans which makes ApoE4 pro-atherogenic lipoprotein than others. Further, ApoE2 and ApoE3 preferentially bind to small, phospholipid-enriched high-density lipoproteins (HDL), whereas ApoE4 preferentially binds to larger, triglyceride-enriched lipoproteins [5, 6]. ApoE isoforms have different binding affinities to different lipoproteins such as ApoE4 that exhibits a better lipid-binding ability with the VLDL particle than apoE3, whereas apoE3 binds preferentially to high-density lipoprotein (HDL) [7].

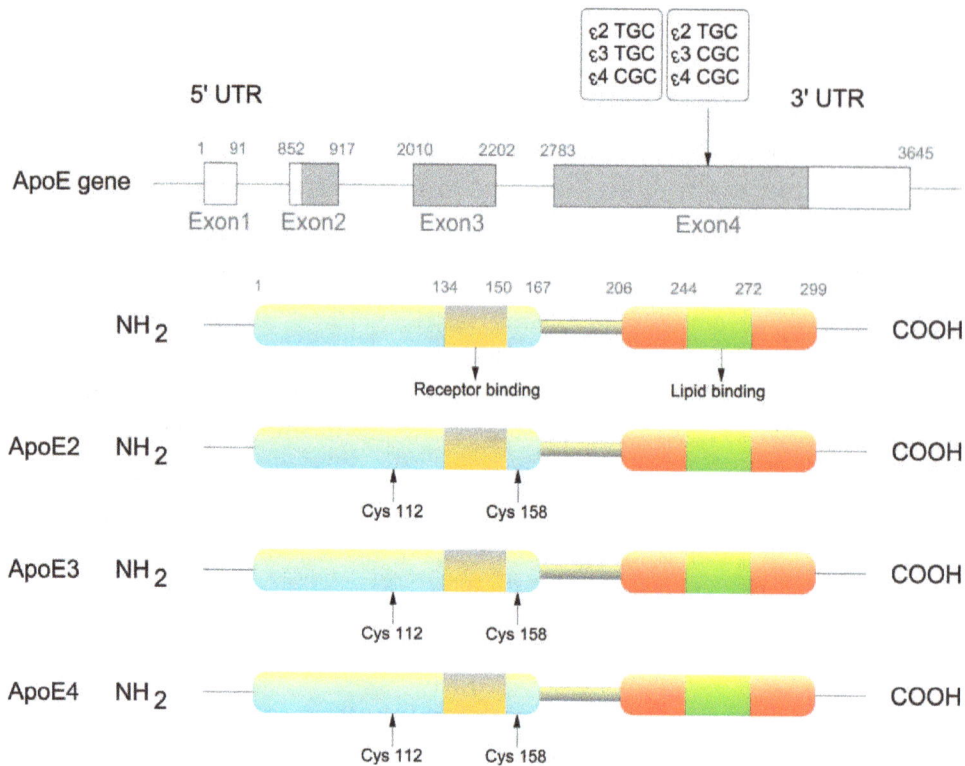

Figure 1. The schematic representation of the structural and functional domains of human apolipoprotein E (ApoE) isoforms.

The three-dimensional structure of apoE differs by Cys-Arg substitution, which causes changes in lipoprotein binding. The human apoE molecule contains the LDLR recognition site in the N-terminal helix bundle domain (residues 1–191) and initiates lipid binding by a C-terminal domain (residues 192–299). The substitution Cys and Arg residues, which differentiates apoE3 and apoE4 in the helix bundle domain, leads to different organizations of the segment spanning residues 261–272 which plays a critical role in the interaction with lipid surfaces; this structural change is the basis for the preferential binding of apoE4 to VLDL than of apoE3 [8–10]. The relative lipid- and lipoprotein-binding abilities of apoE3 and apoE4 have important consequences for the distribution of cholesterol between the VLDL and HDL fractions of plasma [11].

To date, several epidemiological studies have investigated the relationship between apoE polymorphism and coronary artery disease (CAD) risk, with a significant association [12–17]. It has been shown that apoE polymorphism may contribute to the plasma LDL cholesterol level and apolipoprotein B concentration in the various populations. The effects of apoE genotypes on coronary risk might also be explained as not only the receptor affinity or lipid levels but also apolipoprotein concentrations affecting the CAD phenotype. To the best of our knowledge, it has been shown that the ε2 allele is associated with lower levels of total plasma cholesterol (TC), LDL cholesterol (LDL-C), and apolipoprotein B (apo B) and with elevated levels of triglycerides (TG) as compared to the ε3 allele. An elevated level of TG is related with the impaired clearance of remnant particles containing apo ε2, which might be due to a defective receptor recognition of those particles. Reduced levels of apo B and LDL cholesterol in E2/2 and E2/3 individuals are results of impaired conversion of the intestinal VLDL particles to LDL by interfering with normal lipolytic processing [18, 19]. On the other hand, the ε4 allele is associated with higher levels of total and LDL-C and apo B because particles with carriers of that allele have a faster catabolic rate than the ε3 counterparts [20]. Meta-analysis has been emphasized that ε2 carriers had a 20% reduced coronary risk as compared to ε3/ε3 genotype [21]. The precise mechanism may be explained by the binding affinity of apoE2 isoform to heparin and small, phospholipid-enriched HDL. These effective binding mechanisms enhance remnant lipoprotein metabolism and also reverse cholesterol transport [5–22]. Further, apo E2 isoforms bind to LDL receptors much more weakly than apo E3 or apo E4 counterparts. Apo E4 isoforms are also related with an increased cholesterol absorption and statin hyporesponsiveness. However, meta-analysis has been suggested that ApoE genetic testing contributes to little information for statin treatment [23].

Numerous effects of apoE genotypes on coronary risk might also be explained by influences on additional lipid-related phenotypes such as lipoprotein subtypes, markers of inflammation, immunity, or oxidative status.

Recently, the atherogenicity of LDL and HDL subclasses and their relationship to coronary heart disease has taken more attention. Various studies revealed that small, dense LDL is more atherogenic and associated with an increased risk of CHD [24, 25] with a high triglyceride level [26]. Researchers reported confusing results about apoE genotypes and LDL, HDL subtypes. Some studies stated a relationship between ε2 allele and smaller LDL particles compared to ε4 allele carriers [27, 28]; others reported contradictory results [29, 30]. As we know that the relationships between apo E polymorphism, serum lipids, and CHD were differed due to different ethnicities, lifestyles, diet habits, and even to age. Epidemiological studies showed that men have more atherogenic profile than women with a low level of HDL cholesterol and an increased triglyceride level. The incidence of first cardiovascular events is also higher among young men and is increasing very fast along with age, than in women [31]. The effect of apo E allelic variants on lipids and lipoprotein particle sizes has been studied in many populations [28, 30, 32, 33]. Several studies suggested that the apo E polymorphism influences lipoprotein particle size and might indirectly increase the CHD risk differently for each gender. Topic and his friends stated that apo ε carriers and its relationship with lipoprotein subtypes differed among sex; men with ε2 allele had the smaller LDL particles and a higher TG/HDL-C ratio [1]. Further, Dobiasova and Frohlich proposed that the Log (TG/HDL-C) be called "atherogenic index of plasma" and used as a marker of plasma atherogenicity because this ratio showed a strong inverse correlation with LDL size [34]. Some researchers have reported an increased LDL-C concentration and a decreased LDL size in subjects with ε4 allele [30]. On the women side, studies showed an association of the ε4 allele with smaller HDL particle and a higher frequency of small HDL phenotype and Framingham Risk Score ("intermediate"). Further, the presence of the ε4 alleles is found to be the independent factor for HDL size variation in women. Others reported different results with ε4 allele; carrier women had the small HDL particles which relates with the severity of CHD [27, 35, 36].

1.2. Endothelial dysfunction and cardiovascular diseases

Despite the strong evidences about lipoproteins and apolipoproteins, it has been shown that chronic oxidative stress and inflammatory changes in the vascular tissue play a crucial role in coronary atherosclerosis pathogenesis. Endothelium controls the normal vasomotor balance, the inhibition and stimulation of smooth muscle cell proliferation, migration, thrombogenesis, and fibrinolysis. When these functions of endothelium are impaired, endothelial dysfunction occurs and leads to damage of the wall. Damage to the endothelium promotes substantial events and provokes atherosclerosis by increasing endothelial permeability, platelet aggregation, and leukocyte adhesion.

The early lesion of atherosclerosis results in the focal accumulation of lipoproteins in the intimal layer of the artery. The intimal layer contains smooth muscle cell which is embedded in the extracellular matrix, so lipoprotein accumulation often associates with proteoglycans of the arterial extracellular matrix such as heparin sulfate, keratan sulfate, or chondroitin sulfate. These proteoglycan molecules increase the retention of lipoprotein particles in the arterial bed and permit their chemical modification. The extracellular bed of arterial wall is particularly susceptible to oxidative modification. The modification of lipids leads to hydroperoxides, lysophospholipids, oxysterol, and oxidized phospholipids formation which are other stimulators of arterial lesion progression. On the other hand, the apoprotein part of the lipoproteins may undergo similar chemical modification which performs irregular protein moieties that have a pro-inflammatory role during lesion development. The irregular changes of the arterial wall might also activate mononuclear phagocytes. These phagocytes as well as vascular endothelial and smooth muscle cells can produce reactive oxygen species when activated. Then, reactive oxygen species can induce smooth muscle cell growth and trigger inflammatory response.

The second step of the lesion formation is leukocyte recruitment which is the main cell of atheroma of the mononuclear lineage: monocytes and lymphocytes. The vascular endothelium synthesizes certain biomolecules for a regular vascular function. Various adhesion molecules or receptors are synthesized on the endothelial cell surface for leukocytes such as vascular adhesion molecule I (VCAM-I), intercellular adhesion molecule I (ICAM-I), and P-selectin. In normal arteries, the laminar shear stress suppresses the expression of adhesion molecules and stimulates adequate nitric oxide (NO) to maintain vasodilatation. Further, NO production can control adhesion molecules expression such as VCAM-I and show an anti-inflammatory effect. Reactive oxygen species may also react with NO, reduce NO bioavailability, and improve vascular damage indirectly by disrupting adhesion molecule express. In addition to relationship between adhesion molecules and NO, in vitro studies have shown that this relationship is attenuated by apoE [37, 38]. Recently, Ma et al. reported a reduced VCAM-1 and ICAM-1 gene expression in the whole aorta of hyperlipidemic mice at the sub-physiological levels of plasma apoE [39]. As a result of an increased adhesion of certain key molecules to endothelial cells, this leads to the penetration of monocytes and lymphocytes to the subendothelial layer. Besides modified lipoproteins, mediators of inflammation, cytokines can also regulate adhesion molecule expression and promote leukocyte recruitment. For example, VCAM-I and ICAM-I expressions on endothelial cells are stimulated by cytokine interleukin-I (IL-1) and tumor necrosis factor α (TNF-α). As mentioned earlier, the different pathways perform a cumulative effect on endothelial dysfunction and lesion formation. In the intima, the recruitment of mononuclear phagocytes differentiates to macrophages which promote the lipid-loaded foam cell formation. Foam cells have two different features: they either can go to apoptotic pathway or produce cytokines and growth factors which lead to further complicated cellular events in complicated lesion. Growth factors (platelet growth factor, fibroblast growth factor, etc.) and cytokines again stimulate smooth muscle cell proliferation and induce extracellular matrix formation. Among numerous growth factors, some of them solely trigger interstitial collagen production by smooth muscle cells. These mediators induce lesion progression by inducing transformation of fatty streak into a more complicated lesion with a high fibrous tissue and extracellular matrix by using either paracrine or autocrine pathway. As well as the effect of traditional risk factors and local mediators of various cell types, coagulation and thrombosis also contribute to lesion progression.

Endothelium serves as a barrier between circulating blood and its surrounding tissue. A transmembrane receptor tissue factor (TF) is expressed by blood vessels. An injury of the vascular endothelium leads to exposure of TF and activates the clotting cascade. The imbalance of hemodynamics might also effect the normal activity of endothelial cells. Endothelial cells control platelet function via the synthesis and secretion of Von Willebrand factor (vWF). The vWF is an important glycoprotein in the regulation of hemostasis, stored also in platelets, and can be released as a response to prothrombotic and inflammatory factors. It is a bridge between platelet adhesion and coagulation. VWF contains functional domains for collagen, platelet (GPIb binding), and factor VIII binding. At the site of injury, VWF recognizes collagen in the subendothelial matrix, steer platelet adhesion via collagen, and GPIb-binding sites. Its level increases in plasma as a result of endothelial damage. vWF increases platelet adhesion to subendothelial layer and contributes to thrombus formation [40, 41].

The other anticoagulant functions of the endothelium are inhibition of coagulation by TFPI, keeping balance between thrombin- thrombomodulin secretion and regulation of coagulation factors by antitrypsin. On the other hand, the endothelium controls the activation and regulation of fibrinolysis by the secretion of tPA and PAIs. tPA is released in response to thrombin which is controlled by PAI-1. Various complex functions of endothelium are controlled strictly with high fidelity to maintain vascular health.

Based on the robust relationship between lipoprotein metabolism and basic endothelium functions, it has been recommended that different types of inflammatory reactions might be involved in the initiation and progression stages of atherosclerosis and contribute to vascular events.

Numerous epidemiologic studies reported that 20% of the coronary events occurred in the absence of the classical risk factors: hyperlipidemia, diabetes, hypertension, and smoking. In this situation, a question raises whether traditional risk factors are adequate to predict CVD risk. To solve this issue, new biomarkers are proposed for daily practice for better identification of the risk, including hemostatic system markers (the best identified ones, tissue plasminogen activator inhibitor—PAI-I, tissue plasminogen activator—tPA, fibrinogen, von Willebrand Factor—vWF, etc.) and inflammatory markers (high sensitive C reactive protein—HsCRP, lipoprotein-associated phospholipase II—Lp-PLA2, myeloperoxidase, pentraxin III—PTX3, serum amyloid A, etc.). Together with these, interleukins, inflammatory cytokines, adhesion molecules, homocysteine, and heat shock proteins can be used as appropriate. All these factors participate in the atherosclerotic process and show an abnormal behavior in individuals at high risk, or suffered from a cardiovascular event.

1.3. Vascular inflammation as a risk factor for cardiovascular diseases

Among the wide range of markers, C-reactive protein (CRP) was recommended as a comprising marker for the evaluation of CVD risk in 2009 by the common declaration of the Laboratory Medicine Practice Guideline of National Academy of Clinical Biochemistry (NACB) and American Heart Association and the CDC (AHA/CDC) [42]. CRP is an acute-phase protein, which is primarily produced in the liver during acute inflammation or infection. CRP is stimulated by interleukin 6 (IL-6) and also detected at local sites of inflammation or injury. It is not specific for vascular inflammation. Then, more sensitive types of CRP have been developed to detect the small changes of the protein, called hs-CRP. Since hs-CRP has been increased, the predictive accuracy of risk evaluation with other risk-scoring systems is still inadequate. Hs-CRP levels are known to be systemic inflammatory marker and increased by infection and tissue damage, malignancies, obesity, aging, hypertension, diabetes mellitus, smoking, and other cardiovascular risks [43].

As described earlier, the increased expression of endothelial adhesion molecules, which trigger subendothelial penetration of LDL, is more susceptible to oxidation and stimulates inflammatory cytokines. Great attention has been recently given to myeloperoxidase (MPO), released systemically and locally by activated leukocytes. It has been shown that this enzyme is present in atherosclerotic lesions with higher concentrations and also contributes to LDL oxidation by different mechanisms via radical and non-radical mechanisms either lipid or apoprotein moieties [44]. Moreover, MPO limits the bioavailability of nitric oxide ($\bullet$NO) and contributes to endothelial dysfunction [45, 46]. Unlike CRP, MPO is more involved in different stages of atherosclerosis such as foam cells, endothelial dysfunction and apoptosis, the activation of matrix metalloproteinases, and the expression of tissue factor which could address the patients with vulnerable plaques, and the potential burden of such plaques in clinical practice [47]. The members of the inflammatory cytokine family IL-6 and tumor necrosis factor (TNF)-α, released from the main cells of the plaque, vascular smooth muscle cells, endothelial cells, monocytes, and macrophages, are highly involved in atherosclerosis [48]. Ridker and colleagues reported from 14,916 healthy male; blood IL-6 concentrations were significantly elevated in individuals who had myocardial infarction as compared with those who did not [49]. Another prospective study reported a relationship between IL-6 levels and the incidences of ischemic cardiac disease, stroke, and heart failure events from middle-aged participants [50]. The other important player of the inflamed plaque is chemokines, leading to the recruitment of leukocytes to the damaged area of the arterial wall, as well as other systemic inflammatory markers, particularly monocyte chemoattractant protein 1 (MCP-1), which is again non-specific for interpreting CV risk [51].

Lipoprotein-associated phospholipase A_2 (Lp-PLA$_2$) or platelet-activating factor acetylhydrolase is a unique pro-inflammatory biomarker, specific for vascular inflammation and atherosclerosis [52, 53]. Lp-PLA$_2$ was discovered in 1980, and it was classified as a Ca^{2+}-independent PLA$_2$ [54] produced by a wide range of inflammatory and non-inflammatory cells [55] (**Figure 2**).

Lp-PLA$_2$ shows a positive correlation with CV events by various scientific and clinical studies [56–58]. Lavi et al. found that patients with early coronary atherosclerosis had higher

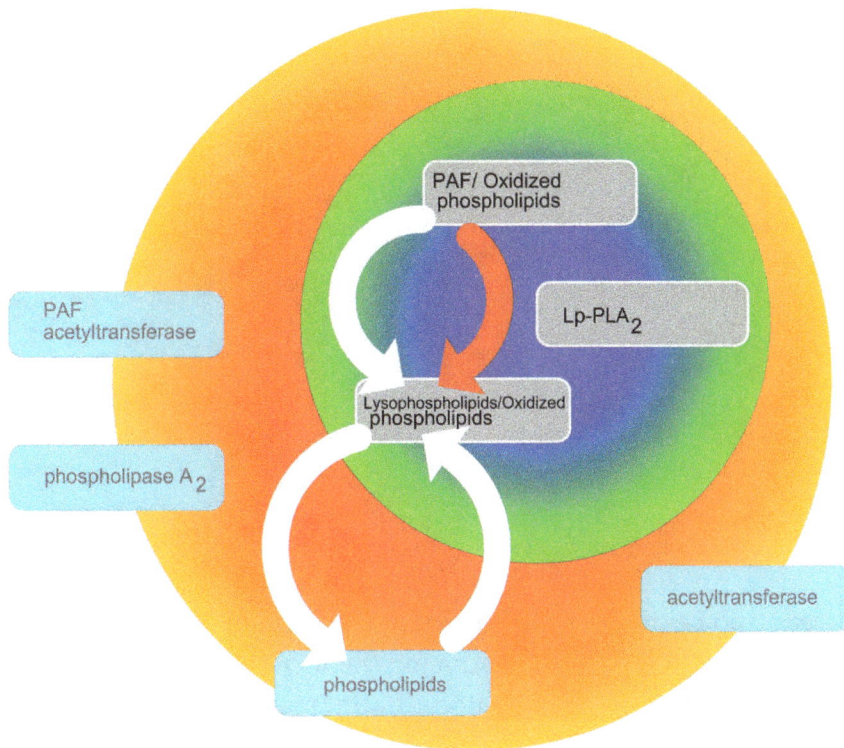

Figure 2. Relationship of Lp-PLA2 action with phospholipids. Platelet-activating factor (PAF) is an active phospholipid related to many pathologic and physiologic reactions. The PAF is formed through two reactions: firstly, the cytosolic phospholipase A2 (cPLA2) acts on membrane phospholipids producing lysophospholipids; then, the lysophospholipids are modified by PAF acetyltransferase, Thus, PAF concentration is modulated by Lp-PLA2 activity.

lysophosphatidylcholine when compared with control subjects [59]. Herrmann et al. showed that carotid artery plaques of patients with cardiac events presented higher Lp-PLA2, lysophospholipids, macrophage, and collagen content when compared to patients without events [60]. Kuniyasu et al. demonstrated that oxLDL and, particularly, the lysophosphatidylcholine present in this particle enhance the plasminogen activator inhibitor-1 expression [61].

Moreover, the difference in the distribution and association of Lp-PLA$_2$ activity and index with apoB containing lipoproteins across lipoprotein subfractions has also been reported [62]. Further, Lp-PLA$_2$ has been recommended as an adjunct to traditional risk factors for individuals at a moderate or a high CV risk by the Adult Treatment Panel III (ATP III) guideline [63].

Lp-PLA$_2$ is synthesized mainly by macrophages of atherosclerotic plaque, then enters the circulation, and binds to LDL, HDL, and Lp(a). In the atherosclerotic plaque, Lp-PLA$_2$ hydrolyzes oxLDL into Lyso-PC and oxidized nonesterified fatty acids (oxNEFAs), both of which have a pro-inflammatory role (**Figure 3**). The degradation products, Lyso-PC and oxNEFAs, hydrolyzed by Lp-PLA$_2$ play crucial roles on the development of atherosclerosis. Both Lyso-PC and oxNEFAs induce the recruiting of leukocytes, upregulating inflammatory cytokine such as TNF-a and IL-6, amplifying oxidation, and increasing matrix metalloproteinase expression. During the process, the presence of OxLDL, as well as lysophospholipids and oxNEFAS, stimulates the growth of the plaque [64, 65]. As mentioned earlier, Lp-PLA2 resides on different types of lipoproteins, so dyslipidemia effects the enzyme mass and activity and alters its

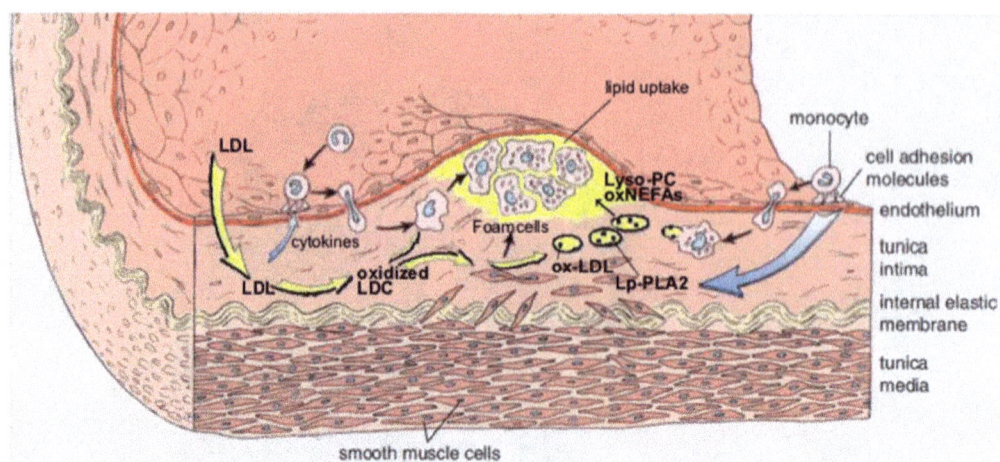

Figure 3. The role of Lp-PLA$_2$ on atherosclerotic plaque.

distribution between apo B- and apo AI-containing lipoproteins, as reported by Tsimihodimos et al. The same study also demonstrated inducing the increase of HDL-Lp-PLA2 activity and the reduction of LDL-Lp-PLA$_2$ activity by atorvastatin treatment [66].

Lp-PLA$_2$ quantitatively reflects the degree of inflammatory reaction of the plaque in the plasma. Lp-PLA$_2$ measurement can be classified into enzyme activity and enzyme mass; however, Berglund and colleagues recommended an integrated measure of Lp-PLA$_2$ activity and mass as Lp-PLA$_2$ index which showed an independent predictor of CAD in different ethnicity [58]. Since the first report, many epidemiological studies and meta-analysis have also proved the significant associations between Lp-PLA$_2$ atherogenesis and CV-risk stratification [52, 67, 68]. A meta-analysis of 32 clinical studies evaluated the association of Lp-PLA$_2$ mass or activity with the future risk of CHD, emphasizing strongly that Lp-PLA$_2$ is a reliable indicator for the future CV-risk assessment. The study also revealed that the association of the enzyme activity with lipid markers is stronger than the association with mass [69]. Further, Gungor et al. demonstrated an association between apoE genotype and Lp-PLA$_2$, for the first time. The Lp-PLA$_2$ index, an integrated measure of Lp-PLA$_2$ mass and activity, was higher in apo E4 carriers irrespective of ethnicity and underlines the importance of assessing the relationship between genetic predisposition and inflammation, in the assessment of cardiovascular disease risk [70]. The genetic variation of Lp-PLA$_2$ activity and mass and relationship with 13 common single nucleotide polymorphisms (SNPs) of the PLA2G7 gene was investigated in the community-based Framingham Heart Study. The study reported that Lp-PLA2 activity is influenced by variation in the genomic region of PLA2G7. Further, it has been underlined that different pathophysiological roles of Lp-PLA$_2$ activity and mass conveyed different clinical outcome. The strong association is seen for Lp-PLA$_2$ activity with cardiovascular risk factors compared to Lp-PLA$_2$ mass [71].

Pentraxin 3 (PTX3) is a protein from acute-phase reactant family. It belongs to long pentraxins and possesses numerous properties in the field of inflammation. Pentraxin 3 transcription is upregulated by tumor necrosis factor and interleukins (IL-1) in different cell types such as endothelial cells, phagocytes, smooth muscle cells, and fibroblasts which are involved in the different stages of atherosclerosis. PTX3 represents a specific and sensitive marker connecting inflammation with CVD.

During inflammation, the blood vessel produces large amounts of PTX3; its high level in circulation related with pathological conditions affects cardiovascular system. Recently, epidemiological and clinical data showed that PTX3 is a valid biomarker for atherosclerosis [72] and its high plasma levels were found to be related with the severity of coronary atherosclerosis [34]. It has been demonstrated that PTX3 increases the tissue factor (TF) expression in mononuclear and endothelial cells. The increased level of TF activates the coagulation cascade and causes the thrombus formation [73]. PTX3 might also bind to growth factor 2 (FGF2) and interfere with plaque stability via effect of the proliferation and migration of smooth muscle cells [74]. Based on such findings, PTX3 is more specific for coronary plaque instability than for atherosclerosis. In addition, the elevated plasma level of PTX3 has been found in patients with high systolic and diastolic blood pressure levels [75]. On the other hand, in patients with acute myocardial infarction, PTX3 was shown to be produced by the neutrophils penetrating into unstable coronary plaques. This underscored the fact that PTX3 might be more accurate predictor of cardiovascular events after myocardial infarction than other markers [76].

As conclusion, it is well known that atherosclerosis is a chronic inflammatory disease of the vessel wall. This chapter reviewed the relationship between atherosclerosis and the various effects of different inflammatory biomarkers and possible roles of genetic predisposition on the development and progression of coronary artery diseases (**Figure 4**). Atherosclerotic disease mostly starts

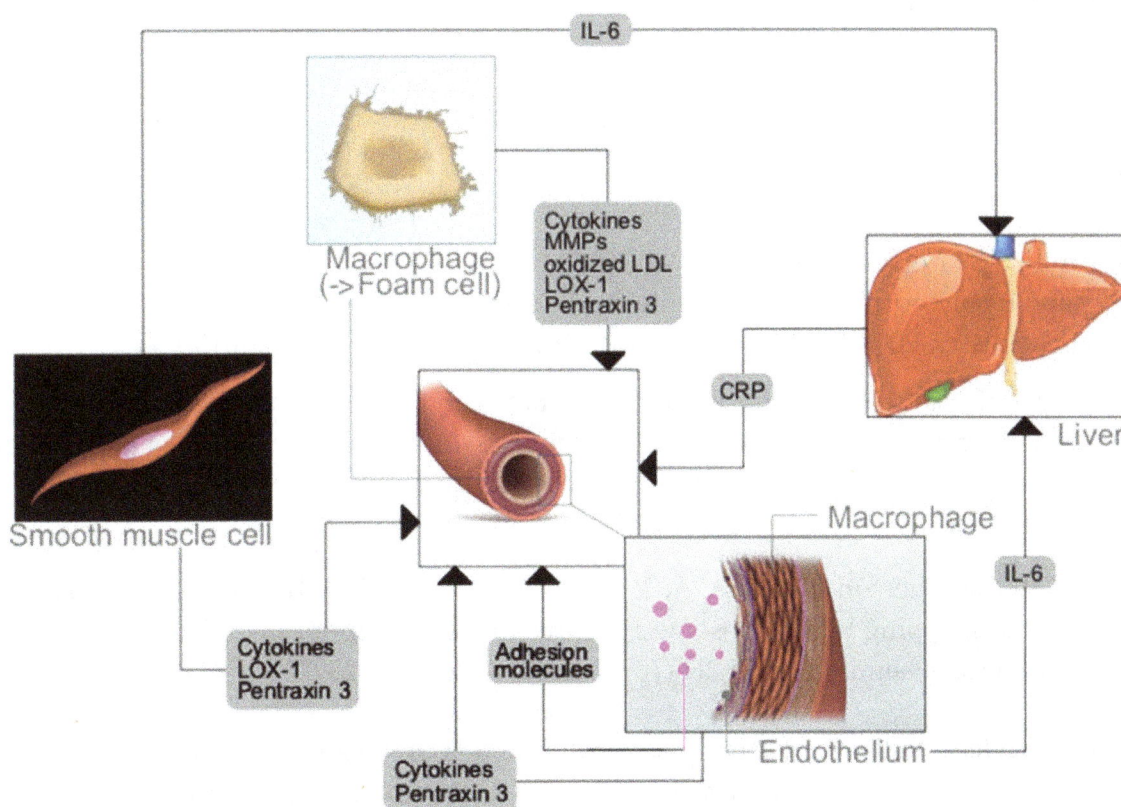

Figure 4. Inflammatory markers secreted from various cells in atherosclerotic lesion. Pro-inflammatory markers such as cytokines, pentraxin-3, MMPs, and LOX-1 are produced by macrophages, endothelial cells, and vascular smooth muscle cells in atherosclerotic lesion. CRP is mainly produced in the liver stimulated by IL-6. CRP indicates C-reactive protein; IL-6, interleukin-6; LDL, low-density lipoprotein; LOX-1, lectin-like oxidized LDL receptor-1; and MMP, matrix metalloproteinase.

as asymptomatic, however, when it gives symptoms; the life quality is effected significantly and sometimes it will be life threatening. In these circumstances, the early detection of the disease or prediction of the individuals with a high CV risk becomes very important. The evaluation of a CV risk or a disease progression by an accurate biomarker either vascular inflammation or genetic markers would be promising and underscores their diagnostic importance in clinical practice.

Acknowledgements

The author would like to thank Zeynep Erdem and Berna Kavas for reviewing the English of this chapter and Gizem Ozturk for drawing the figures.

Author details

Zeynep Banu Gungor

Address all correspondence to: zbozturk@gmail.com

Department of Medical Biochemistry, Cerrahpasa Medical School, University of Istanbul, Istanbul, Turkey

References

[1] Topic A, Spasojevic Kalimanovska V, Zeljkovic A, Vekic J, Jelic IZ. Gender-related effect of apo E polymorphism on lipoprotein particle sizes in the middle-aged subjects. Clinical Biochemistry. 2008;**41**:361-367. DOI: 10.1016/j.clinbiochem.2007.11.013

[2] Frieden C, Garai K. Structural differences between apoE3 and apoE4 may be useful in developing therapeutic agents for Alzheimer's disease. Proceedings of the National Academy of Sciences of the United States of America. 2012;**109**:8913-8918. DOI: 10.1073/pnas.1207022109

[3] Das HK, McPherson J, Bruns GA, Karathanasis SK, Breslow JL. Isolation, characterization, and mapping to chromosome 19 of the human apolipoprotein E gene. The Journal of Biological Chemistry. 1985;**260**(10):6240-6247 PMID: 3922972

[4] Mahley RW, Rall SC Jr. Apolipoprotein E: Far more than a lipid transport protein. Annual Review of Genomics and Human Genetics. 2000;**1**:507-537. DOI: 10.1146/annurev.genom.1.1.507

[5] Weisgraber KH, Innerarity TL, Mahley RW. Abnormal lipoprotein receptor-binding activity of the human E apoprotein due to cysteine-arginine interchange at a single site. The Journal of Biological Chemistry. 1982;**257**:2518-2521 PMID: 6277903

[6]   Davignon J, Gregg RE, Sing CF. Apolipoprotein E polymorphism and atherosclerosis. Arteriosclerosis. 1988;**8**(1):1-21. DOI: 10.1161/01.ATV.8.1.1

[7]   Nguyen D, Dhanasekaran P, Nickel M, Nakatani R, Saito H, Phillips MC, Lund-Katz S. Molecular basis for the differences in lipid and lipoprotein binding properties of human apolipoproteins E3 and E4. Biochemistry. 2010;**49**:10881-10889. DOI: 10.1021/bi1017655

[8]   Saito H, Lund-Katz S, Phillips MC. Contributions of domain structure and lipid interaction to the functionality of exchangeable human apolipoproteins. Progress in Lipid Research. 2004;**43**:350-380. DOI: 10.1016/j.plipres.2004.05.002

[9]   Nguyen D, Dhanasekaran P, Phillips MC, Lund-Katz S. Molecular mechanism of apolipoprotein E binding to lipoprotein particles. Biochemistry. 2009;**48**:3025-3032. DOI: 10.1021/bi9000694

[10] Sakamoto T, Tanaka M, Vedhachalam C, Nickel M, Nguyen D, Dhanasekaran P, Phillips MC, Lund-Katz S, Saito H. Contributions of the carboxyl-terminal helical segment to the self-association and lipoprotein preferences of human apolipoprotein E3 and E4 isoforms. Biochemistry. 2008;**47**:2968-2977. DOI: 10.1021/bi701923h

[11] Li H, Dhanasekaran P, Alexander ET, Rader DJ, Phillips MC, Lund-Katz S. Molecular mechanisms responsible for the differential effects of apoE3 and apoE4 on plasma lipoprotein-cholesterol levels. Arteriosclerosis, Thrombosis, and Vascular Biology. 2013;**33**:687-693. DOI: 10.1161/ATVBAHA.112.301193

[12] Utermann G, Hees M, Steinmetz A. Polymorphism of apolipoprotein E and occurrence of dysbetalipoproteinaemia in man. Nature. 1977;**269**:604-607 PMID: 199847

[13] van Bockxmeer FM, Mamotte CD. Apolipoprotein epsilon 4 homozygosity in young men with coronary heart disease. Lancet. 1992;**340**:879-880. 10.1016/0140-6736(92)93288-X

[14] Stengård JH, Pekkanen J, Ehnholm C, Nissinen A, Sing CF. Genotypes with the apolipoprotein epsilon4 allele are predictors of coronary heart disease mortality in a longitudinal study of elderly Finnish men. Human Genetics. 1996;**97**:677-684. DOI: 10.1007/s004390050115

[15] Anuurad E, Rubin J, Lu G, Pearson TA, Holleran S, Ramakrishnan R, Berglund L. Protective effect of apolipoprotein E2 on coronary artery disease in African Americans is mediated through lipoprotein cholesterol. Journal of Lipid Research. 2006;**47**:2475-2481. DOI: 10.1194/jlr.M600288-JLR200

[16] Chen Q, Reis SE, Kammerer CM, McNamara DM, Holubkov R, Sharaf BL, Sopko G, Pauly DF, Bairey Merz CN, Kamboh MI. Women's Ischemia Syndrome Evaluation (WISE) Study. APOE polymorphism and angiographic coronary artery disease severity in the Women's Ischemia Syndrome Evaluation (WISE) study. Atherosclerosis. 2003;**169**:159-167. DOI: 10.1016/S0021-9150(03)00160-6

[17] Koopal C, Geerlings MI, Muller M, de Borst GJ, Algra A, van der Graaf Y, Visseren FL; SMART Study Group. The relation between apolipoprotein E (APOE) genotype and peripheral artery disease in patients at high risk for cardiovascular disease. Atherosclerosis 2016;**246**:187-192. 10.1016/j.atherosclerosis.2016.01.009

[18] Havel RJ, Chao Y, Windler EE, Kotite L, Guo LS. Isoprotein specificity in the hepatic uptake of apolipoprotein E and the pathogenesis of familial dysbetalipoproteinemia. Proceedings of the National Academy of Sciences of the United States of America. 1980;**77**:4349-4353 PMCID: PMC349832

[19] Ehnholm C, Mahley RW, Chappell DA, Weisgraber KH, Ludwig E, Witztum JL. Role of apolipoprotein E in the lipolytic conversion of beta-very low density lipoproteins to low density lipoproteins in type III hyperlipoproteinemia. Proceedings of the National Academy of Sciences of the United States of America. 1984;**81**:5566-5570 PMCID: PMC391747

[20] Gregg RE, Zech LA, Schaefer EJ, Stark D, Wilson D, Brewer HB Jr. Abnormal in vivo metabolism of apolipoprotein E4 in humans. The Journal of Clinical Investigation. 1986;**78**:815-821. DOI: 10.1172/JCI112645

[21] Bennet AM, Di Angelantonio E, Ye Z, Wensley F, Dahlin A, Ahlbom A, Keavney B, Collins R, Wiman B, de Faire U, Danesh J. Association of apolipoprotein E genotypes with lipid levels and coronary risk. Journal of the American Medical Association. 2007;**298**:1300-1311. DOI: 10.1001/jama.298.11.1300

[22] Weisgraber KH. Apolipoprotein E distribution among human plasma lipoproteins: Role of the cysteine-arginine interchange at residue 112. Journal of Lipid Research. 1990;**31**:1503-1511. PMID: 2280190

[23] Remaley AT, Dayspring TD, Warnick GR. Lipids, lipoproteins, apolipoproteins and other cardiovascular risk factors. In: Rifai N, Horvarth AR, Wittwer CT. Tietz Textbook of Clinical Chemistry and Molecular Diagnostics. 6th ed. USA: Elsevier; 2018. p. 556-teitz sh 555-560. ISBN: 978-0-323-35921-4

[24] Sacks FM, Campos H. Cardiovascular endocrinology: Low-density lipoprotein size and cardiovascular disease: a reappraisal. The Journal of Clinical Endocrinology and Metabolism. 2003;**88**:4525-4532. DOI: 10.1210/jc.2003-030636

[25] Williams PT, Superko HR, Haskell WL, Alderman EL, Blanche PJ, Holl LG, Krauss RM. Smallest LDL particles are most strongly related to coronary disease progression in men. Arteriosclerosis, Thrombosis, and Vascular Biology. 2003;**23**:314-321. DOI: 10.1161/01.ATV.0000053385.64132.2D

[26] Coresh J, Kwiterovich PO Jr, Smith HH, Bachorik PS. Association of plasma triglyceride concentration and LDL particle diameter, density, and chemical composition with premature coronary artery disease in men and women. Journal of Lipid Research. 1993;**34**:1687-1697. PMID: 8245719

[27] Dart AM, Cooper B. Independent effects of Apo E phenotype and plasma triglyceride on lipoprotein particle sizes in the fasting and postprandial states. Arteriosclerosis, Thrombosis, and Vascular Biology. 1999;**19**:2465-2473. DOI: 10.1161/01.ATV.19.10.2465

[28] Adams HP Jr, Kappelle LJ, Biller J, Gordon DL, Love BB, Gomez F, Heffner M. Ischemic stroke in young adults. Experience in 329 patients enrolled in the Iowa Registry of stroke in young adults. Archives of Neurology. 1995;**52**:491-495. DOI: 10.1001/archneur.1995.00540290081021

[29] Schaefer EJ, Lamon-Fava S, Johnson S, Ordovas JM, Schaefer MM, Castelli WP, Wilson PW. Effects of gender and menopausal status on the association of apolipoprotein E phenotype with plasma lipoprotein levels. Results from the Framingham Offspring Study. Arteriosclerosis and Thrombosis. 1994;**14**:1105-1113. DOI: 10.1161/01.ATV.14.7.1105

[30] Haffner SM, Stern MP, Miettinen H, Robbins D, Howard BV. Apolipoprotein E polymorphism and LDL size in a biethnic population. Arteriosclerosis, Thrombosis, and Vascular Biology. 1996;**16**:1184-1188. DOI: 10.1161/01.ATV.16.9.1184

[31] Mosca L, Benjamin EJ. Effectiveness-based guidelines for the prevention of cardiovascular disease in women—2011 update. A guideline from the American Heart Association. Circulation. 2011;**123**:1243-1262. DOI: 10.1161/CIR.0b013e31820faaf8

[32] Jarvik GP, Austin MA, Fabsitz RR, Auwerx J, Reed T, Christian JC, Deeb S. Genetic influences on age- related change in total cholesterol, low density lipoprotein-cholesterol, and triglyceride levels: Longitudinal apolipoprotein E genotype effects. Genetic Epidemiology. 1994;**11**:375-384. DOI: 10.1002/gepi.1370110407

[33] Skoglund AC, Ehrenborg E, Fisher RM, Olivecrona G, Hamsten A, Karpe F. Influence of common variants in the CETP, LPL, HL and APO E genes on LDL heterogeneity in healthy, middle-aged men. Atherosclerosis. 2003;**167**:311-317. DOI: 10.1016/S0021-9150(03)00016-9

[34] Dobiásová M, Frohlich J. The plasma parameter log (TG/HDL-C) as an atherogenic index: Correlation with lipoprotein particle size and esterification rate in apoB-lipoprotein-depleted plasma (FER(HDL)). Clinical Biochemistry. 2001;**34**:583-588. DOI: 10.1016/S0009-9120(01)00263-6

[35] Cheung MC, Brown BG, Wolf AC, Albers JJ. Altered particle size distribution of apolipoprotein A-I-containing lipoproteins in subjects with coronary artery disease. Journal of Lipid Research. 1991;**32**:383-394 PMID: 1906084

[36] Yang Y, Yan B, Fu M, Xu Y, Tian Y. Relationship between plasma lipid concentrations and HDL subclasses. Clinica Chimica Acta. 2005;**354**:49-58. DOI: 10.1016/j.cccn.2004.11.015

[37] Stannard AK, Riddell DR, Sacre SM, Tagalakis AD, Langer C, von Eckardstein A, Cullen P, Athanasopoulos T, Dickson G, Owen JS. Cell-derived apolipoprotein E (ApoE) particles inhibit vascular cell adhesion molecule-1 (VCAM-1) expression in human endothelial cells. The Journal of Biological Chemistry. 2001;**276**:46011-46016. DOI: 10.1074/jbc.M104812200

[38] Mullick AE, Powers AF, Kota RS, Tetali SD, Eiserich JP, Rutledge JC. Apolipoprotein E3- and nitric oxide-dependent modulation of endothelial cell inflammatory responses. Arteriosclerosis, Thrombosis, and Vascular Biology. 2007;**27**:339-345. DOI: 10.1161/01.ATV.0000253947.70438.99

[39] Ma Y, Malbon CC, Williams DL, Thorngate FE. Altered gene expression in early atherosclerosis blocked by low level apolipoprotein E. PLoS One. 2008;**3**:e2503. DOI: 10.1371/journal.pone.0002503

[40] Brill A, Fuchs TA, Chauhan AK, Yang JJ, De Meyer SF, Köllnberger M, Wakefield TW, Lämmle B, Massberg S, Wagner DD. von Willebrand factor-mediated platelet adhesion is critical for deep vein thrombosis in mouse models. Blood. 2011;117:1400-1407. DOI: 10.1182/blood-2010-05-287623

[41] Güngör ZB, Ekmekçi H, Tüten A, Toprak S, Ayaz G, Çalışkan O, Sönmez H, Madazlı R, Donma O, Kucur M, Ulutin T, Ekmekçi OB. Is there any relationship between adipocytokines and angiogenesis factors to address endothelial dysfunction and platelet aggregation in untreated patients with preeclampsia? Archives of Gynecology and Obstetrics. 2017;296:495-502. DOI: 10.1007/s00404-017-4461-2

[42] Remaley AT, Dayspring TD, Warnick GR. Lipids, lipoproteins, apolipoproteins and other cardiovascular risk factors. In: Rifai N, Horvarth AR, Wittwer CT. Tietz Textbook of Clinical Chemistry and Molecular Diagnostics. 6th ed. USA: Elsevier; 2018. p. 556-teitz sh 594-596. ISBN: 978-0-323-35921-4

[43] Goldstein JA, Chandra HR, O'Neill WW. Relation of number of complex coronary lesions to serum C-reactive protein levels and major adverse cardiovascular events at one year. The American Journal of Cardiology. 2005;1:56-60. DOI: 10.1016/j.amjcard.2005.02.044

[44] Carr AC, McCall MR, Frei B. Oxidation of LDL by myeloperoxidase and reactive nitrogen species: Reaction pathways and antioxidant protection. Arteriosclerosis, Thrombosis, and Vascular Biology. 2000;20:1716-1723. DOI: 10.1161/01.ATV.20.7.1716

[45] Stocker R, Huang A, Jeranian E, Hou JY, Wu TT, Thomas SR, Keaney JF Jr. Hypochlorous acid impairs endothelium-derived nitric oxide bioactivity through a superoxide-dependent mechanism. Arteriosclerosis, Thrombosis, and Vascular Biology. 2004;24:2028-2033. DOI: 10.1161/01.ATV.0000143388.20994.fa

[46] Kataoka Y, Shao M, Wolski K, Uno K, Puri R, Murat Tuzcu E, Hazen SL, Nissen SE, Nicholls SJ. Myeloperoxidase levels predict accelerated progression of coronary atherosclerosis in diabetic patients: Insights from intravascular ultrasound. Atherosclerosis. 2014;232:377-383. DOI: 10.1016/j.atherosclerosis.2013.11.075

[47] Teng N, Maghzal GJ, Talib J, Rashid I, Lau AK, Stocker R. The roles of myeloperoxidase in coronary artery disease and its potential implication in plaque rupture. Redox Report. 2017;22:51-73. DOI: 10.1080/13510002.2016.1256119

[48] Miranda LG, Pedrosa HC, Falleiros RK, Oliveira Rde M, Tolentino M, Casulari LA. Evaluation of diabetic patients after three month use of continuous subcutaneous insulin infusion, dispensed by a protocolled form at outpatient reference clinic of Taguatinga Regional Hospital. The Archives of Endocrinology and Metabolism. 2015;59:23-28. DOI: 10.1590/2359-3997000000005

[49] Ridker PM, Rifai N, Stampfer MJ, Hennekens CH. Plasma concentration of interleukin-6 and the risk of future myocardial infarction among apparently healthy men. Circulation. 2000;101:1767-1772. DOI: 10.1161/01.CIR.101.15.1767

[50] Cesari M, Penninx BW, Newman AB, Kritchevsky SB, Nicklas BJ, Sutton-Tyrrell K, Rubin SM, Ding J, Simonsick EM, Harris TB, Pahor M. Inflammatory markers and onset of cardiovascular events: Results from the Health ABC study. Circulation. 2003;108:2317-2322. DOI: 10.1161/01.CIR.0000097109.90783.FC

[50] Cesari M, Penninx BW, Newman AB, Kritchevsky SB, Nicklas BJ, Sutton-Tyrrell K, Rubin SM, Ding J, Simonsick EM, Harris TB, Pahor M. Inflammatory markers and onset of cardiovascular events: Results from the Health ABC study. Circulation. 2003;**108**:2317-2322. DOI: 10.1161/01.CIR.0000097109.90783.FC

[51] Weber C, Schober A, Zernecke A. Chemokines: Key regulators of mononuclear cell recruitment in atherosclerotic vascular disease. Arteriosclerosis, Thrombosis, and Vascular Biology. 2004;**24**:1997-2008. DOI: 10.1161/01.ATV.0000142812.03840.6f

[52] Packard CJ, O'Reilly DS, Caslake MJ, McMahon AD, Ford I, Cooney J, Macphee CH, Suckling KE, Krishna M, Wilkinson FE, Rumley A, Lowe GD. Lipoprotein-associated phospholipase A2 as an independent predictor of coronary heart disease. West of Scotland Coronary Prevention Study Group. The New England Journal of Medicine. 2000;**343**:1148-1155. DOI: 10.1056/NEJM200010193431603

[53] Corson MA, Jones PH, Davidson MH. Review of the evidence for the clinical utility of lipoprotein-associated phospholipase A2 as a cardiovascular risk marker. The American Journal of Cardiology. 2008;**101**:41F-50F. DOI: 10.1016/j.amjcard.2008.04.018

[54] Silva IT, Mello APQ, Damasceno NRT. Antioxidant and inflammatory aspects of lipoprotein-associated phospholipase A(Lp-PLA2). Lipids in Health and Disease. 2011;**10**:170. DOI: 10.1186/1476-511X-10-170

[55] Snyder F. Platelet-activating factor and its analogs: Metabolic pathways and related intracellular processes. Biochimica et Biophysica Acta. 1995;**1254**:231-249. DOI: 10.1016/0005-2760(94)00192-2

[56] Koenig W, Twardella D, Brenner H, Rothenbacher D. Lipoprotein-associated phospholipase A2 predicts future cardiovascular events in patients with coronary heart disease independently of traditional risk factors, markers of inflammation, renal function, and hemodynamic stress. Arteriosclerosis, Thrombosis, and Vascular Biology. 2006;**26**:1586-1593. DOI: 10.1161/01.ATV.0000222983.73369.c8

[57] Gerber Y, McConnell JP, Jaffe AS, Weston SA, Killian JM, Roger VL. Lipoprotein-associated phospholipase A2 and prognosis after myocardial infarction in the community. Arteriosclerosis, Thrombosis, and Vascular Biology. 2006;**26**:2517-2522. DOI: 10.1161/01.ATV.0000240406.89440.0c

[58] Anuurad E, Ozturk Z, Enkhmaa B, Pearson TA, Berglund L. Association of lipoprotein-associated phospholipase A2 with coronary artery disease in African-Americans and Caucasians. The Journal of Clinical Endocrinology and Metabolism. 2010;**95**:2376-2383. DOI: 10.1210/jc.2009-2498

[59] Lavi S, McConnell JP, Rihal CS, Prasad A, Mathew V, Lerman LO, Lerman A. Local production of lipoprotein-associated phospholipase A2 and lysophosphatidylcholine in the coronary circulation: Association with early coronary atherosclerosis and endothelial dysfunction in humans. Circulation. 2007;**115**:2715-2721. DOI: 10.1161/CIRCULATIONAHA.106.671420

[60] Herrmann J, Mannheim D, Wohlert C, Versari D, Meyer FB, McConnell JP, Gössl M, Lerman LO, Lerman A. Expression of lipoprotein-associated phospholipase A(2) in carotid artery plaques predicts long-term cardiac outcome. European Heart Journal. 2009;**30**:2930-2938. DOI: 10.1093/eurheartj/ehp309

[61] Kuniyasu A, Tokunaga M, Yamamoto T, Inoue S, Obama K, Kawahara K, Nakayama H. Oxidized LDL and lysophosphatidylcholine stimulate plasminogen activator inhibitor-1 expression through reactive oxygen species generation and ERK1/2 activation in 3T3-L1 adipocytes. Biochimica et Biophysica Acta. 2011;**1811**:153-162. DOI: 10.1016/j.bbalip.2010.11.011

[62] Saougos VG, Tambaki AP, Kalogirou M, Kostapanos M, Gazi IF, Wolfert RL, Elisaf M, Tselepis AD. Differential effect of hypolipidemic drugs on lipoprotein-associated phospholipase A2. Arteriosclerosis, Thrombosis, and Vascular Biology. 2007;**27**:2236-2243. DOI: 10.1161/ATVBAHA.107.147280

[63] Third Report of the National Cholesterol Education Program (NCEP) Expert Panel on Detection, Evaluation, and Treatment of High Blood Cholesterol in Adults (Adult Treatment Panel III) final report. National Cholesterol Education Program (NCEP) Expert Panel on Detection, Evaluation, and Treatment of High Blood Cholesterol in Adults (Adult Treatment Panel III). Circulation. 2002;**106**:3143-3421

[64] Benítez S, Camacho M, Arcelus R, Vila L, Bancells C, Ordóñez-Llanos J, Sánchez-Quesada JL. Increased lysophosphatidylcholine and non-esterified fatty acid content in LDL induces chemokine release in endothelial cells. Relationship with electronegative LDL. Atherosclerosis. 2004;**177**:299-305. DOI: 10.1016/j.atherosclerosis.2004.07.027

[65] Shi Y, Zhang P, Zhang L, Osman H, Mohler ER, Macphee C, Zalewski A, Postle A, Wilensky RL. Role of lipoprotein-associated phospholipase A2 in leukocyte activation and inflammatory responses. Atherosclerosis. 2007;**191**:54-62. DOI: 10.1016/j.atherosclerosis.2006.05.001

[66] Tsimihodimos V, Karabina SA, Tambaki AP, Bairaktari E, Goudevenos JA, Chapman MJ, Elisaf M, Tselepis AD. Atorvastatin preferentially reduces LDL-associated platelet-activating factor acetylhydrolase activity in dyslipidemias of type IIA and type IIB. Arteriosclerosis, Thrombosis, and Vascular Biology. 2002;**22**:306-311 Print ISSN: 1079-5642. Online ISSN: 1524-4636

[67] Ballantyne CM, Hoogeveen RC, Bang H, Coresh J, Folsom AR, Heiss G, Sharrett AR. Lipoprotein-associated phospholipase A2, high-sensitivity C-reactive protein, and risk for incident coronary heart disease in middle-aged men and women in the Atherosclerosis Risk in Communities (ARIC) study. Circulation. 2004;**109**:837-842. DOI: 10.1161/01.CIR.0000116763.91992.F1

[68] Wilensky RL, Hamamdzic D. The molecular basis of vulnerable plaque: Potential therapeutic role for immunomodulation. Current Opinion in Cardiology. 2007;**22**:545-551. DOI: 10.1097/HCO.0b013e3282f028fe

[69] Lp-PLA(2) Studies Collaboration, Thompson A, Gao P, Orfei L, Watson S, Di Angelantonio E, Kaptoge S, Ballantyne C, Cannon CP, Criqui M, Cushman M, Hofman A, Packard C, Thompson SG, Collins R, Danesh J. Lipoprotein-associated phospholipase A (2) and risk of coronary disease, stroke, and mortality: Collaborative analysis of 32 prospective studies. Lancet. 2010;**375**:1536-1544. DOI: 10.1016/S0140-6736(10)60319-4

[70] Gungor Z, Anuurad E, Enkhmaa B, Zhang W, Kim K, Berglund L. Apo E4 and lipoprotein-associated phospholipase A2 synergistically increase cardiovascular risk. Atherosclerosis. 2012;**223**(1):230-234. DOI: 10.1016/j.atherosclerosis.2012.04.021

[71] Schnabel R, Dupuis J, Larson MG, Lunetta KL, Robins SJ, Zhu Y, Rong J, Yin X, Stirnadel HA, Nelson JJ, Wilson PW, Keaney JF, Vasan RS, Benjamin EJ. Clinical and genetic factors associated with lipoprotein-associated phospholipase A2 in the Framingham Heart Study. Atherosclerosis. 2009;**204**:601-607. DOI: 10.1016/j.atherosclerosis.2008.10.030

[72] Savchenko A, Imamura M, Ohashi R, Jiang S, Kawasaki T, Hasegawa G, Emura I, Iwanari H, Sagara M, Tanaka T, Hamakubo T, Kodama T, Naito M. Expression of pentraxin 3 (PTX3) in human atherosclerotic lesions. The Journal of Pathology. 2008;**215**:48-55. DOI: 10.1002/path.2314 DOI:10.1002/path.2314

[73] Fornai F, Carrizzo A, Forte M, Ambrosio M, Damato A, Ferrucci M, Biagioni F, Busceti C, Puca AA, Vecchione C. The inflammatory protein Pentraxin 3 in cardiovascular disease. Immunity & Ageing. 2016;**13**:25. DOI: 10.1186/s12979-016-0080-1

[74] Napoleone E, di Santo A, Peri G, Mantovani A, de Gaetano G, Donati MB, Lorenzet R. The long pentraxin PTX3 up-regulates tissue factor in activated monocytes: Another link between inflammation and clotting activation. Journal of Leukocyte Biology. 2004; **76**:203-209. DOI: 10.1189/jlb.1003528

[75] Jylhävä J, Haarala A, Kähönen M, Lehtimäki T, Jula A, Moilanen L, Kesäniemi YA, Nieminen MS, Hurme M. Pentraxin 3 (PTX3) is associated with cardiovascular risk factors: The Health 2000 Survey. Clinical and Experimental Immunology. 2011;**164**:211-217. DOI: 10.1111/j.1365-2249.2011.04354.x

[76] Nebuloni M, Pasqualini F, Zerbi P, Lauri E, Mantovani A, Vago L, Garlanda C. PTX3 expression in the heart tissues of patients with myocardial infarction and infectious myocarditis. Cardiovascular Pathology. 2011;**20**:e27-e35. DOI: 10.1016/j.carpath.2010.02.005

8

Role of Cholesterol as a Risk Factor in Cardiovascular Diseases

Eyup Avci, Ahmet Dolapoglu and Didar Elif Akgun

Abstract

Cardiovascular disease is the most common cause of death in adult population in the world. The disease includes numerous problems, many of which are related to a process called atherosclerosis. Atherosclerosis is a condition that develops when a substance called plaque builds up in the walls of the arteries. This plaque narrows the arteries, making it harder for blood to flow through. If a blood clot forms, it can stop the blood flow. This can cause a heart attack or stroke. There are many risk factors associated with cardio vascular disease (CVD). While some risk factors cannot be changed, such as family history, some of them can be modified with treatment such as abnormal blood lipid and sugar levels, obesity, smoking, and high blood pressure. Research makes it clear that abnormal blood lipid (fat) levels have a strong correlation with the risk of coronary artery disease, heart attack and coronary death. Cholesterol plays detrimental roles in the pathogenesis of atherosclerosis and CVD. In this chapter, we aim to summarize the relationship between blood cholesterol levels and CVD.

Keywords: cholesterol, cardiovascular disease, atherosclerosis

1. Introduction

Atherosclerotic cardiovascular disease is a group of disease which contains coronary artery disease, carotid artery disease, upper and lower extremity disease, and renal arterial diseases. The main cause of atherosclerotic cardiovascular diseases is the atherothrombotic process that occurs with atherosclerotic plaque rupture. Atherosclerosis is a chronic lipid-associated inflammatory disease concomitant with intimal thickening, especially involving bifurcation regions where endothelial damage is particularly high. Hypertension, hyperlipidemia, diabetes, and smoking are the main risk factors for atherosclerosis. Fibrinogen, hsCRP, and interleukin-6 (IL-6) which are markers for inflammation have been found elevated in atherosclerosis. Atherosclerotic diseases are also common with systemic inflammatory diseases such as lupus and rheumatoid arthritis.

2. Pathogenesis of atherosclerosis

Atherogenesis starts early in life. Subintimal lipoprotein accumulation and leukocyte adhesion occurs as a result of increased endothelial permeability due to endothelial damage. Intimal neovascularization is seen with the migration of vasa vasorum into the intima. There is a structure in the luminal side of the atherosclerotic plaque that is called fibrous cap which contains molecules such as smooth muscle, collagen, and elastin. External elastic lamina is placed adjacent to the atherosclerotic plaque and tunica media and the lipid core is found between these two structures and it is made from the cholesterol crystals, smooth muscle cells, vascular structures, and foam cells.

Atherosclerotic plaques create luminal stenosis in the advanced stage. The first study in this subject was conducted by Glagov et al. in autopsy material of a patient with 136 left main coronary artery (LMCA) lesions. In this study, there is a positive correlation between internal elastic membrane area and plaque area, and luminal stenosis is prevented by expansion of the compensator at the atheromatous load of less than 40% [1]. In the REVERSAL trial, statin therapy was performed in patients with asymptomatic coronary artery disease. Atheroma volume, percentage of atheroma volume, and atheromatous change in the diseased segment were evaluated and progression of coronary atherosclerosis was observed in the pravastatin receiving group compared to baseline but no progression of atherosclerosis was observed in the atorvastatin group [2].

3. Lipoprotein structure

The lipid core that carries triglycerides and cholesterol esters has a hydrophobic structure and is coated with polar capsules which contain apolipoproteins, phospholipids, and nonesterified cholesterol crystals. When the lipoproteins were classified according to their migration rates in lipoprotein electrophoresis, the band closest to the origin formed the chylomicron band; low-density lipoprotein (LDL) in the beta band, very-low-density lipoproteins (VLDL) in the pre-beta band, and high-density lipoprotein (HDL) in the alpha band, respectively.

Chylomicron is synthesized in liver from dietary fat molecules. Since chylomicrons and VLDL molecules larger than 70 nanometers cannot reach the subintimal region through the transcytotic transport system, chylomicrons do not have atherogenic potential. But chylomicron remnants are atherogenic and cannot be removed from circulation when they are present in high quantities [3]. Hydrolysis of the chylomicrons with lipoprotein lipase results in the formation of VLDL. The majority of VLDL is converted to LDL. Chylomicrons are attached to ApoB48. Chylomicron remnants, LDL, and VLDL are connected to apoB100 and are called non-HDL cholesterol.

4. Atherosclerosis and cholesterol hypothesis

The hypothesis of cholesterol suggests that lipids play a major role in the development of atherosclerosis. The 4S trial (Scandinavian Simvastanin Survival Study) showed that while there was significant reduction in total cholesterol level, LDL cholesterol level, and decrease in major coronary events, HDL cholesterol level was elevated in simvastatin receiving group [4]. After 4S study, REVERSAL, ASTEROID, and SATURN studies revealed that parallel plaque regression was observed with aggressive lipid-lowering therapy and reduction in major cardiovascular events was achieved. These similar studies have proven the relationship between hyperlipidemia and atherosclerosis [2, 5, 6].

Statins reduce macrophages and extracellular lipid accumulation in atherosclerotic plaque region and increase the content of collagen in the extracellular matrix which result in intimal calcification. Statins also stabilize inflammation and coagulation cascade after plaque rupture.

5. LDL and total cholesterol

LDL is the particle that is responsible for transporting cholesterol to tissues. Cholesterol transportation is achieved by binding of the LDL receptor and apoB. There are three separate fractions of LDL: LDL (large/floating), IDL, and small dense LDL. The most atherogenic LDL is small dense LDL.

In the WOSCOP trial and the AFCAPS/TeXCAPS trial which used pravastatin and lovastatin, respectively, the effect of hyperlipidemic therapy on the primary prevention of coronary artery disease was shown [7, 8]. The ASCOT-LLA study was terminated early in hypertensive individuals because atorvastatin significantly reduced nonfatal MI and CAD-induced mortality [9]. Similarly, the CARDS study was terminated early in diabetic individuals because atorvastatin decreased 37% in major cardiovascular events and 48% in stroke [10].

LIPID study compared low-dose and high-dose atorvastatin in patients with stable coronary artery disease and mortality was similar in both groups, but there was a significant decrease in major cardiovascular events in the high-dose atorvastatin group. The HPS study has shown that statin therapy protects high-risk patients with LDL cholesterol levels below 116 mg/dL [11]. CARE study with pravastatin in acute MI and MIRACLE study with atorvastatin in USAP or MI have shown early initiation of statins have a positive affect [12, 13].

In the ASTEROID trial, high-dose statin therapy (rosuvastatin 40 mg/day) was shown to reduce 53% LDL cholesterol, 15% increase in HDL cholesterol, and regression in 78% atheroma [5].

Proprotein convertase subtilisin/kexin type 9 (PCSK9) inhibitors inhibit the PCSK9 protein, which is effective in LDL receptor synthesis and provide 50–70% reduction in LDL-C levels.

In the ACCELERATE study, it was shown that the CETP inhibitor (Evacetrapib) did not reduce major cardiovascular events despite a 39% reduction in cholesterol level [14].

6. HDL

HDL is a molecule that is antioxidant, antiinflammatory, antiapoptotic and increases macrophage cholesterol excretion and endothelial healing. The removal of cholesterol from the body by the liver via HDL is called reverse cholesterol transport. ABCA-1, ABCG-1, and SR-B1 are effective in reverse cholesterol transport.

ApoA1 and ApoA2 are mainly found in the structure of HDL, and also HDL includes apoCs, ApoE, apoD, apoJ, lecithin-cholesterol acyltransferase (LCAT), serum paraoxonase (PON1) and platelet-activating factor acetylhydrolase (PAF-AH) molecules. Enzymes carried by HDL prevent oxidative modification of LDL.

Pentraxin 3 (PTX-3) in HDL controls leukocyte level. Defective PTX-3 was associated with large atherosclerotic plaques and higher level of inflammation [15, 16].

The association between low HDL and atherosclerotic cardiovascular disease was first shown by the Framingham study. Hypertension, diabetes mellitus, elevated total cholesterol, low HDL cholesterol, smoking, and age is considered as risk factor for coronary artery disease. The association between a low HDL cholesterol and atherosclerosis has been proven, but the increase in HDL has not been associated with a reduction in the incidence of atherosclerotic cardiovascular disease. Due to HDL being a molecule that prevents inflammation, some changes in HDL structure occur in chronic inflammatory processes.

7. Lipoprotein (a)

Lipoprotein (a) (Lp (a)) consists of an LDL molecule bound to apolipoprotein (a). Lipoprotein (a) is structurally similar to plasminogen and is thought to play a role in atherothrombosis with antifibrinolytic properties. In a study with patients with normal LDL and elevated Lp(a) levels, it was determined that increased Lp(a) levels was associated with high cardiovascular risk [17].

Cholesterol ester transfer protein (CETP) is responsible for transferring cholesterol esters. CETP inhibitors are associated with increased HDL and decreased LDL levels. In the study conducted with anacetrapib, there was no significant difference in mortality despite a significant increase in HDL and a significant decrease in non-HDL cholesterol compared to placebo [18].

8. Atherogenic dyslipidemia

In atherogenic dyslipidemia which is the result of an increase in triglyceride levels, triglyceride content is increased. The primary source of triglycerides is the VLDL. While LDL molecules are more easily oxidized, HDL molecules are more easily eliminated from the kidneys. Metabolic syndrome, type 2 diabetes, insulin resistance, abdominal obesity, and polycystic ovary syndrome are associated with atherogenic dyslipidemia.

In the case of atherogenic dyslipidemia, since chylomicrons have no effect on atherosclerosis, non-HDL cholesterol level is used rather than triglyceride level. Although levels of

LDL, VLDL, and chylomicron residues can be determined by detecting Apo B levels, there is limited access and standardization for the detection of Apo B level. In the ESC dyslipidemia guide, non-HDL cholesterol calculation is recommended instead of measuring ApoB levels in the presence of hypertriglyceridemia. (Class 2a) In a study conducted by Puri et al., the level of non-HDL cholesterol rather than LDL cholesterol significantly correlated with atheromatous progression when the triglyceride level rises above 200 mg/dl. In the NICE guideline, all individuals are focused on evaluating non-HDL cholesterol exclusively from LDL cholesterol.

9. Familial hypercholesterolemia

Familial hypercholesterolemia is a metabolic disorder that occurs as a result of the absence or lack of LDL receptors in the liver. Since LDL molecules are removed from the circulation, very high LDL levels and premature atherosclerosis are observed. Familial hypercholesterolemia is thought to be approximately 1/500 of the homozygous form and approximately 1/1 million of the heterozygous form. Tendon xanthomas are pathognomonic signs for familial hypercholesterolemia. There is also an increase in the frequency of corneal arcus, xanthelasma.

10. Sitosterolemia

Sitosterol is a plant-derived molecule and its structure resembles cholesterol. Cytosterolemia is a progressive disease with an increase in the absorption and a decrease in biliary secretion of cholesterol and sitosterol molecules. Sitosterolemia is also called pseudohomozygous familial hyperlipidemia.

Recommendations for ESC 2016:

- Total cholesterol should be used to predict cardiovascular risk via the SCORE system. (1-C)

- LDL-C should be used primarily in screening, diagnosis, risk estimation, and treatment. (1-C)

- HDL-C should be used in the Heart Score algorithm. (1-C)

- TG provides additional information in the risk estimation. (1-C)

- Non-HDL cholesterol should be considered as a risk indicator, especially in individuals with high triglyceride levels. (1-C)

- ApoB should be considered as an alternative risk marker in patients with high triglyceride values. (2a-C)

- Lp (a) may be considered in individuals with high-risk, early family history of CVD and in the reclassification of individuals with borderline risk. (2a-C)

- ApoB1/ApoA1 ratio can be considered as an alternative analysis in risk prediction. (2b-C)

- The ratio of non-HDL cholesterol/HDL cholesterol can be considered as an alternative, but the HDL cholesterol used in the HEART SCORE provides a better risk estimate. (2b-C)

- LDL cholesterol is the main treatment target. (1-A)

- When available, apoB should be an alternative to non-HDL-C. (2a-C)

- Lp(a) should be recommended in selected case at high-risk, for reclassification at border-line risk, and in subjects with a family history of premature CVD. (2a-C)

- TC may be considered but is usually not enough for the characterization of dyslipidemia before initiation of treatment. (2a-C)

- HDL cholesterol and non-HDL cholesterol/HDL cholesterol levels are not recommended as treatment targets (Class 3).

11. Epidemiology

More than 30% of worldwide deaths are thought to be cardiovascular based and the frequency tends to increase due to changes in lifestyle and prolonged life. According to AHA 2016 statistics, in the United States, one in every 42 seconds loses his/her life due to cardiovascular reasons [19]. In Europe, the cardiovascular mortality rate is 4.1 million a year. A total of 1.8 million deaths, in other words 20% of all deaths, are due to ischemic heart disease. This is followed by cerebrovascular events with an annual death of 1.1 million. According to ESC data, 1.5 million deaths before the age of 75 and 710,000 deaths before the age of 65 are cardiovascular sources; half is due to coronary artery disease [20]. Deaths in all age groups, 51% of women and 42% of men are cardiovascular.

12. Coronary artery disease and cholesterol

Acute coronary syndrome is a clinical event that occurs when the coronary blood flow is reduced by thrombus on the rupture plaque and the myocardial oxygen requirement cannot be met. Acute coronary syndrome is broad spectrum which contains STEMI, nonSTEMI, unstable angina pectoris, and sudden cardiac death. In many cases, the thrombosis process begins with plaque rupture. Up to 25% of cases of acute coronary syndromes can begin with plaque erosion. Lymphocyte and macrophage activation and the inflammatory response is accompanied by atherothrombosis. There are clinical differences according to coronary collateral reserve and obstruction severity. This process occurs after a plaque rupture and is called Type 1 MI.

Atherosclerotic plaques that play an essential role in acute coronary syndrome are divided according to their structural characteristics: Plaque structure is with thin fibrous cap, dense necrotic core, high inflammatory cell density, and low smooth muscle content; it is called vulnerable plaque. Vulnerable plaque increases with hypertension, diabetes mellitus, elevated LDL, decreased HDL, and elevated ACE. Conversely, stabilized plaques with thick fibrous caps, poor necrotic cells, and dense extracellular matrix with low inflammatory content are observed in individuals with low risk factors (**Figure 1**).

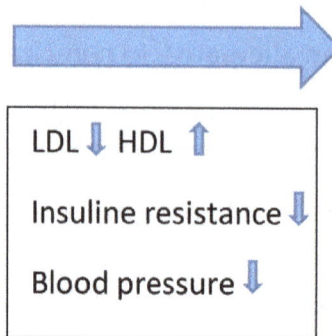

VULNERABLE PLAQUE   STABLE PLAQUE

Thin fibrous cap   Thick fibrous cap

Large lipit pool   Smaller lipid pool

Many inflammatory cells   Few inflammatory cells

Few smooth muscle cells   LDL ⇩ HDL ⇧   Dense extracellular matrix

                                 Insuline resistance ⇩

                                 Blood pressure ⇩

Figure 1. Structural differences between vulnerable and stable plaques.

In a meta-analysis involving 90,056 patients, a reduction of 38.6 mg/dl in LDL was shown to be associated with a 20% reduction in major cardiovascular events [21]. In MIRACLE study: increased plaque stability with statin therapy reduces death, incidence of acute coronary syndrome and frequency of recurrent coronary ischemia [13]. In the PROVE IT TIMI-22 trial, atorvastatin 80 mg and pravastatin 40 mg were compared and it was determined that high-dose statin therapy was more effective than low-dose statin therapy in reducing cardiovascular events. The 2017 ESC STEMI guidelines recommended that high-dose statin therapy was independent of cholesterol level. In the FOURIER study, it has been shown that the addition of the evolocumab in patient with LDL level ≥ 70 mg/dl, despite the use of high dose statin, is associated with a decrease in cardiovascular deaths [22].

13. Coronary calcium score

The coronary calcium score began to be used in the 1990s and the method was prepared by Agatson et al. Zero coronary calcium score has a high negative predictive value. It is the most commonly used method. In the 2016 ESC Guidelines for Cardiovascular Disease Prevention, the use of coronary calcium scoring has been proposed for predicting cardiovascular risk in individuals with a SCORE risk threshold of 5–10%.

CARDIA study showed a correlation between elevated LDL or non-HDL cholesterol and coronary calcium score [23].

14. Peripheral arterial diseases and cholesterol

Peripheral arterial disease is a concept that involves diseases of arteries other than coronary arteries. It most commonly occurs as a result of atherosclerotic process. In addition to atherosclerosis, vasculitis, and injuries, trapping syndromes are also effective in the formation of peripheral arterial disease. Approximately one-third of the individuals with peripheral artery disease are accompanied by coronary artery disease. Peripheral artery disease should be considered as equivalent to coronary artery disease risk. Deaths are mostly of cardiac origin.

According to the REACH study, 3-year vascular-induced deaths were more common in patients with peripheral arterial disease than in those with coronary and carotid artery disease [24]. The use of statin has reduced both symptoms and cardiovascular mortality in a variety of studies on peripheral arterial disease [25, 26].

15. Carotid diseases, stroke, and cholesterol

Ischemic stroke should be investigated in two groups as embolic and thrombotic stroke.

Smoking and age are the most important risk factors for carotid atherosclerosis. The atherosclerotic plaque is located in the bifurcation area and often extends on the outer wall of the carotid bulb.

When stenotic plague increases, the risk of emboli increases. Carotid stenosis is defined as a stenosis of 50% or more in the extracranial portion of the internal carotid artery. In addition to the luminal narrowing, the lesion's edge irregularity, the presence of intraplate plaque hemorrhage, whether the lesion is unilateral or not, also determines the severity of the disease. Symptomatic carotid stenosis is the occurrence of symptoms related to carotid stenosis in the last 6 months.

In the heart protection study with simvastatin, a reduction of 39 mg/dL at the LDL level resulted in a 20% reduction in major cardiovascular events, 25% reduction in stroke, and 38% reduction in ischemic stroke [11].

In the SPARCLE trial (stroke prevention by aggressive reduction in cholesterol levels), patients who had stroke and TIA within the last 1–6 months were evaluated for 5 years. In patients receiving high-dose atorvastatin, a reduction of 43% in LDL levels resulted in a 20% reduction in major cardiovascular events and a 16% reduction in stroke. Despite the increase in hemorrhagic stroke rates in the high-dose statin group, there was no difference in lethal hemorrhagic stroke [27, 28].

It has been suggested that statin therapy initiated after stroke also improves neurological function with a decrease in infarct area. According to the information obtained from the meta-analyses, the use of statin before and after stroke is associated with improvement in neurological function. However, there was a relationship between statin therapy and hemorrhagic transformation in cases treated with thrombolytic therapy [29].

Carotid intima media thickness is a subclinical atherosclerosis indicator and it is recommended to use it in addition to classical cardiovascular risk indicators, especially in individuals with hypertensive middle cardiovascular risk (SCORE risk 1–5%). Values above 0.9 mm or values above normal 75th percentile should be considered pathological. According to the American Society of Echocardiography, these individuals should be considered as having increased CV risk. Individuals between 75 and 25% have expected cardiovascular risk. Individuals below the 25th percentile have low cardiovascular risk [30].

16. Renal artery stenosis hypertension and cholesterol

Renovascular hypertension is about 5% of all hypertension cases. In the presence of peripheral artery disease, the frequency of renal artery stenosis reaches up to 14%. There is an increase in the frequency of renal artery stenosis and peripheral artery disease association in the presence of diffuse peripheral artery disease [31]. Atherosclerotic renal artery disease is the most common cause of renovascular hypertension. Atherosclerotic renal artery disease is often defined as having ≥60% stenosis in the osteal or proximal one-third of the renal artery. The second most common cause is fibromuscular dysplasia in younger individuals with no atherosclerotic risk factors. There is a "string of beats" view at the distal one-third of the renal artery. Renal artery stenosis can be tolerated by autoregulation mechanisms until the renal perfusion pressure reaches 70 mmHg. Renal revascularization has not been shown to reduce hypertension, renal, or cardiovascular events. Antihypertensive therapy, antiplatelet therapy, and statins are the main treatments.

17. Lower extremity peripheral artery diseases and cholesterol

A common cause of lower extremity peripheral artery disease is atherosclerosis. It is common in men who have cigarette use at a young age. Diabetes and smoking are the most common causes of amputation in peripheral artery diseases. In the atherosclerotic process, progressive narrowing of the vessel wall occurs. Clinical signs are observed in the later stages of the disease. Clinical disease severity is determined by Fontaine and Rutherford classifications. There are studies that argue that the ankle brachial index (ABI) used in lower extremity diseases should be used as a risk factor for coronary artery disease. When ABI is above 0.9, it is considered normal but below 0.40 is considered as serious disease.

The 2017 ESC guidelines for peripheral arterial disease recommended LDL cholesterol lowering to 70 mg/dL or 50% reduction in LDL levels in patients with an initial LDL level of 70–135 mg/dL. Studies in lower extremity arterial disease patients have shown that statin therapy decreases all-cause mortality and cardiovascular mortality.

18. Aortic aneurysm and cholesterol

Aneurysm is defined as enlarging the diameter of artery, local or diffuse, by 50% or more relative to normal. According to localization, it is divided into thoracic and abdominal. Aortic aneurysms are 80% in abdominal location [32]. It is a chronic disease associated with inflammation of the aortic wall. It is suggested that the vessel is formed as a result of elasticity and power loss of the aortic wall after occlusion of vasa vasorum.

In the population with abdominal aortic aneurysm, association with other atherosclerotic cardiovascular diseases was frequently observed. The presence of abdominal aortic aneurysm was frequently associated with other atherosclerotic cardiovascular diseases. Smoking, age, and male sex increases the risk of aortic aneurysm. While intimal atheroma and thrombosis process are present in both diseases, elastin fragmentation and adventitial chronic inflammation are limited to aortic aneurysms [33, 34].

In the tromsø study, there was a relation between the intima media thickness and the incidence of coronary artery disease and abdominal aortic aneurysm, but no correlation with aortic diameter [35]. The relationship between lipid level and aortic aneurysm has not been clearly elucidated [36]. The data for the studies are based on the similarity of risk factors for atherosclerosis and aortic aneurysm risk factors.

19. Retinal vascular diseases and cholesterol

Hyperlipidemia is associated with retinal vascular diseases. In old age, structures called "druzen" in tissue are similar to atherosclerotic lesions. Ischemic optic neuropathy can be seen as a result of stenosis in the retinal arteries and venules. In the ACCORD Eye trial, although strict treatment for diabetes and hyperlipidemia was beneficial, there was no significant benefit from strict blood pressure regulation [37, 38].

Author details

Eyup Avci[1]*, Ahmet Dolapoglu[2] and Didar Elif Akgun[1]

*Address all correspondence to: dreyupavci@gmail.com

1 Faculty of Medicine, Department of Cardiology, Balikesir University, Turkey

2 Cardiovascular Surgery Clinic, Balikesir Ataturk State Hospital, Turkey

References

[1] Glagov S et al. Compensatory enlargement of human atherosclerotic coronary arteries. New England Journal of Medicine. 1987;**316**(22):1371-1375

[2] Nicholls SJ et al. Effects of obesity on lipid-lowering, anti-inflammatory, and antiatherosclerotic benefits of atorvastatin or pravastatin in patients with coronary artery disease (from the REVERSAL Study). The American Journal of Cardiology. 2006;**97**(11):1553-1557

[3] Kenneth C-W, John CL. Chylomicron-remnant-induced foam cell formation and cytotoxicity: A possible mechanism of cell death in atherosclerosis. Clinical Science. 2000;**98**(2):183-192

[4] Scandinavian Simvastatin Survival Study Group. Randomised trial of cholesterol lowering in 4444 patients with coronary heart disease: The Scandinavian simvastatin survival study (4S). The Lancet. 1994;**344**(8934):1383-1389

[5]   Wiviott SD et al. Safety and efficacy of achieving very low low-density lipoprotein cho-
      lesterol levels with rosuvastatin 40 mg daily (from the ASTEROID study). The American
      Journal of Cardiology. 2009;**104**(1):29-35

[6]   Nicholls SJ et al. Impact of statins on progression of atherosclerosis: Rationale and
      design of SATURN (Study of coronary atheroma by in travascular ultrasound: Effect
      of Rosuvastatin versus AtorvastatiN). Current Medical Research and Opinion. 2011;
      27(6):1119-1129

[7]   West of Scotland Coronary Prevention Study Group. Influence of pravastatin and
      plasma lipids on clinical events in the West of Scotland Coronary Prevention Study
      (WOSCOPS). Circulation. 1998;**97**(15):1440-1445

[8]   Downs JR et al. Primary prevention of acute coronary events with lovastatin in men
      and women with average cholesterol levels: results of AFCAPS/TexCAPS. JAMA. 1998;
      279(20):1615-1622

[9]   Sever PS et al. Prevention of coronary and stroke events with atorvastatin in hyper-
      tensive patients who have average or lower-than-average cholesterol concentrations, in
      the Anglo-Scandinavian Cardiac outcomes trial—Lipid lowering arm (ASCOT-LLA): A
      multicentre randomised controlled trial. The Lancet. 2003;**361**(9364):1149-1158

[10] Colhoun HM et al. Primary prevention of cardiovascular disease with atorvastatin in
      type 2 diabetes in the Collaborative Atorvastatin Diabetes Study (CARDS): Multicentre
      randomised placebo-controlled trial. The Lancet. 2004;**364**(9435):685-696

[11] Heart Protection Study Collaborative Group. MRC/BHF heart protection study of cho-
      lesterol lowering with simvastatin in 20 536 high-risk individuals: A randomised place-
      bocontrolled trial. The Lancet. 2002;**360**(9326):7-22

[12] Ridker PM et al. Inflammation, pravastatin, and the risk of coronary events after myocar-
      dial infarction in patients with average cholesterol levels. Circulation. 1998;**98**(9):839-844

[13] Schwartz GG et al. Effects of atorvastatin on early recurrent ischemic events in acute
      coronary syndromes: The MIRACL study: A randomized controlled trial. JAMA.
      2001;**285**(13):1711-1718

[14] Nicholls SJ et al. Assessment of the clinical effects of cholesteryl ester transfer protein
      inhibition with evacetrapib in patients at high-risk for vascular outcomes: Rationale and
      design of the ACCELERATE trial. American Heart Journal. 2015;**170**(6):1061-1069

[15] Norata GD et al. Long pentraxin 3, a key component of innate immunity, is modulated
      by high-density lipoproteins in endothelial cells. Arteriosclerosis, Thrombosis, and
      Vascular Biology. 2008;**28**(5):925-931

[16] Norata GD, Garlanda C, Catapano AL. The long pentraxin PTX3: A modulator of the
      immunoinflammatory response in atherosclerosis and cardiovascular diseases. Trends
      in Cardiovascular Medicine. 2010;**20**(2):35-40

[17] Aim-High Investigators. The role of niacin in raising high-density lipoprotein choles-
      terol to reduce cardiovascular events in patients with atherosclerotic cardiovascular

disease and optimally treated low-density lipoprotein cholesterol: Rationale and study design. The atherothrombosis intervention in metabolic syndrome with low HDL/high triglycerides: Impact on Global Health outcomes (AIM-HIGH). American Heart Journal. 2011;**161**(3):471-477

[18] Bowman L et al. Effects of anacetrapib in patients with atherosclerotic vascular disease. Journal of Vascular Surgery. 2018;**67**(1):356

[19] Writing, Group Members, et al. Heart disease and stroke statistics-2016 update: A report from the American Heart Association Circulation. 2016;**1334**:e38

[20] Nichols M et al. Cardiovascular disease in Europe: Epidemiological update. European Heart Journal. 2013;**34**(39):3028-3034

[21] Trialists, Cholesterol Treatment. Efficacy and safety of cholesterol-lowering treatment: Prospective meta-analysis of data from 90 056 participants in 14 randomised trials of statins. The Lancet. 2005;**366**(9493):1267-1278

[22] Mikhail N. Effects of evolocumab on cardiovascular events. Current Cardiology Reviews. 2017;**13**(4):319-324

[23] Wilkins JT et al. Discordance between apolipoprotein B and LDL-cholesterol in young adults predicts coronary artery calcification: The CARDIA study. Journal of the American College of Cardiology. 2016;**67**(2):193-201

[24] Bhatt DL et al. International prevalence, recognition, and treatment of cardiovascular risk factors in outpatients with atherothrombosis. JAMA. 2006;**295**(2):180-189

[25] Aung, Phyu Phyu, et al. Lipid-lowering for peripheral arterial disease of the lower limb. The Cochrane Database of Systemic Reviews. 17 Oct 2007;(4):CD000123

[26] Mohler ER, Hiatt WR, Creager MA. Cholesterol reduction with atorvastatin improves walking distance in patients with peripheral arterial disease. Circulation. 2003;**108**(12):1481-1486

[27] Stroke Prevention by Aggressive Reduction in Cholesterol Levels (SPARCL) Investigators. High-dose atorvastatin after stroke or transient ischemic attack. The New England Journal of Medicine. 2006;**355**(2006):549-559

[28] Adams RJ et al. Update to the AHA/ASA recommendations for the prevention of stroke in patients with stroke and transient ischemic attack. Stroke. 2008;**39**(5):1647-1652

[29] Hong K-S, Ji SL. Statins in acute ischemic stroke: A systematic review. Journal of Stroke. 2015;**17**(3):282

[30] Stein JH et al. Use of carotid ultrasound to identify subclinical vascular disease and evaluate cardiovascular disease risk: A consensus statement from the American Society of Echocardiography Carotid Intima-Media Thickness Task Force endorsed by the Society for Vascular Medicine. Journal of the American Society of Echocardiography. 2008;**21** 2 :93-111

[31] Aboyans V et al. Renal artery stenosis in patients with peripheral artery disease: Prevalence, risk factors and long-term prognosis. European Journal of Vascular and Endovascular Surgery. 2017;**53**(3):380-385

[32] Aggarwal S et al. Abdominal aortic aneurysm: A comprehensive review. Experimental and Clinical Cardiology. Spring; 2011;**16**(1):11-15

[33] Golledge J et al. Abdominal aortic aneurysm. Arteriosclerosis, Thrombosis, and Vascular Biology. 2006;**26**(12):2605-2613

[34] Cornuz J et al. Risk factors for asymptomatic abdominal aortic aneurysm: Systematic review and meta-analysis of population-based screening studies. The European Journal of Public Health. 2004;**14**(4):343-349

[35] Johnsen SH et al. Atherosclerosis in abdominal aortic aneurysms: A causal event or a process running in parallel? The Tromsø study. Arteriosclerosis, Thrombosis, and Vascular Biology. 2010;**30**(6):1263-1268

[36] Ferguson CD et al. Association of statin prescription with small abdominal aortic aneurysm progression. American Heart Journal. 2010;**159**(2):307-313

[37] Chew EY et al. The effects of medical management on the progression of diabetic retinopathy in persons with type 2 diabetes: The Action to Control Cardiovascular Risk in Diabetes (ACCORD) eye study. Ophthalmology. 2014;**121**(12):2443-2451

[38] Tsao SW, Fong DS. Do statins have a role in the prevention of age-related macular degeneration? Drugs & Aging. 2013;**30**(4):205-213

9

The Role of Cholesterol in the Pathogenesis of Hypertension-Associated Nonalcoholic Steatohepatitis

Yuan Yuan, Hisao Naito and Tamie Nakajima

Abstract

Dietary cholesterol is a crucial risk factor for nonalcoholic steatohepatitis (NASH). Our recent studies indicated that high cholesterol intake was associated with the pathogenesis of hypertension-associated NASH. We developed a novel hypertensive rat model of NASH by feeding stroke-prone spontaneously hypertensive rats (SHRSP5/Dmcr) a high fat and cholesterol (HFC) diet. Histological features resembling human NASH were observed in this model. Furthermore, we investigated the kinetics of cholesterol in the rats fed an HFC diet and determined that suppression of bile acid (BA) detoxification led by HFC feeding results in cytotoxic BA accumulation in hepatocytes, which induces inflammatory response and liver damage. Sex differences in fibrogenesis were also observed in this model, and we found this was associated with a different ability in BA detoxification. Since SHRSP5/Dmcr rats are hypertensive, we investigated the role of hypertension in NASH progression by comparing NASH development among SHRSP5/Dmcr rats, spontaneously hypertensive rats and their original strain, Wistar Kyoto, with normal blood pressure. HFC diet induced more severe hepatic fibrosis in the hypertensive strains compared with the normotensive one. In conclusion, dietary cholesterol plays an essential role in the pathogenesis of NASH, and the combined action of cholesterol and hypertension further aggravates its progression.

Keywords: cholesterol, hypertension, nonalcoholic steatohepatitis, spontaneously hypertensive rat, Wistar Kyoto rat, CYP7A1, kinetics of bile acids, gender differences in fibrogenesis

1. Introduction

High dietary cholesterol intake may lead to increased risk of diseases such as cardiovascular disease and diabetes [1, 2]. Although the recommendation to restrict daily dietary cholesterol intake (300 mg) was removed from the 2015–2020 Dietary Guidelines for Americans [3], it is still recommended that individuals minimize cholesterol consumption. Animal foods such as egg yolk, meats, dairy products, fish, and poultry are major sources of dietary cholesterol. Meanwhile, dietary cholesterol is not found in plant foods. Instead, many plants contain phytosterols, which are chemically similar to cholesterol, and can therefore compete with it and decrease its absorption in the intestinal tract [4]. The effect of dietary cholesterol on plasma cholesterol levels remains undetermined, since the body may suppress endogenous cholesterol synthesis in response to additional cholesterol ingestion [1]. Some studies have suggested that dietary cholesterol increases serum total cholesterol (TC), low-density lipoprotein (LDL) cholesterol, as well as the ratio of LDL to high-density lipoprotein cholesterol [5–8], which are considered to be associated with risk of vascular diseases.

Dietary cholesterol is also linked to the pathogenesis of nonalcoholic fatty liver disease (NAFLD)/nonalcoholic steatohepatitis (NASH) [9, 10]. NAFLD is one of the most common chronic liver diseases worldwide and comprises a spectrum of liver damage, from simple steatosis (a benign non-progressive condition) to NASH, the advanced form that may progress to hepatic cirrhosis or hepatocellular carcinoma [11]. The pathological characteristics of NASH include steatosis, hepatocellular ballooning, lobular inflammation, and hepatic fibrosis. Cholesterol may contribute to NASH development by being catabolized in the liver into bile acids (BAs), which are hepatotoxic and cause liver damage [12]. Li et al. demonstrated that dietary cholesterol exacerbates liver damage and hepatic inflammation in mice fed a high-fat diet [13]. Subramanian et al. reported that an LDL receptor-deficient mouse fed a high-fat, high-carbohydrate diet was a good animal model of NAFLD/NASH, and showed that dietary cholesterol worsened hepatic steatosis and inflammation in this model [9].

In addition, NAFLD/NASH was described as a hepatic manifestation of metabolic syndrome, and its development was associated with hypertension, obesity, diabetes, and hyperlipidemia [14, 15]. Some studies have shown an increased prevalence of NAFLD/NASH among hypertensive patients [16–18]. Using spontaneously hypertensive (SHR) rats fed a choline-deficient diet as a hypertensive animal model of NASH, and its normotensive control, the Wistar Kyoto (WKY) rat [19], Ikuta et al. revealed that hypertension enhances the progression of NASH. We previously developed a novel animal model of hypertension-associated NASH by feeding stroke-prone spontaneously hypertensive5/Dmcr (SHRSP5/Dmcr) rats a high fat and cholesterol (HFC) diet [20]. Further studies from our group suggested that dietary cholesterol may have a potential effect on the development of hypertension-associated NASH (unpublished).

In this chapter, we will discuss the crucial role of dietary cholesterol in the progression of hypertension-associated NASH.

2. The development of a novel animal model of NASH and the mechanism underlying the progression of NASH in this model

The mechanisms of the pathogenesis of NASH are not completely understood, partly due to a lack of ideal animal models with histological patterns that resemble human NASH. Matsuzawa et al. showed that an HFC diet (an atherogenic, high-fat diet containing 1.25%

cholesterol and 60% fat) induced steatohepatitis, cellular ballooning, and fibrosis in the livers of male C57Bl/6J mice [21]. We previously established an HFC diet-induced NASH model using hypertensive SHRSP5/Dmcr rats [20].

SHRSP5/Dmcr rats are the fifth substrain of the stroke-prone spontaneously hypertensive (SHRSP) rat [20, 22], which is derived from the SHR strain [23]. To establish this strain, SHRSP rats were fed an HFC diet for 1 week, then those with high serum cholesterol levels (600–900 mg/dL in females and 300–600 mg/dL in males) were selected for brother–sister inbreeding. Selective inbreeding was repeated and offspring with increased hypercholes-terolemic responses were obtained. Although the SHRSP5/Dmcr rats, formally known as arteriolipidosis-prone rats, were developed as an animal model of arteriosclerosis, marked enlargement and an abnormal whitish color of the liver were noted in the 47th generation. These findings prompted our studies on HFC diet-induced liver damage in this strain.

In order to determine whether the HFC diet-fed SHRSP5/Dmcr strain was a suitable model of NASH, we investigated hepatic histopathological changes following HFC feeding [20]. Male SHRSP5/Dmcr rats at 10 weeks of age were fed either an HFC (35.3% crude lipid and 5% choles-terol) or control diet (4.8% crude lipid and no additional cholesterol) for 2, 8, and 14 weeks. We found that the HFC diet induced microvesicular steatosis and lymphocyte infiltration at 2 weeks. Macrovesicular steatosis, ballooned hepatocytes with eosinophilic Mallory-Denk bodies, and multilobular necrosis were observed in the livers of rats fed an HFC diet at 8 weeks. The severity of steatosis and hepatocyte ballooning was further increased at 14 weeks. Meanwhile, a progressive deterioration of hepatic fibrosis occurred during HFC feeding. Slight pericellular and perivenular fibrotic changes, bridging fibrosis, and end-stage honeycomb fibrosis were observed at 2, 8, and 14 weeks, respectively. In addition, the HFC diet induced a progressive increase in indicators of liver damage, including serum levels of alanine transaminase (AST), aspartate transaminase (ALT), and γ-glutamyltranspeptidase (γ-GTP). Matteoni et al. classified human NAFLD into four types according to histological analysis of liver biopsy specimens: type 1, fatty liver alone; type 2, fat accumulation and lobular inflammation; type 3, fat accumulation and ballooning degenera-tion; and type 4, fat accumulation, ballooning degeneration, and hepatic fibrosis [24]. The histo-logical characteristics observed in the liver of the SHRSP5/Dmcr strain at 2, 8, and 14 weeks of HFC feedings were very similar to those in type 2, type 3 or 4, and type 4 human NAFLD, respec-tively. Therefore, all pathological stages of NAFLD can be observed in the SHRSP5/Dmcr strain during HFC feeding. In addition, obesity, insulin resistance, and diabetes were not observed in this model. Therefore, it represents an excellent model of NAFLD/NASH without obesity and diabetes, and is useful for studying the pathogenesis and therapeutics of this disease.

We further investigated the molecular mechanisms underlying the progression of HFC-induced NASH in the SHRSP5/Dmcr strain [25]. Rats were fed either an HFC or control diet for 2, 8, and 16 weeks, and expression of genes involved in inflammation and hepatic fibrosis was evaluated. Tumor necrosis factor α (TNF-α), a proinflammatory cytokine, was reported to be upregulated in the livers of NASH patients [26]. We showed that the HFC diet increased the hepatic expression of TNF-α in SHRSP5/Dmcr rats at all time points. Nuclear factor κB (NF-κB; p50/p65) and inhibitor of κBα, the proteins involved in NF-κB signaling, which is regulated by TNF-α and plays an important role in inflammatory response, were also upregulated by the HFC diet. Hepatocyte injury and inflammation led to hepatic fibrosis via hepatic stellate cell (HSC) activation, which results in the production and deposition of extracellular matrix (ECM) [27]. The HFC diet induced the upregulation of transforming growth factor-β1 (TGF-β1), a profibrotic cytokine that promotes HSC activation, prior to the appearance of obvious hepatic fibrosis (at 2 weeks). Its upregulation was also observed at subsequent stages (at 8 and 16 weeks). Expression of alpha smooth muscle actin (α-SMA) and platelet-derived growth factor-B, involved in hepatic fibrosis, were elevated at 8 weeks of HFC feeding, indicating extensive activation of HSC at this time point. Alpha-1 type I collagen, the major component of ECM, was produced by activated HSC (myofibroblast) and was markedly elevated at 8 and 16 weeks, corresponding to the appearance of extensive liver fibrosis observed at the same time points.

In order to investigate the role of dietary cholesterol in the pathogenesis of HFC diet-induced NASH in SHRSP5/Dmcr rats, we compared hepatic histological changes induced by a high fat (HF) diet and those by an HFC diet (unpublished). As described above, the HFC diet induced severe steatosis, lymphocyte infiltration, ballooned hepatocytes, and fibrosis in the livers of the rats. In contrast, HF feeding only led to mild hepatic steatosis and lymphocyte infiltration, while liver fibrosis was not observed. It was suggested that dietary cholesterol may play a key role in the transition from simple steatosis to fibrotic steatohepatitis, the progressive stage, during the progression of NAFLD/NASH.

3. The role of hypertension in the progression of NASH

SHRSP5/Dmcr rats are hypertensive, making this strain an ideal model in which to study the correlation between hypertension and NASH. In our previous study, we investigated the mechanism underlying the development of hypertension-associated NASH using three strains of a rat: normotensive WKY, hypertensive SHR and SHRSP5/Dmcr [28]. As mentioned previously, SHRSP5/Dmcr was established from the SHRSP strain, which was derived from SHR strain that was developed from normotensive WKY rats by selective inbreeding of the rats with spontaneously high systolic blood pressure in normal conditions [29]. Male rats with a blood pressure of 150–175 mmHg persisting for more than 1 month, and females with a blood pressure of 130–140 mmHg were mated, and the offspring with high blood pressure (over 150 mmHg persisting for more than 1 month) were selected for further inbreeding. The severity of hypertension was elevated from generation to generation, and all the rats from the third to sixth generation developed spontaneous hypertension by 15 weeks of age. Since the SHR and WKY originated from the same parental outbred Wistar rats, the WKY strain was used as the normotensive control for the SHR and SHRSP5/Dmcr strains. The blood pressure in the adult male rats of the three strains, WKY, SHR, and SHRSP5/Dmcr, were 130, 235, and 180 mmHg, respectively [28].

In our study, the normotensive WKY strain, and two hypertensive SHR and SHRSP5/Dmcr strains were fed either the HFC or control diet for 8 weeks. Changes to liver pathology and expression of proteins associated with inflammation and oxidative stress were determined [28]. We evaluated serum levels of AST, ALT, and γ-GTP, and confirmed that mild liver damage occurred in the hypertensive strains in the absence of HFC feeding, suggesting that hypertension may be a risk factor for chronic liver disease. The HFC diet induced more severe lobular inflammation and hepatic fibrosis in the hypertensive strains compared with the normotensive strain. The severity of the hepatic fibrosis observed in the SHRSP5/Dmcr strain was even higher compared with that of the SHR strain. The HFC diet induced elevation of serum inflammatory cytokines, TNF-α and TGF-β1, in the hypertensive strains, whereas an increase in TGF-β1 was not observed in the normotensive rats. The combination of TNF-α and TGF-β1 may trigger a more severe inflammatory response in the hypertensive rats by regulating the activation of downstream inflammatory signaling such as NF-κB and mitogen-activated protein kinase (MAPK) pathways. Increased activation of NF-κB and MAPK (p38 and JNK) signaling occurred in the hypertensive strains, which may have contributed to the more severe lobular inflammation observed in these rats. In addition, oxidative stress, defined as an imbalance between the production of reactive oxygen species (ROS) and their elimination by antioxidant defenses, may lead to cellular injury and chronic inflammation [30]. An increase in oxidative stress in NASH patients was previously reported [31, 32]. We measured serum thiobarbituric acid reactive substances levels and found that oxidative stress was significantly elevated in hypertensive strains fed an HFC diet but not in normotensive rats (unpublished data). Meanwhile, in hypertensive rats, the HFC diet suppressed the nuclear factor erythroid 2-related factor 2 (Nrf2)/ Kelch-like ECH-associated protein 1 (Keap1) pathway, involved in antioxidative defenses [33]. We also found that hepatic levels of superoxide dismutase-1 (SOD-1) [25] and SOD-2 [28], that contribute to antioxidant defense by catalyzing the dismutation of superoxide anions [34], were decreased in hypertensive SHRSP5/Dmcr rats fed the HFC diet. The decrease in SOD-2 expression induced by HFC feeding was not observed in normotensive WKY and hypertensive SHR strains [28]. This could suggest that an increase in oxidative stress and a lower antioxidative capacity may trigger a more severe inflammatory response and liver damage in hypertensive rat strains following HFC feeding, compared with normotensive strains.

4. The role of cholesterol in the development of hypertension-associated NASH

As previously stated, dietary cholesterol intake is considered a risk factor for NAFLD/NASH. The liver is a crucial organ implicated in the regulation of cholesterol metabolism, including the synthesis and secretion of cholesterol, as well as the synthesis of BAs from cholesterol (a major pathway for hepatic cholesterol catabolism) and BA detoxification [35]. Disturbed cholesterol homeostasis in the liver is thought to be associated with the pathogenesis of NAFLD/NASH [35]. Our study showed that the HFC diet increased serum and hepatic levels of TC in the hypertensive SHR and SHRSP5/Dmcr strains, as well as the normotensive WKY strain [28]. It is worth noting that the increase in hepatic TC levels in the hypertensive rats was significantly lower than those in the normotensive WKY strain. Therefore, we postulated that more cholesterol was consumed for the synthesis of BAs in the livers of the hypertensive rats. In addition, serum TC levels in the hypertensive strains fed the control diet were markedly lower compared with those of the normotensive WKY strain, suggesting that the dysregulation of cholesterol metabolism may play an important role in the progression of hypertension-associated NASH.

In order to investigate the kinetics of cholesterol during the development of HFC-induced NASH in our hypertensive SHRSP5/Dmcr rat model, we evaluated the expression of proteins involved in de novo cholesterol synthesis, cholesterol uptake from bloodstream in the form of LDL, cholesterol secretion into blood in the form of very-low-density lipoprotein, and BA synthesis and detoxification [36].

4.1. De novo cholesterol synthesis and its uptake from blood

Excessive intake of cholesterol may suppress de novo cholesterol synthesis via a feedback mechanism dependent on the transcriptional factor sterol regulator element-binding protein 2 (SREBP-2) [35]. SREBP-2 resides in the endoplasmic reticulum and remains there when cholesterol is abundant in hepatocytes; however, SREBP-2 is activated in response to low levels of cholesterol and translocated to the nucleus, where it triggers the expression of various genes, including low-density lipoprotein receptor (LDLR) and 3-hydroxy-3-methylglutaryl coenzyme A reductase (HMGCR). HMGCR is the rate-limiting enzyme for cholesterol biosynthesis. Our study showed that HMGCR was downregulated in the livers of SHRSP5/Dmcr rats during consumption of the HFC diet (2, 8, and 14 weeks), although SREBP-2 expression remained unchanged [36]. It was proposed that additional signaling, except SREBP-2, may be required for cholesterol synthesis in our rat model. The HFC diet decreased the expression of LDLR and LDLR-related protein 1, which are required for clearing cholesterol-contained lipoproteins from the blood by the liver [37]. Therefore, excessive intake of dietary cholesterol led to accumulation in the liver and consequently resulted in suppression of cholesterol synthesis and uptake.

4.2. BA synthesis and excretion

There are two major pathways of BA synthesis. The classic pathway is initiated by cholesterol 7 alpha-hydroxylase (CYP7A1), the rate-limiting enzyme, followed by the catalytic action of sterol 12 alpha-hydroxylase (CYP8B1) [38]. On the other hand, the initial step in the alternative (acidic) pathway is catalyzed by sterol 27-hydroxylase (CYP27A1), followed by oxysterol 7alpha-hydroxylase (CYP7B1). The major primary BAs, cholic acid (CA) and chenodeoxycholic acid (CDCA), are produced from cholesterol in the liver, while the secondary BAs, lithocholic acid (LCA) and deoxycholic acid (DCA), are generated from CDCA and CA in the intestines, respectively. After synthesis, conjugation of Bas is required for effective transport and detoxification [39]. BAs are conjugated with amino acids (taurine or glycine) or sulfate, mediated by BA coenzyme A synthase and BA amino acid transferase, and sulfotransferase (SULT2A1), respectively. Some BAs are glucuronidated by UDP-glucuronosyl N-transferases (UGT1A1, 2B4, and 2B7). Amino acid-conjugated BAs are excreted from the liver into the bile canaliculi via the bile salt export pump (BSEP), an ATP-binding cassette (ABC) transporter protein located in the canalicular membrane of hepatocytes [40]. Multidrug-resistant protein 2 (MRP2) is another ABC transporter implicated in the transport of sulfated or glucuronidated BAs to bile, while MRP3, located in the basolateral membrane of hepatocyte, is responsible for the transport of BAs from the liver to the blood. In addition, bile acid-activated nuclear receptors (a group of transcriptional factors), such as farnesoid X receptor (FXR), pregnane X receptor (PXR), and constitutive androstane receptor (CAR), are implicated in the regulation of BA metabolism, including synthesis, transport, and detoxification [39]. Several studies have reported that activation of FXR, PXR, and CAR inhibits transcription of the CYP7A1 gene in hepatocytes, and therefore suppress BA synthesis [41–43]. Activation of FXR and PXR also induces expression of the BA transporter proteins, BSEP and MRP2 [44–46].

Increased levels of hepatic BA were observed in NASH patients and were correlated with inflammation and fibrosis in the liver [47]. In our SHRSP5/Dmcr model, the HFC diet increased hepatic levels of CYP7A1 but decreased levels of CYP8B1, while CYP27A1 was downregulated and CYP7B1 was upregulated [36]. We used ultra-performance liquid chromatography–tandem mass spectrometry (UPLC-MS/MS) to further determine the hepatic levels of 21 types of BA in rats fed the HFC or control diet [48]. The HFC diet significantly increased total BA levels in the liver at 2 weeks, but decreased it at 8 weeks. We also investigated the composition of the total BA in the rats' livers. In the total BA pool, the relative proportions of CDCA species, which are hydrophobic and show high cytotoxicity [49], were markedly elevated at 8 and 14 weeks, whereas hydrophilic CA species, with lower toxicity, were significantly decreased at 14 weeks. The ratio of total CA to CDCA was prominently reduced by HFC feeding at 8 and 14 weeks. Most BAs (about 90% of the total) in the livers of rats fed the control diet were taurine-conjugated. In contrast, glycine-conjugated BAs were predominant in HFC-fed rats. In addition, canalicular transporters, BSEP and MRP2, were reduced in the livers of the rats during HFC feeding (2, 8, and 14 weeks), whereas MRP3, the basolateral transporter, was significantly increased at 8 and 14 weeks [36]. Therefore, the accumulation of total BAs in the rats' liver at 2 weeks of HFC feeding may have resulted from suppressed BA excretion to the bile duct, mediated by BSEP and MRP2 transporter proteins. Meanwhile, the decrease in total BA levels in the liver at 8 weeks may have been triggered by an increase in MRP3-mediated BA excretion to the blood. Furthermore, we demonstrated that the ratio of CA to CDCA was negatively correlated with liver injury (macrovesicular steatosis, serum ALT levels, and fibrotic area), whereas total glycol-BA/total tauro-BA was positively correlated. Therefore, the accumulation of BAs at 2 weeks of HFC-feeding, led by dysregulated BA synthesis and excretion, may trigger liver damage during the initial stages of NAFLD/NASH. Furthermore, a decrease in nuclear FXR, PXR, and CAR was observed in the livers of rats following HFC feeding. The downregulation of these nuclear receptors may be responsible for the increase in CYP7A1, as well as the decrease in BSEP and MRP2.

4.3. BA detoxification

Toxic BA accumulation in the liver induces hepatocyte injury, and BA hydrophobicity is correlated with cytotoxicity [12]. The order of BA hydrophobicity was reported to be CA < CDCA < DCA < LCA [12]. Hydrophobic BAs are potent inflammatory agents, whereas the hydrophilic BAs are anti-inflammatory [38]. Hydrophobic BAs stimulate ROS generation in hepatic mitochondria and lead to oxidative stress, hepatocyte apoptosis, and subsequent liver damage [50, 51]. BAs with detergent properties may also induce damage in hepatocyte membranes by binding to membrane components and disrupting the integrity of the plasma membrane [12, 52].

BA metabolism is tightly regulated to prevent the retention of excessive BAs in the liver [12]. Sulfation and glucuronidation of BAs, catalyzed by SULT2A1 and UGT, respectively, are major detoxification pathways of Bas [53, 54]. These reactions increase the solubility of BAs, enhance their fecal and urinary excretion, and reduce their toxicity. In addition, the nuclear receptors, PXR and CAR, protect hepatocytes from BA toxicity by regulating the transcription of genes involved in BA detoxification, including SULT and UGT [55, 56]. Our study showed that the HFC diet impaired BA detoxification by inducing the downregulation of PXR and CAR and further suppressing SULT2A1-catalyzed sulfation and UGT-catalyzed glucuronidation in the hypertensive SHRSP5/Dmcr rats [36].

5. CYP7A1

Our previous study showed that dysregulated expression of enzymes involved in BA synthesis led to the accumulation of BA in the livers of SHRSP5/Dmcr rats fed an HFC diet [36]. We further investigate the role of CYP7A1 in the pathogenesis of hypertension-associated NASH, and evaluated its hepatic levels in hypertensive SHR and SHRSP5/Dmcr rats, and the normotensive WKY strain [28]. Constitutive CYP7A1 levels were markedly higher (over 300-fold) in the hypertensive strains compared with those in the normotensive WKY strain. Upregulation of CYP7A1 may result in an excessive accumulation of toxic BAs, such as hydrophobic BAs, which may lead to oxidative stress and liver damage. In addition, Kamisako et al. showed that the Nrf2 pathway may regulate the expression of genes associated with BA synthesis and fatty acid metabolism, including CYP7A1 [57]. Our study showed increased activation of Nrf2 signaling in the livers of hypertensive rats fed a control diet compared with the normotensive WKY, which might be the responsible for the overexpression of CYP7A1 in the hypertensive strains [28].

6. Gender differences in NASH development

The prevalence and severity of human NAFLD/NASH varies with gender and age [58]. Yatsuji et al. studied 193 Japanese patients with NASH (86 women and 107 men) and showed a predominance of the disease in women over 50 years old, yet a greater prevalence in men aged 30–40 years [59]. Williams et al. reported that NAFLD patients were more likely to be male, older, and hypertensive [60]. The incidence of NAFLD/NASH is higher in men than premenopausal women (less than 50 years of age), while this immediately increases in women after menopause. Therefore, sex hormones such as estradiol may influence gender differences in NASH. In our study, we regarded female SHRSP5/Dmcr rats aged 12–24 weeks to correspond to the menopausal age in women. We also found female rats were less susceptible to HFC diet-induced liver damage compared with males [61]. Hence, our rat model may be useful for studies into gender differences in HFC-induced NASH. In order to investigate the related mechanisms, mature female and male SHRSP5/Dmcr rats (10 weeks old) were fed either an HFC or control diet for 2, 8, and 14 weeks. The severity of hepatic fibrosis was markedly lower in the female rats compared with the males. Although HFC feeding significantly reduced serum estradiol levels in female rats at 2 weeks, these levels were still much higher in females compared with males during HFC feeding, suggesting that this female hormone may contribute to the gender difference in NASH. In addition, only minor gender differences were noted in the expression of CYP7A1, CYP8B1, CYP27A1, and CYP7B1, the enzymes involved in BA synthesis, as well as MRP3 and BSEP, the proteins associated with BA transport. On the other hand, the enzymes implicated in BA detoxification, UGT and SULT2A1, as well as the nuclear receptors, CAR and PXR, were significantly suppressed in the male rats fed the HFC diet, whereas expression of these proteins was only slightly changed in females following HFC feeding. Since estradiol, which markedly decreases in women after menopause, may stabilize CAR and PXR proteins [61, 62], these results suggested a stronger capacity of BA detoxification associated with higher estradiol levels may be responsible for the resistance to HFC-induced liver damage and hepatic fibrosis in female rats compared with males.

7. Treatment of NAFLD/NASH

NAFLD/NASH is related to poor lifestyle, including unhealthy diet habit and lack of exercise, which may, in turn, lead to excessive weight gain. Therefore, dietary intervention and exercise, targeted at weight loss, are the primary therapies for obesity-related NAFLD/NASH [63]. Vilar-Gomezet al. evaluated the effect of weight loss through lifestyle modifications on the improvement of NASH-related histologic features [64]. The study included 293 patients with NASH who followed a recommended lifestyle over 52 weeks to reduce body weight, including a low-fat, hypocaloric diet (750 kcal per day) and walking (200 min per week). Among these patients, 30% lost ≥5% of their weight at 52 weeks, 25% showed resolution of steatohepatitis, and 47% showed reduced nonalcoholic fatty liver disease activity score (NAS). This study also reported that the extent of weight loss was associated with histologic improvement. A higher proportion of patients with ≥5% weight loss had NASH resolution compared with those with ≤5% weight loss. Furthermore, 45% of patients with ≥10% weight loss showed regression of hepatic fibrosis.

Although NAFLD/NASH is closely linked with obesity and diabetes, it may also occur in the absence of these diseases [65]. As described before, the hypertensive SHRSP5/Dmcr rat represents a good model of NAFLD/NASH without obesity and diabetes [20]. We used this model to investigate the efficacy of dietary intervention for improving HFC-induced NASH [66]. Rats were fed an HFC diet for 2 weeks (before the appearance of hepatic fibrosis) or 8 weeks (after the appearance of fibrosis), then subsequently fed a control diet for 6 or 12 weeks. We found that dietary intervention prior to the appearance of fibrosis markedly improved steatosis and suppressed the HFC-induced increase in serum AST, ALT, and TC. On the other hand, dietary intervention after the appearance of fibrosis was unable to suppress the increase in serum ALT and hepatic TC. Although the dietary intervention (in both cases) reset the increased expression of fibrosis-relative proteins, TGF-β1 and α-SMA, it only slightly reduced the fibrotic area compared with continuous HFC feeding. Taken together, dietary intervention was able to completely or partially improve steatosis, inflammation, and cholesterol accumulation in the livers of rats fed an HFC diet, although this was not enough to improve hepatic fibrosis.

In addition, several pharmacological agents use in the treatment of NASH, including vitamin E and pioglitazone, have been tested [67, 68]. Oxidative stress and insulin resistance are considered as key factors implicated in the progression of NASH, and are, therefore, attractive targets for the treatment of NASH [69]. Sanyal et al. tested the efficacy of vitamin E, a lipid-soluble antioxidant, and pioglitazone, an insulin sensitizer, in NASH patients without diabetes [69]. The 247 patients included in this study received 800 IU vitamin E (84 subjects), 30 mg pioglitazone (80 subjects), or placebo (83 subjects) daily for 96 weeks. Both vitamin E and pioglitazone were associated with improvements in hepatic steatosis and lobular inflammation, as well as a reduction of serum AST and ALT, compared with the placebo. However, neither drug had a significant effect on hepatic fibrosis. In conclusion, lifestyle intervention (controlled dietary intake as well as exercise) may be the first choice for NAFLD/NASH treatment and should be optimized, while pharmacological management can be used as an auxiliary method, and should be further tested in large studies with long-term outcomes.

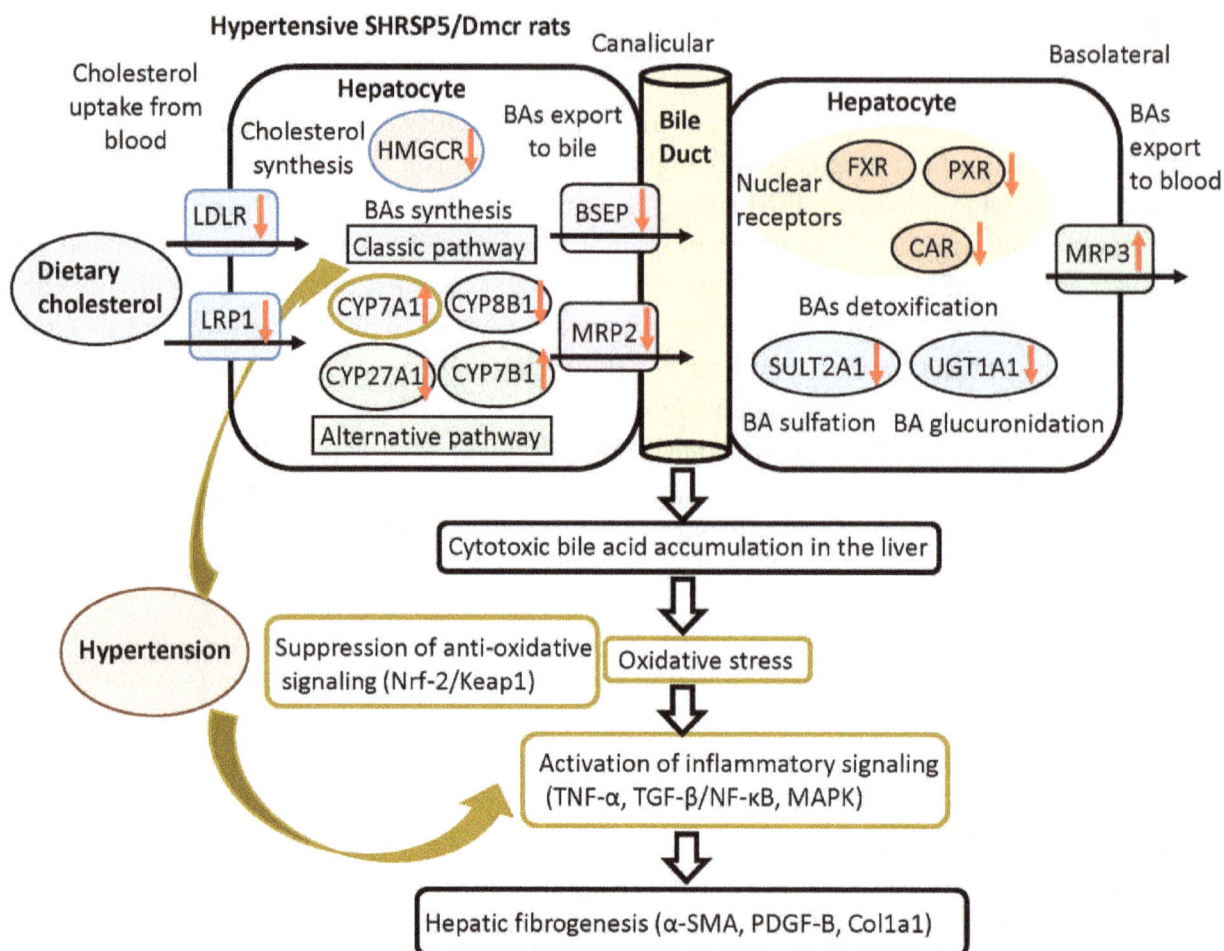

Figure 1. Possible mechanism underlying pathogenesis of HFC diet-induced fibrotic steatohepatitis in hypertensive SHRSP5/Dmcr rats [25, 35, 47]. In response to cholesterol accumulation in the liver triggered by HFC feeding, de novo cholesterol synthesis and its uptake were suppressed, indicated by a reduction in HMGCR, as well as LDLR and LPR1. The HFC diet induced dysregulated BA synthesis (upregulated CYP7A1 and CYP7B1, as well as downregulated CYP8B1 and CYP27A1) and export (downregulated BSEP and MRP2, as well as upregulated MRP3), and led to BA accumulation in hepatocytes. In addition, the HFC diet suppressed BA detoxification by decreasing the expression of nuclear receptors (PXR and CAR), and further downregulating SULT2A1 and UGT1A1, BA detoxification enzymes. Furthermore, cytotoxic BA accumulation in hepatocytes-induced oxidative stress, which activated inflammatory signaling (TNF-α, TGF-β/NF-κB, MAPK) and resulted in hepatitis. Hepatic inflammation-induced upregulation of fibrosis-related genes (α-SMA, PDGF-β, Col1a1) and led to hepatic fibrosis. Additionally, hypertension enhanced the deterioration of HFC-induced fibrotic steatohepatitis by upregulating CYP7A1, further leading to BA accumulation in hepatocytes and increased oxidative stress. On the other hand, hypertension induced the suppression of anti-oxidative signaling (Nrf-2/Keap1) following HFC feeding. Therefore, elevated oxidative stress and suppressed anti-oxidative capacity triggered a more severe inflammatory response in the hypertensive rats fed an HFC diet, as indicated by increased activation of inflammatory signaling (TNF-α, TGF-β/NF-κB, MAPK). BA, bile acid; HMGCR, 3-hydroxy 3-methyl-glutaryl-coenzyme A reductase; LDLR, low density lipoprotein receptor; LRP1, LDLR-related protein 1; CYP7A1, cholesterol 7α-hydroxylase; CYP8B1, sterol 12α-hydroxylase; CYP27A1, sterol 27-hydroxylase; CYP7B1, oxysterol 7α-hydroxylase; BSEP, bile salt export pump; MRP2, multidrug resistance-associated protein 2; MRP3, multidrug resistance-associated protein 3; FXR, farnesoid X receptor; PXR, pregnane X receptor; CAR, constitutive adrostane receptor; SULT2A1, sulfotransferase 2A1; UGT1A1, UDP-glucoronosyltransferase 1A1; TNF-α, tumor necrosis factor-α; TGF-β, transforming growth factor; NF-κB, nuclear factor kappa B; MAPK, mitogen-activated protein kinase; α-SMA, α-smooth muscle actin; PDGF-B, platelet-derived growth factor subunit B; Col1a1, alpha 1 type 1 collagen; Nrf-2, nuclear factor erythroid 2-related factor 2; Kea 1, Kelch-like ECH-associated rotein 1.

8. Conclusions

In our previous study, we established a novel model of fibrotic steatohepatitis by feeding hypertensive SHRSP5/Dmcr rats an HFC diet. Histological features resembling human NASH were observed in the rats, suggesting that this model is useful for studying hypertension-associated NASH. We compared NASH development among hypertensive strains (SHRSP5/Dmcr and SHR) and the normotensive WKY strain, and showed that hypertension accelerates progression of HFC-induced NASH by elevating BA synthesis (CYP7A1), inducing increased activation of inflammatory signaling (MAPK and NF-κB), and suppressing signaling associated with antioxidant defense (Nrf2/Keap1). To elucidate the role of cholesterol in NASH development, we investigated the kinetics of cholesterol in this model, and found that the HFC diet induced dysregulation of BA synthesis and suppression of BA detoxification, therefore resulting in cytotoxic BA accumulation in hepatocytes, which further induced oxidative stress, followed by activation of signaling involved in hepatic inflammation and fibrosis (**Figure 1**). Sex differences in fibrogenesis were also observed in this model and were associated with a different sensitivity to BA toxicity. More sustained expression of nuclear receptors, CAR and PXR, and the enzymes involved in BA detoxification, UGT and SULT, contributed to the stronger resistance to HFC-induced liver damage in female rats compared with males. In conclusion, our studies demonstrate that dietary cholesterol may play a crucial role in the progression of NASH-associated hypertension and provide a basis for NAFLD/NASH treatment involving restriction of cholesterol intake.

Author details

Yuan Yuan[1], Hisao Naito[2] and Tamie Nakajima[1]*

*Address all correspondence to: tnasu23@med.nagoya-u.ac.jp

1 College of Life and Health Sciences, Chubu University, Kasugai, Japan

2 Department of Public Health, Fujita Health University School of Medicine, Toyoake, Japan

References

[1] Lecerf JM, de Lorgeril M. Dietary cholesterol: From physiology to cardiovascular risk. The British Journal of Nutrition. 2011;**106**(1):6-14

[2] Lajous M, Bijon A, Fagherazzi G, Balkau B, Boutron-Ruault MC, Clavel-Chapelon F. Egg and cholesterol intake and incident type 2 diabetes among French women. The British Journal of Nutrition. 2015;**114**(10):1667-1673

[3] Rouen PA, Wallace BR. The 2015-2020 dietary guidelines: Overview and implications for nursing ractice. Home Healthc Now. 2017;**35**(2):72-82

[4] Ostlund RE Jr. Phytosterols and cholesterol metabolism. Current Opinion in Lipidology. 2004;**15**(1):37-41

[5] Berger S, Raman G, Vishwanathan R, Jacques PF, Johnson EJ. Dietary cholesterol and cardiovascular disease: A systematic review and meta-analysis. The American Journal of Clinical Nutrition. 2015;**102**(2):276-294

[6] Bowman MP, Van Doren J, Taper LJ, Thye FW, Ritchey SJ. Effect of dietary fat and cholesterol on plasma lipids and lipoprotein fractions in normolipidemic men. The Journal of Nutrition. 1988;**118**(5):555-560

[7] Clifton PM, Kestin M, Abbey M, Drysdale M, Nestel PJ. Relationship between sensitivity to dietary fat and dietary cholesterol. Arteriosclerosis. 1990;**10**(3):394-401

[8] Ginsberg HN, Karmally W, Siddiqui M, Holleran S, Tall AR, Blaner WS, et al. Increases in dietary cholesterol are associated with modest increases in both LDL and HDL cholesterol in healthy young women. Arteriosclerosis, Thrombosis, and Vascular Biology. 1995;**15**(2):169-178

[9] Subramanian S, Goodspeed L, Wang S, Kim J, Zeng L, Ioannou GN, et al. Dietary cholesterol exacerbates hepatic steatosis and inflammation in obese LDL receptor-deficient mice. Journal of Lipid Research. 2011;**52**(9):1626-1635

[10] Wouters K, van Gorp PJ, Bieghs V, Gijbels MJ, Duimel H, Lutjohann D, et al. Dietary cholesterol, rather than liver steatosis, leads to hepatic inflammation in hyperlipidemic mouse models of nonalcoholic steatohepatitis. Hepatology. 2008;**48**(2):474-486

[11] Takahashi Y, Fukusato T. Histopathology of nonalcoholic fatty liver disease/nonalcoholic steatohepatitis. World Journal of Gastroenterology. 2014;**20**(42):15539-15548

[12] Perez MJ, Briz O. Bile-acid-induced cell injury and protection. World Journal of Gastroenterology. 2009;**15**(14):1677-1689

[13] Li S, Zeng XY, Zhou X, Wang H, Jo E, Robinson SR, et al. Dietary cholesterol induces hepatic inflammation and blunts mitochondrial function in the liver of high-fat-fed mice. The Journal of Nutritional Biochemistry. 2016;**27**:96-103

[14] Marchesini G, Brizi M, Bianchi G, Tomassetti S, Bugianesi E, Lenzi M, et al. Nonalcoholic fatty liver disease: A feature of the metabolic syndrome. Diabetes. 2001;**50**(8):1844-1850

[15] Angulo P. GI epidemiology: Nonalcoholic fatty liver disease. Alimentary Pharmacology & Therapeutics. 2007;**25**(8):883-889

[16] Donati G, Stagni B, Piscaglia F, Venturoli N, Morselli-Labate AM, Rasciti L, et al. Increased prevalence of fatty liver in arterial hypertensive patients with normal liver enzymes: Role of insulin resistance. Gut. 2004;**53**(7):1020-1023

[17] Wang Y, Zeng Y, Lin C, Chen Z. Hypertension and non-alcoholic fatty liver disease proven by transient elastography. Hepatology Research. 2016;**46**(13):1304-1310

[18] Brookes MJ, Cooper BT. Hypertension and fatty liver: Guilty by association? Journal of Human Hypertension. 2007;**21**(4):264-270

[19] Ikuta T, Kanno K, Arihiro K, Matsuda S, Kishikawa N, Fujita K, et al. Spontaneously hypertensive rats develop pronounced hepatic steatosis induced by choline-deficient diet: Evidence for hypertension as a potential enhancer in non-alcoholic steatohepatitis. Hepatology Research. 2012;**42**(3):310-320

[20] Kitamori K, Naito H, Tamada H, Kobayashi M, Miyazawa D, Yasui Y, et al. Development of novel rat model for high-fat and high-cholesterol diet-induced steatohepatitis and severe fibrosis progression in SHRSP5/Dmcr. Environmental Health and Preventive Medicine. 2012;**17**(3):173-182

[21] Matsuzawa N, Takamura T, Kurita S, Misu H, Ota T, Ando H, et al. Lipid-induced oxidative stress causes steatohepatitis in mice fed an atherogenic diet. Hepatology. 2007;**46**(5):1392-1403

[22] Yamori Y. Selection of arteriolipidosis-prone rats (ALR) [proceedings]. Japanese Heart Journal. 1977;**18**(4):602-603

[23] Ogata J, Fujishima M, Tamaki K, Nakatomi Y, Ishitsuka T, Omae T. Stroke-prone spontaneously hypertensive rats as an experimental model of malignant hypertension. A pathological study. Virchows Archiv. A, Pathological Anatomy and Histology. 1982;**394**(3):185-194

[24] Matteoni CA, Younossi ZM, Gramlich T, Boparai N, Liu YC, McCullough AJ. Nonalcoholic fatty liver disease: A spectrum of clinical and pathological severity. Gastroenterology. 1999;**116**(6):1413-1419

[25] Moriya T, Kitamori K, Naito H, Yanagiba Y, Ito Y, Yamagishi N, et al. Simultaneous changes in high-fat and high-cholesterol diet-induced steatohepatitis and severe fibrosis and those underlying molecular mechanisms in novel SHRSP5/Dmcr rat. Environmental Health and Preventive Medicine. 2012;**17**(6):444-456

[26] Crespo J, Cayon A, Fernandez-Gil P, Hernandez-Guerra M, Mayorga M, Dominguez-Diez A, et al. Gene expression of tumor necrosis factor alpha and TNF-receptors, p55 and p75, in nonalcoholic steatohepatitis patients. Hepatology. 2001;**34**(6):1158-1163

[27] Koyama Y, Brenner DA. Liver inflammation and fibrosis. The Journal of Clinical Investigation. 2017;**127**(1):55-64

[28] Yuan Y, Naito H, Jia X, Kitamori K, Nakajima T. Combination of hypertension along with a high fat and cholesterol diet induces severe hepatic inflammation in rats via a signaling network comprising NF-kappaB, MAPK, and Nrf2 pathways. Nutrients. 2017;**9**(9). DOI: 10.3390/nu9091018

[29] Okamoto K, Aoki K. Development of a strain of spontaneously hypertensive rats. Japanese Circulation Journal. 1963;**27**:282-293

[30] Reuter S, Gupta SC, Chaturvedi MM, Aggarwal BB. Oxidative stress, inflammation, and cancer: How are they linked? Free Radical Biology & Medicine. 2010;**49**(11):1603-1616

[31] Chalasani N, Deeg MA, Crabb DW. Systemic levels of lipid peroxidation and its metabolic and dietary correlates in patients with nonalcoholic steatohepatitis. The American Journal of Gastroenterology. 2004;**99**(8):1497-1502

[32] Kojima H, Sakurai S, Uemura M, Fukui H, Morimoto H, Tamagawa Y. Mitochondrial abnormality and oxidative stress in nonalcoholic steatohepatitis. Alcoholism, Clinical and Experimental Research. 2007;**31**(1 Suppl):S61-S66

[33] Sajadimajd S, Khazaei M. Oxidative stress and cancer: The role of Nrf2. Current Cancer Drug Targets. 2017. DOI: 10.2174/1568009617666171002144228

[34] Birben E, Sahiner UM, Sackesen C, Erzurum S, Kalayci O. Oxidative stress and antioxidant defense. World Allergy Organization Journal. 2012;**5**(1):9-19

[35] Arguello G, Balboa E, Arrese M, Zanlungo S. Recent insights on the role of cholesterol in non-alcoholic fatty liver disease. Biochimica et Biophysica Acta. 2015;**1852**(9): 1765-1778

[36] Jia X, Naito H, Yetti H, Tamada H, Kitamori K, Hayashi Y, et al. Dysregulated bile acid synthesis, metabolism and excretion in a high fat-cholesterol diet-induced fibrotic steatohepatitis in rats. Digestive Diseases and Sciences. 2013;**58**(8):2212-2222

[37] van de Sluis B, Wijers M, Herz J. News on the molecular regulation and function of hepatic low-density lipoprotein receptor and LDLR-related protein 1. Current Opinion in Lipidology. 2017;**28**(3):241-247

[38] Chiang JY. Bile acid metabolism and signaling. Comprehensive Physiology. 2013;**3**(3): 1191-1212

[39] Li T, Chiang JY. Nuclear receptors in bile acid metabolism. Drug Metabolism Reviews. 2013;**45**(1):145-155

[40] Alrefai WA, Gill RK. Bile acid transporters: Structure, function, regulation and pathophysiological implications. Pharmaceutical Research. 2007;**24**(10):1803-1823

[41] Goodwin B, Jones SA, Price RR, Watson MA, McKee DD, Moore LB, et al. A regulatory cascade of the nuclear receptors FXR, SHP-1, and LRH-1 represses bile acid biosynthesis. Molecular Cell. 2000;**6**(3):517-526

[42] Li T, Chiang JY. Mechanism of rifampicin and pregnane X receptor inhibition of human cholesterol 7 alpha-hydroxylase gene transcription. American Journal of Physiology. Gastrointestinal and Liver Physiology. 2005;**288**(1):G74-G84

[43] Miao J, Fang S, Bae Y, Kemper JK. Functional inhibitory cross-talk between constitutive and rostane receptor and hepatic nuclear factor-4 in hepatic lipid/glucose metabolism is mediated by competition for binding to the DR1 motif and to the common coactivators, GRIP-1 and PGC-1alpha. The Journal of Biological Chemistry. 2006;**281**(21):14537-14546

[44] Ananthanarayanan M, Balasubramanian N, Makishima M, Mangelsdorf DJ, Suchy FJ. Human bile salt export pump promoter is transactivated by the farnesoid X receptor/ bile acid receptor. The Journal of Biological Chemistry. 2001;**276**(31):28857-28865

[45] Kast HR, Goodwin B, Tarr PT, Jones SA, Anisfeld AM, Stoltz CM, et al. Regulation of multidrug resistance-associated protein 2 (ABCC2) by the nuclear receptors pregnane X receptor, farnesoid X-activated receptor, and constitutive androstane receptor. The Journal of Biological Chemistry. 2002;**277**(4):2908-2915

[46] Kliewer SA, Willson TM. Regulation of xenobiotic and bile acid metabolism by the nuclear pregnane X receptor. Journal of Lipid Research. 2002;**43**(3):359-364

[47] Aranha MM, Cortez-Pinto H, Costa A, da Silva IB, Camilo ME, de Moura MC, et al. Bile acid levels are increased in the liver of patients with steatohepatitis. European Journal of Gastroenterology & Hepatology. 2008;**20**(6):519-525

[48] Jia X, Suzuki Y, Naito H, Yetti H, Kitamori K, Hayashi Y, et al. A possible role of chenodeoxycholic acid and glycine-conjugated bile acids in fibrotic steatohepatitis in a dietary rat model. Digestive Diseases and Sciences. 2014;**59**(7):1490-1501

[49] Monte MJ, Marin JJ, Antelo A, Vazquez-Tato J. Bile acids: Chemistry, physiology, and pathophysiology. World Journal of Gastroenterology. 2009;**15**(7):804-816

[50] Sokol RJ, Devereaux M, Khandwala R, O'Brien K. Evidence for involvement of oxygen free radicals in bile acid toxicity to isolated rat hepatocytes. Hepatology. 1993;**17**(5):869-881

[51] Sokol RJ, Dahl R, Devereaux MW, Yerushalmi B, Kobak GE, Gumpricht E. Human hepatic mitochondria generate reactive oxygen species and undergo the permeability transition in response to hydrophobic bile acids. Journal of Pediatric Gastroenterology and Nutrition. 2005;**41**(2):235-243

[52] Schubert R, Schmidt KH. Structural changes in vesicle membranes and mixed micelles of various lipid compositions after binding of different bile salts. Biochemistry. 1988;**27**(24):8787-8794

[53] Alnouti Y. Bile acid sulfation: A pathway of bile acid elimination and detoxification. Toxicological Sciences. 2009;**108**(2):225-246

[54] Perreault M, Bialek A, Trottier J, Verreault M, Caron P, Milkiewicz P, et al. Role of glucuronidation for hepatic detoxification and urinary elimination of toxic bile acids during biliary obstruction. PLoS One. 2013;**8**(11):e80994

[55] Wagner M, Halilbasic E, Marschall HU, Zollner G, Fickert P, Langner C, et al. CAR and PXR agonists stimulate hepatic bile acid and bilirubin detoxification and elimination pathways in mice. Hepatology. 2005;**42**(2):420-430

[56] Guo GL, Lambert G, Negishi M, Ward JM, Brewer HB Jr, Kliewer SA, et al. Complementary roles of farnesoid X receptor, pregnane X receptor, and constitutive androstane receptor in protection against bile acid toxicity. The Journal of Biological Chemistry. 2003;**278**(46):45062-45071

[57] Kamisako T, Tanaka Y, Kishino Y, Ikeda T, Yamamoto K, Masuda S, et al. Role of Nrf2 in the alteration of cholesterol and bile acid metabolism-related gene expression by dietary cholesterol in high fat-fed mice. Journal of Clinical Biochemistry and Nutrition. 2014;**54**(2):90-94

[58] Pan JJ, Fallon MB. Gender and racial differences in nonalcoholic fatty liver disease. World Journal of Hepatology. 2014;**6**(5):274-283

[59] Yatsuji S, Hashimoto E, Tobari M, Tokushige K, Shiratori K. Influence of age and gender in Japanese patients with non-alcoholic steatohepatitis. Hepatology Research. 2007;**37**(12):1034-1043

[60] Williams CD, Stengel J, Asike MI, Torres DM, Shaw J, Contreras M, et al. Prevalence of nonalcoholic fatty liver disease and nonalcoholic steatohepatitis among a largely middle-aged population utilizing ultrasound and liver biopsy: A prospective study. Gastroenterology. 2011;**140**(1):124-131

[61] Yetti H, Naito H, Yuan Y, Jia X, Hayashi Y, Tamada H, et al. Bile acid detoxifying enzymes limit susceptibility to liver fibrosis in female SHRSP5/Dmcr rats fed with a high-fat-cholesterol diet. PLoS One. 2018;**13**(2):e0192863

[62] Rando G, Wahli W. Sex differences in nuclear receptor-regulated liver metabolic pathways. Biochimica et Biophysica Acta. 2011;**1812**(8):964-973

[63] Hannah WN Jr, Harrison SA. Lifestyle and dietary interventions in the management of nonalcoholic fatty liver disease. Digestive Diseases and Sciences. 2016;**61**(5):1365-1374

[64] Vilar-Gomez E, Martinez-Perez Y, Calzadilla-Bertot L, Torres-Gonzalez A, Gra-Oramas B, Gonzalez-Fabian L, et al. Weight loss through lifestyle modification significantly reduces features of nonalcoholic steatohepatitis. Gastroenterology. 2015;**149**(2):367-378 e5; quiz e14-5

[65] Wei JL, Leung JC, Loong TC, Wong GL, Yeung DK, Chan RS, et al. Prevalence and severity of nonalcoholic fatty liver disease in non-obese patients: A population study using proton-magnetic resonance spectroscopy. The American Journal of Gastroenterology. 2015;**110**(9):1306-1314; quiz 15

[66] Tamada H, Naito H, Kitamori K, Hayashi Y, Yamagishi N, Kato M, et al. Efficacy of dietary lipid control in healing high-fat and high-cholesterol diet-induced fibrotic steatohepatitis in rats. PLoS One. 2016;**11**(1):e0145939

[67] Barb D, Portillo-Sanchez P, Cusi K. Pharmacological management of nonalcoholic fatty liver disease. Metabolism. 2016;**65**(8):1183-1195

[68] Gitto S, Vitale G, Villa E, Andreone P. Treatment of nonalcoholic steatohepatitis in adults: Present and future. Gastroenterology Research and Practice. 2015;**2015**:732870

[69] Sanyal AJ, Chalasani N, Kowdley KV, McCullough A, Diehl AM, Bass NM, et al. Pioglitazone, vitamin E, or placebo for nonalcoholic steatohepatitis. The New England Journal of Medicine. 2010;**362**(18):1675-1685

10

Role of Membrane Cholesterol in Modulating Actin Architecture and Cellular Contractility

Barbara Hissa and Bruno Pontes

Abstract

Atherosclerosis is a chronic inflammatory process that initiates with accumulation of apolipoprotein B containing lipoproteins (LPs) in the subendothelium (intima), especially in areas where the laminar flow is disturbed. LP retention triggers an inflammatory response leading to activation of endothelial and vascular smooth muscle cells that culminates with recruitment of leukocytes. Atherosclerosis is the leading cause of vascular disease worldwide being its major clinical manifestations ischemic heart disease, ischemic stroke, and peripheral arterial disease. Even though a lot has been done to unravel the role of turbulent flow and mechanotransduction for atherosclerosis development, little is known about the role of plasma membrane (PM) cholesterol in this process. This chapter is going to be focused on exploring what has been done so far to decipher the role of PM cholesterol in regulating actin architecture, cellular mechanical properties, and cellular contractility in muscle and nonmuscle cells.

Keywords: cholesterol, actin, myosin, cytoskeleton, contractility

1. Introduction

The role that cholesterol plays in cardiovascular diseases is widely known and studied [1]. However, less appreciated is the importance that cholesterol has in orchestrating other important cellular functions, such as cellular contractility and cytoskeleton organization. Cellular contractility is the ability of a cell to exert mechanical work on a substrate or on a neighboring cell due to actomyosin cytoskeleton enzymatic activity [2]. In muscle and nonmuscle cells, most of the cholesterol content is localized at the plasma membrane [3] where it can partition into microdomains called lipid rafts. Lipid rafts are highly dynamic regions of the plasma membrane that contain sphingolipids and cholesterol and are responsible for compartmentalizing and regulating several intracellular signaling events [4–6]. One way of studying the importance of cholesterol for a specific cellular function is to decrease its concentration by either interfering directly with its synthesis, through the mevalonate pathway, or by chelating the molecule directly through the use of cyclodextrins [7]. However, depending on how one does the cholesterol depletion, the effects on cellular contractility can be opposite. Differences in muscle versus nonmuscle cell contractile behavior are observed upon cholesterol depletion using cyclodextrins. Muscle cells get impairment in their contractile machinery [8] whereas nonmuscle cells get more contractile [9]. This book chapter gives an overview about how cholesterol is organized at the plasma membrane and how its depletion changes cellular contractile properties.

2. Lipid rafts and membrane heterogeneity

Even though the Cell Theory started to be developed in the nineteenth century [10], it was not until the first quarter of the twentieth century that the idea of a membrane encompassing the cell was experimentally observed. In 1924, the Dutch physiologists Gorter and Grendel elegantly demonstrated, for the first time, the existence of a lipid bilayer surrounding red blood cells of various animals [11]. They isolated erythrocytes from humans and different mammals (rabbit, dog, guinea pig, sheep, and goat), extracted their lipids using acetone, and let those lipids spread on an air-water interface of a Langmuir-Adam apparatus. By knowing the number and area of the erythrocytes used in their experiment, they concluded that those cells were surrounded by a layer of lipids whose thickness was equivalent to two molecules [11], hence a lipid bilayer. The Gorter and Grendel model for cellular plasma membrane considered only the lipid nature of this cellular component and, because of that and due to other experimental and theoretical inaccuracies, it failed in explaining satisfactorily experimental results for membrane thickness [12], membrane tension [13], membrane electrical capacitance [14], and membrane permeability [15].

In order to explain those membrane properties, another model, called the paucimolecular model, was proposed by Danielli and coworkers in 1935 [12, 16, 17]. By examining the surface tension of a single drop of mackerel egg oil, Danielle and Harvey found that the value they measured was lower than the equivalent obtained for nonliving pure water-oil systems. They hypothesized that the difference observed for surface tension in living versus nonliving water-oil systems was due to the fact that the plasma membrane not only contained lipids but also proteins adsorbed in the lipid bilayer [16]. In the same year, Danielli and Davson [17] extended the paucimolecular model in order to explain permeability experiments. In that model, the layer of proteins adsorbed on top of a lipid film was able to discern size of molecules and charge of ions that were penetrating the membrane. This lipid film containing adsorbed proteins was considered to be relatively stable with mosaics consisting of practically impenetrable regions and hydrated areas where anions could move through [17].

For the next 30 years, the paucimolecular model was the most accepted one among the scientific community. However, with the advancement of microscopy techniques and structural studies, a new and more robust model, named the fluid mosaic model, was proposed in 1972 by Singer and Nicolson [18]. According to that model, integral transmembrane proteins are arranged in the plasma membrane of living cells such that the polar regions are facing the aqueous phase and the hydrophobic regions are embedded on a viscous phospholipid bilayer and those proteins are able to move freely on that two-dimensional, approximately homogeneous fluid "sea" of phospholipids [18]. One year later, in 1973, Bretscher published a Science paper in which he discusses overall membrane organization based on evidences collected from experiments performed in red blood cells [19]. According to that paper, the plasma membrane of mammalian cells was not as simple as depicted by the fluid mosaic model. Some of the integral proteins span the membrane and their glycosylation is responsible for locking them at the membrane impeding their migration to the cytoplasm. Another important contribution from this paper is that proteins not only interact with the outer layer of the plasma membrane but also with the inner layer, and membrane proteins are a subtype of cytoplasmic proteins that are not secreted [19]. In the same year, Yu and collaborators, also performing experiments in red blood cells, showed that when those cells are incubated with the nonionic detergent Triton X-100, there are some fractions of the cellular proteins that are resistant to the detergent extraction and seem to form oligomeric complexes with some of the lipid components, which were preferentially composed by nonglycosylated proteins and sphingolipids [20].

2.1. Lipid rafts

The idea of possible membrane microdomains started to be speculated in the early 1970s [20, 21] and experimentally demonstrated in 1982 by Karnovsky [22], who showed that there were multiple phases in the lipid environment of a membrane. One type of microdomain can be formed by cholesterol and sphingolipids [23]. These microdomains were already shown to be present in cell membranes [24]. In 1988, after several experimental demonstrations, Simons and van Meer called these microdomains as lipid rafts [25]. Thus, lipid rafts are defined as small, heterogeneous, and highly dynamic microdomains enriched in cholesterol, glycosphingolipids, and proteins that are much more organized than the surrounding lipid bilayer [26]. These membrane microdomains serve as organizing clusters capable of influencing several cellular processes such as membrane trafficking and neurotransmission [26].

The most striking difference between lipid rafts and the plasma membrane from which they are derived from is the lipid composition. Experiments have shown that rafts contain much more cholesterol than the surrounding bilayer [27, 28]. Cholesterol, therefore, works as a sort of "dynamic glue" that maintains the raft together [29], serving as a molecular spacer and filling the empty spaces between sphingolipids [30]. One of the main challenges when studying lipid rafts in living cells is their size. They are small microdomains ranging from 10 to 200 nm, below the classical diffraction limit of the optical microscope [28]. The first studies in the field considered methods to extract and separate rafts from the surrounding membrane. The procedure would take advantage of lipid raft resistance to nonionic detergents. When detergents are added to cells, the fluid membrane will dissolve while the lipid rafts may remain intact and could be extracted [31]; however, the validity of this methodology has been called into question due to ambiguities in the lipids and proteins obtained after extraction [32]. Other methods, based on synthetic membranes, were also used, however with many drawbacks. Firstly, synthetic membranes either lack or have lower protein concentration when compared to cell membranes [26]. Secondly, it is very difficult to simulate, in synthetic membranes, the membrane-cytoskeletal interactions that occur in cell membranes, although some recent studies have been able to overcome these limitations [33–35]. Finally, another problem includes the lack of natural asymmetry between the bilayer leaflets [36].

Although lipid rafts present sizes below the classical diffraction limit of the optical microscope, fluorescence microscopy has been extensively used in the field. For example, fluorophores conjugated to cholera-toxin B-subunit, which binds to the raft constituent ganglioside GM1, is used. Also, lipophilic membrane dyes (such as Laudran) that either partition between rafts and the surrounding membrane or change their fluorescent properties in response to membrane phase are used. Finally, lipid rafts can also be fluorescently labeled in cells after genetic expression of fluorescent fusion proteins [35].

Another methodology, which has been widely used in the study of lipid rafts, is the manipulation of cholesterol contents in membranes. Sequestration (using filipin, nystatin, or amphotericin), depletion and removal (using methyl-β-cyclodextrin, MβCD), or inhibition of cholesterol synthesis (using 3-hydroxy-3-methyl-glutaryl-coenzyme A, HMG-CoA, reductase inhibitors) are great examples of how cholesterol can be manipulated in lipid raft studies [26]. Several questions, however, have been raised against the effectiveness of the experimental design when disrupting lipid rafts. Acute methods of cholesterol depletion, which disrupt the rafts, can also disrupt another lipid, called PI(4,5)P2, which plays an important role in cytoskeletal regulation [37]. Thus, the loss of a particular cellular function after cholesterol depletion cannot necessarily be attributed only to raft disruption, since other processes are also being affected.

Despite these limitations, more sophisticated methods have been applied in order to fight against the problems of small size and dynamic nature of lipid rafts. These methods include single particle and molecule tracking using very sensitive CCD cameras together with total internal reflection microscopy. These combined techniques provide information of the diffusion coefficient of particles in the membrane and also reveal membrane corrals, barriers, and sites of confinement [38]. Finally, other optical techniques have been used to elucidate other features of lipid rafts: fluorescence correlation spectroscopy, to gain information of fluorophore mobility in the membrane [39]; fluorescence resonance energy transfer, to detect when fluorophores are in close proximity [40], and optical tweezers, to give information about the membrane mechanical parameters [8, 41]. In the future, it is expected that other super-resolution microscopy techniques, such as stimulated emission depletion microscopy [42] or various forms of structured illumination microscopy may overcome the problems imposed by the diffraction limit.

Apart from the different imaging methods, research over the last decades have demonstrated the existence of two types of rafts: (1) planar lipid rafts (also known as noncaveolar or glycolipid rafts) and caveolae. Planar rafts are known to be continuous with the plane of the plasma membrane (not invaginated) and contain flotillin proteins. Caveolae are flask shaped invaginations of the plasma membrane that contain caveolin proteins. Both types are enriched in cholesterol and sphingolipids. Flotillin and caveolins can either recruit or separate other molecules from lipid rafts and caveolae, respectively, thus playing an essential role in signal transduction [43].

2.2. Caveolae

Caveolae are plasma membrane invaginations with a diameter ranging from 60 to 80 nm and were first identified in the early 1950s by electron microscopy [44]. These invaginations are

expressed in various cell types such as smooth muscle, fibroblasts, endothelial cells and adipocytes, among several others. Their functions are diverse and include endocytosis, calcium signaling as well as regulation of various cell signaling pathways [45].

The major constituent of caveolae is caveolin1 [46], followed by two other isoforms: caveolin2 [47] and the muscle-specific caveolin3 [48]. All three caveolin proteins share a common topology with both their N and C terminal domains in the cytoplasm and a long hairpin transmembrane domain. All three types of caveolin are formed inside the cells, more precisely in the Golgi apparatus, as monomers [49]. However, as soon as they enter in the secretory pathway, they start to be structured as oligomers [50]. For caveolin1, for example, its exit from the Golgi apparatus is accelerated upon addition of cholesterol [49]. The oligomerization ability of caveolin1 is crucial for caveolae formation [51]. Caveolin2 has also been implicated in caveolae formation [52], and although caveolin1 null mouse shows a significant decrease in caveolae assembly, they are still present in the caveolin2 mouse [53]. In muscle, caveolin3 is crucial for caveolae formation. Mutations or loss of caveolin3 result in dystrophic phenotypes [54, 55].

Caveolin expression at the plasma membrane is not the only inducer of caveolae formation. Cholesterol extraction has been extensively shown to disrupt caveolae at the plasma membrane [46] since it is required for caveolin incorporation into raft domains at the plasma membrane, a critical event for caveolae formation [56].

Although caveolins and cholesterol were initially thought to be necessary and sufficient for caveolae formation, several studies have shown additional molecular players called cavins. This protein family has four different members already described: cavin-1 (also called PTRF) [57], cavin-2 (also called SDPR) [58], cavin-3 (also called SRBC) [59], and the muscle-specific cavin-4 (also called MURC) [60]. These four proteins are essential to caveolae formation and functions. Thus, caveolae formation is a highly complex and regulated cellular process. It has been estimated that ~150–200 caveolin monomers are necessary to associate with ~50–60 cavins in order to form a single caveola [61, 62]. Moreover, caveolae architecture was recently proposed to be a dodecahedron formed by cavins aligned with their vertices and also in the caveolin oligomers located at each of the pentagonal faces [61, 62].

As already mentioned, caveolae represent a subdomain of lipid rafts [43]. Confocal microscopy has shown that the distribution of GM1, a well characterized raft marker, do not merge with caveolin1 [63]. Another raft marker, flotillin, defines noncaveolar rafts and merges with GM1 [63]. Thus, rafts exhibit a heterogeneous distribution over the plasma membrane changing between caveolar (invaginated) and noncaveolar (planar) regions.

3. Actomyosin cytoskeleton: the contractile machinery of muscle and nonmuscle cells

The cytoskeleton constitutes a dynamic network of filaments that exists in the inner space of a cell. This network not only provides scaffolding but is also responsible for transporting organelles, generating and transducting mechanical forces. The cytoskeleton maintains cellular organization by linking together several cellular components in such a way that it mediates communication across the entire cell and, therefore, has a tremendous impact on cellular functions [64]. Three main filaments constitute the cytoskeleton, each one with its distinct protein composition and function: the microtubules, intermediate filaments, and microfilaments.

Microfilaments, also known as actin filaments, are ~7 nm in width. They are primarily composed of actin, the most abundant protein in cells. Actin filaments can create a huge number of arrays, such as bundles, two-dimensional networks, and three-dimensional gels. These different structural organizations are controlled by several actin-binding proteins and are found, for example, at the leading edge of a moving cell, particularly in filopodia and lamellipodia (**Figure 1B**), which causes the actin filaments to be the primary cytoskeletal component to drive cell motility [64]. Actin filaments also allow the cell to probe or sense its microenvironment. More stable networks of actin filaments, known as stress fibers, allow cells to brace against the underlying surface [65]. Thus, microfilaments can either be alone, as simple filaments, or together with the myosin filaments, which are part of the actomyosin contractile apparatus, in muscle and nonmuscle cells. Myosin filaments, associated with actin filaments, use ATP hydrolysis to exert forces against stress fibers during cytoskeletal contractility [65].

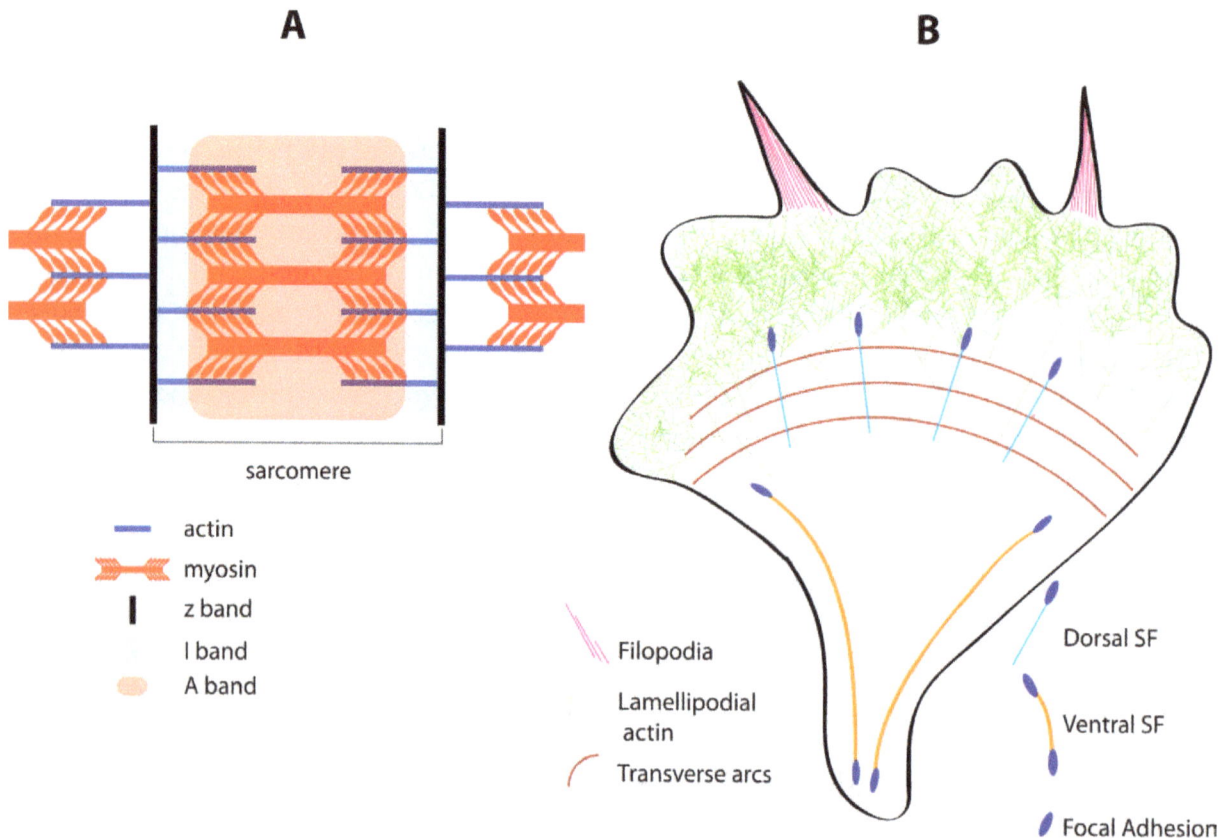

Figure 1. Actomyosin cytoskeleton schematic of striated muscle cell (A) and smooth muscle/nonmuscle cells. Striated muscle cells have the sarcomeric organization, which is shown in A and consists of actin and myosin filaments overlapping. Smooth muscle and nonmuscle cells (B) have different populations of actin stress-fibers that can be found in distinct parts of the cell. There are stress fibers that form filopodia (pink), lamellipodia (green), contractile transverse arcs (red), dorsal stress fibers (light-blue) and ventral stress fibers (orange) that terminate into one or two focal adhesions (navy-blue).

The actomyosin contractile machinery is relatively well conserved, despite some differences in organization and dynamics among different cell types. Actin filaments are polarized as barbed ends (fast-growing end) and pointed ends (slow-growing ends) and serve as scaffold for myosin filaments, which vary in size ranging from a few heads, in nonmuscle cells, to hundreds of heads in thick filaments of striated muscle cells. The myosin filaments drive the translocation of actin filaments toward their barbed ends. This event can trigger either the contraction or extension of two actin filaments [64].

The most well understood example of a contractile actomyosin apparatus is found in striated muscles and is called sarcomere. The sarcomeres are what give the striated muscles their appearance. It is known that a sarcomere is defined as a segment between two neighboring Z-lines. The Z-lines (from the German "Zwischenscheibe") are "dark" lines that appear in both extremities of a sarcomere (**Figure 1A**). They act as anchoring points for actin filaments. Surrounding two Z-lines, there are two regions called I-bands, regions of actin filaments that are not superimposed by myosin filaments (**Figure 1A**). Between the two I-bands is an A-band, which contains the entire length of myosin filaments and part of actin filaments that extend from I-bands (**Figure 1A**). The barbed ends of actin filaments are localized at the Z-line. The myosin filaments are segregated toward the pointed ends of actin filaments. Several other proteins are present and allow the stability of a sarcomere. The interaction between actin and myosin filaments in the A-band of a sarcomere is responsible for muscle contraction (**Figure 1A**) [64].

The contraction starts when a motor neuron releases acetylcholine, a neurotransmitter that binds to a postsynaptic nicotinic acetylcholine receptor on the muscle fiber, causing a change in receptor conformation and allowing an influx of sodium ions followed by postsynaptic action potential initiation. The action potential travels through T-tubules until it reaches the sarcoplasmic reticulum, where it activates voltage-gated L-type calcium channels. The initial inward flow of calcium from the L-type calcium channels activates ryanodine receptors, which releases a huge amount of calcium ions from the sarcoplasmic reticulum toward the cytoplasm of muscle cells. This mechanism is called calcium-induced calcium-release [64]. Inside muscle cells, the protein tropomyosin covers the myosin binding sites of actin filaments in the sarcomere. In order to allow contraction, tropomyosin must be moved from its original place. Initially, tropomyosin is attached to the actin filaments, covering myosin binding sites. When calcium ions enter in the muscle cell cytoplasm, they immediately bind to troponin-C and trigger a change in the structure of tropomyosin. This change in conformation forces tropomyosin to reveal the myosin-binding sites on actin filaments and allows myosin filaments to pull antiparallel actin filaments together. Muscle contraction ends when calcium ions are pumped back from the muscle cell cytoplasm into the sarcoplasmic reticulum, allowing the contractile machinery to relax [64].

The actomyosin cytoskeleton in nonmuscle and smooth muscle cells is organized in similar ways, both different from sarcomeres of striated muscles. Nonmuscle and smooth muscle cells use myosin to generate contractility during migration, cytokinesis, as well as cell-cell and cell-matrix junctions, for example [66]. Nonaligned actomyosin networks, with actin filaments and clusters of bipolar myosin filaments interacting with each other at their ends, represent the simplest contractile machinery in nonmuscle and smooth muscle cells, especially in cytoskeletal regions that do not have stress fibers [67, 68]. Smooth muscle and nonmuscle cells also contain more organized actomyosin bundles, such as transverse arcs, radial stress fibers, peripheral bundles, and ventral stress fibers (**Figure 1B**) [65]. Transverse stress fibers or arcs (**Figure 1B**) are formed after reorganization of lamellipodial actin filaments [69] during lamellipodium retraction [70]. This process is driven by myosin filaments, which become co-aligned with actin filaments and form stacks separated by alfa-actinin [68]. Radial stress fibers (**Figure 1B**), on the other hand, are anchored to focal adhesions in one end. Myosin molecules are recruited to the tips of focal adhesions, where nascent radial stress fibers start to form [71]. Contractility of the radial-transverse-stress fiber network leads to the formation of ventral stress fibers (**Figure 1B**) attached to focal adhesions on both ends [72]. Also, actomyosin filaments from nonmuscle and smooth muscle cells are highly dynamic when compared to striated muscle cells. Both actin and myosin can frequently undergo turnover or cycles of assembly/disassembly [73, 74].

Based on all above-described features, the most striking differences between stress fibers and sarcomeres are: (1) the molecular composition is cell-specific [75], (2) stress fiber contraction is regulated by phosphorylation of myosin light chain (pMLC) (see pMLC regulation in Section 4), while sarcomere contraction is regulated by troponin switching [76], (3) stress fibers are approximately one order of magnitude thinner, less organized (with different directions and lengths) and with less coordinated contraction when compared to sarcomeres [75], (4) the magnitude of the force they produce is different, while the stress fiber contractile forces come from individual cells and are applied, through focal adhesions, to the extracellular environment in which these cells are located [77], the sarcomeres from striated muscles can transmit contractile forces over macroscopic lengths. Finally, (5) striated muscles can rapidly contract and relax based on action potentials and Ca^{2+} release [64, 78] while stress fibers from smooth muscle and nonmuscle cells respond much slower and do not depend solely on electrical pulses [78].

While striated muscle cells present different actomyosin organization and features when compared to nonmuscle and smooth muscle cells, these three cell types share a common actomyosin structure: the actin cortex, also known as cell cortex or actomyosin cortex. This is a thin and highly disordered contractile actomyosin network underling the plasma membrane of cells [79]. It was first discovered in large cells, like amoeba and animal eggs and subsequently, extrapolated to all animal cells [79]. Non-adherent cells [80], cells during mitosis [81], or cells performing amoeboid-like migration [82] present a well distributed and uniform actin cortex. Cells spread over flat surfaces, although more difficult to be observed, also present a cortical layer of actomyosin, as shown by electron microscopy [83]. The actomyosin appears as an isotropic network parallel (and some perpendicular) to the plasma membrane with a width of 20–250 nm [83, 84]. Numerous actin-binding proteins have already been described to be part of the actin cortex [84], most of them are classical actin-binding proteins; however, little is known about how actin cortex is assembled.

The actin cortex plays a major role in cell mechanics as the main determinant of cell surface tension [79]. Biophysical methods like micropipette aspiration and membrane tether pulling assays (using either optical tweezers or atomic force microscopy) have been used to measure cell surface mechanics [85]. Micropipette aspiration is a suitable technique to measure the overall cellular tension, which is a combination of the tension in the plasma membrane together with the tension in the underlying actin cytoskeleton [86]. Moreover, membrane tether pulling assays also bring information about the membrane itself and its attachment with the cortical cytoskeleton [86, 87]. During bleb formation, for example, a momentary separation between the plasma membrane and the actin cortex occurs [88].

Biophysical methods show that the membrane-cortex attachment is the major determinant in cell surface tension [89, 90] and that different cells have different surface tension values, indicating that there may have different mechanisms to maintain surface tension homeostasis among cells [90]. Modifications of specific cross-linking proteins, whose function is to link the plasma membrane to the actin cortex, can induce changes in cell surface tension [91–94]. Also, actin filament disruption or myosin inhibition can reduce cell surface tension [90, 95–97]. Changes in membrane composition, particularly in cholesterol content, have also been shown to influence cell surface tension. MβCD causes an increase in tension in embryonic kidney cells [98], fibroblasts [9] and cardiomyocytes [99]. This increase is not only due to changes in membrane composition, but it also affects the actomyosin cytoskeleton. In fibroblasts, MβCD treatment shows an increase in stress fiber formation [9] whereas cardiomyocytes show sarcomeric disorganization together with contraction abnormalities [99].

4. Cellular contractility in nonmuscle cells: the role of Rho and pleiotropic effects of statins

In order to divide, migrate, and undergo tissue morphogenesis, cells change shape and exert forces either on the substrate that they are attached to or on the neighboring cells. Nonmuscle cells generate contractile stresses via molecular motors, such as myosin, that are able to convert chemical energy into mechanical work [2]. Myosin activity is controlled through phosphorylation of its light chain via myosin light chain kinase (MLCK) [100, 101] which, in turn, is activated by Rho kinase ROCK and the small GTPase Rho A upstream. In 1985, the Rho gene was first isolated, from abdominal ganglia of the Aplysia, and identified as a member of the Ras family [102]. In 1990, after injecting a constitutively active form of Rho (Vall4rho), Paterson and collaborators verified that active Rho is able to cause changes in cellular morphology inducing formation of stress fibers [103]. In 1992, Ridley and Hall showed that active RhoA induces formation of stress fibers and focal adhesions upon growth factor stimulation [104]. Being a GTPase, Rho can switch back and forth between its active state, when bound to GTP, and its inactive state, when bound to GDP. The switching process is finely regulated by guanine nucleotide exchange factors (GEFs), which promote activation, and GTPase-activating proteins (GAPs), which promote inactivation. There are approximately 60 GEFs and 70 GAPs that were already identified in the human genome [105]. In order to be activated, Rho goes through some posttranslational modifications that are essential to induce Rho migration toward the plasma membrane, where it gets activated. Prenylation is a posttranslational modification that is known to be pivotal for Rho translocation to the membrane [106]. Protein prenylation is essentially an insertion of a prenyl group, which is a hydrophobic group, to the c-terminal of a protein. That way, the protein has a lipid anchor that allows it to stay membrane bound. There are two types of prenylation: farnesylation and geranyl-geranylation, which are regulated by farnesyltransferase and geranylgeranyltransferase I, respectively [107]. In the case of RhoA, the protein gets geranyl-geranylated before it goes to the membrane to get activated and trigger downstream effectors [108, 109] (**Figure 2**).

Both isoprenoids, farnesyl pyrophosphate and geranylgeranyl pyrophosphate, are synthe-tized by the mevalonate pathway. Interestingly, cholesterol is the end product of this pathway [110] (**Figure 3**). Therefore, by manipulating the mevalonate pathway, one can perturb both cholesterol synthesis and prenylation of important target proteins such as RhoA, and, as a consequence, cellular contractility (**Figure 3**).

The rate-limiting step of the mevalonate pathway is regulated by the enzyme HMG-CoA reductase. The activity of HMG-CoA reductase is precisely governed by the amount of cholesterol available. There are basically two different sources of cholesterol in the body: the exogenous one (obtained through intestinal absorption of cholesterol from the diet) and the endogenous one (through the *de novo* synthesis via the mevalonate pathway), being the endogenous source down regulated when enough cholesterol is obtained from nutri-tion [111]. During the early 1970s, a lot of effort was put into identifying pharmacological candidates that were able to reduce the HMG-CoA reductase activity especially in patients with high LDL cholesterol. In 1984, on a National Institutes of Health (NIH) Consensus Conference for Coronary Primary Prevention Trial, it was demonstrated the importance of a balance diet and drug treatment in order to lower LDL-cholesterol to prevent coronary heart disease [112]. After 1987, statins, that are essentially very specific drug inhibitors of HMG-CoA reductase activity, started to be prescribed for patients with high cholesterol

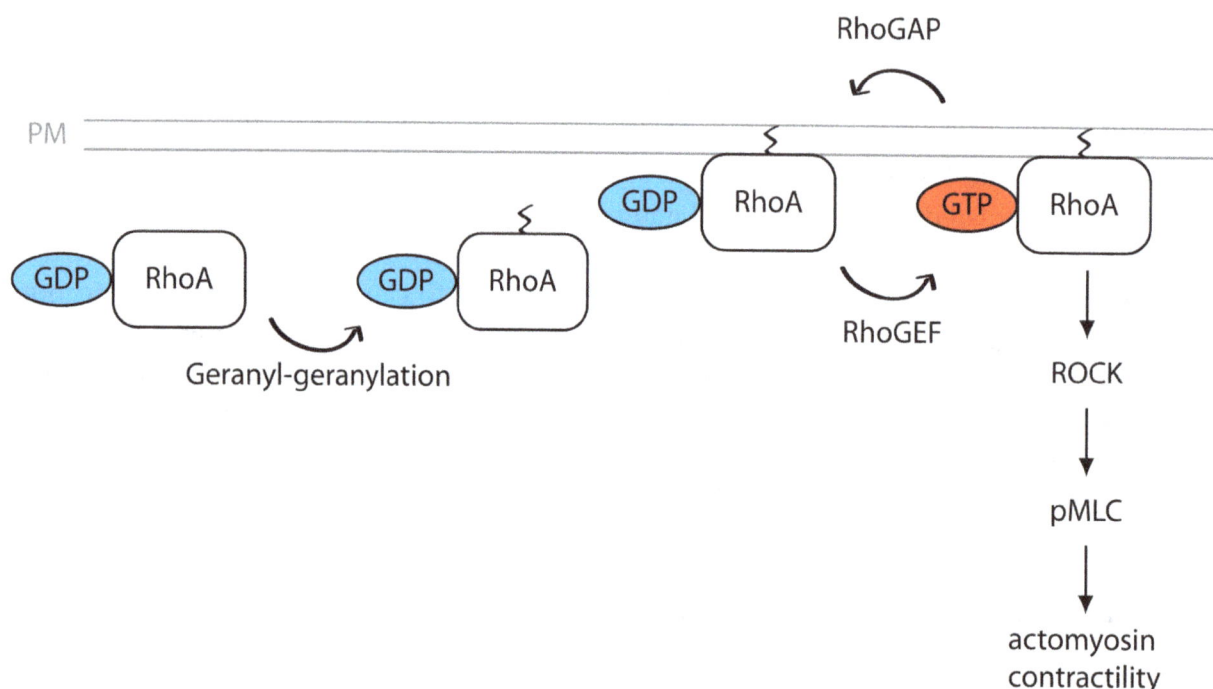

Figure 2. RhoA requires geranyl-geranylation in order to go to the membrane and be activated by RhoGEFs. Active RhoA triggers actomyosin contractility by inducing ROCK phosphorylation of myosin light chain (pMLC).

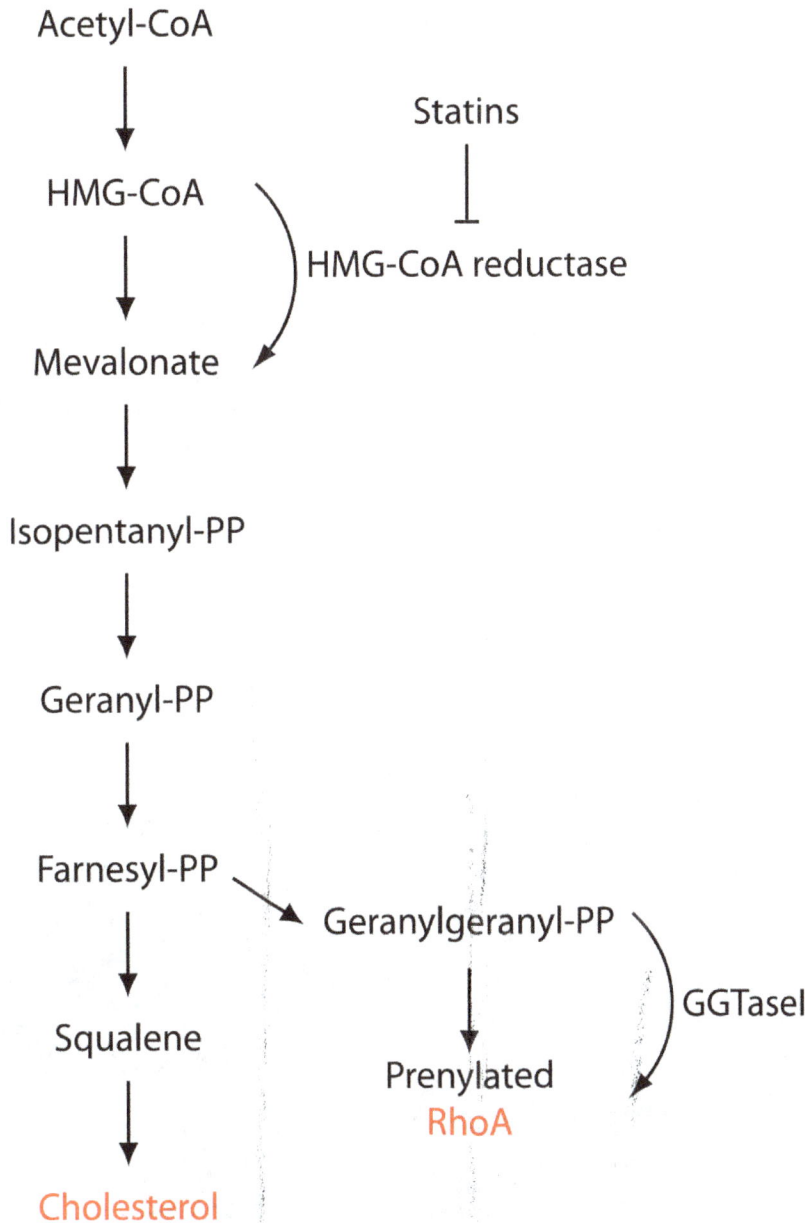

Figure 3. Simple schematic of the mevalonate pathway showing that posttranslational modifications pivotal for RhoA (red) activation and cholesterol (red) synthesis are part of the same intracellular pathway.

values [113]. By reducing the activity of HMG-CoA reductase, statins not only lower the amount of circulating cholesterol but also the amount of isoprenoid, both synthesized the mevalonate pathway, as one can see in **Figure 3**. Active RhoA as well as RhoA downstream effectors, such as ROCK, are inhibited upon statin treatment [114]. In endothelial cells, for example, a combination of flow and simvastatin exposure led to cell rounding and disorganization of the actin cytoskeleton [115]. In order to mimic atherosclerosis and aging effects on vessel walls, endothelial cells were plated in a series of substrates with low (physiological) and high stiffness values. High stiffness substrates increased both RhoA and ROCK activities. However, upon simvastatin incubation, contractility was abrogated in those cells [116].

Interestingly, when cholesterol is directly depleted by MβCD, an opposite trend is observed regarding nonmuscle cellular contractility. Human skin fibroblasts, after MβCD treatment, showed a reduction in the mobility of plasma membrane proteins being that reduction in motion a direct result of cytoskeleton reorganization [117]. It was also shown, for bovine aortic endothelial cells, that MβCD-dependent cholesterol depletion increased cortical stiffness [118]

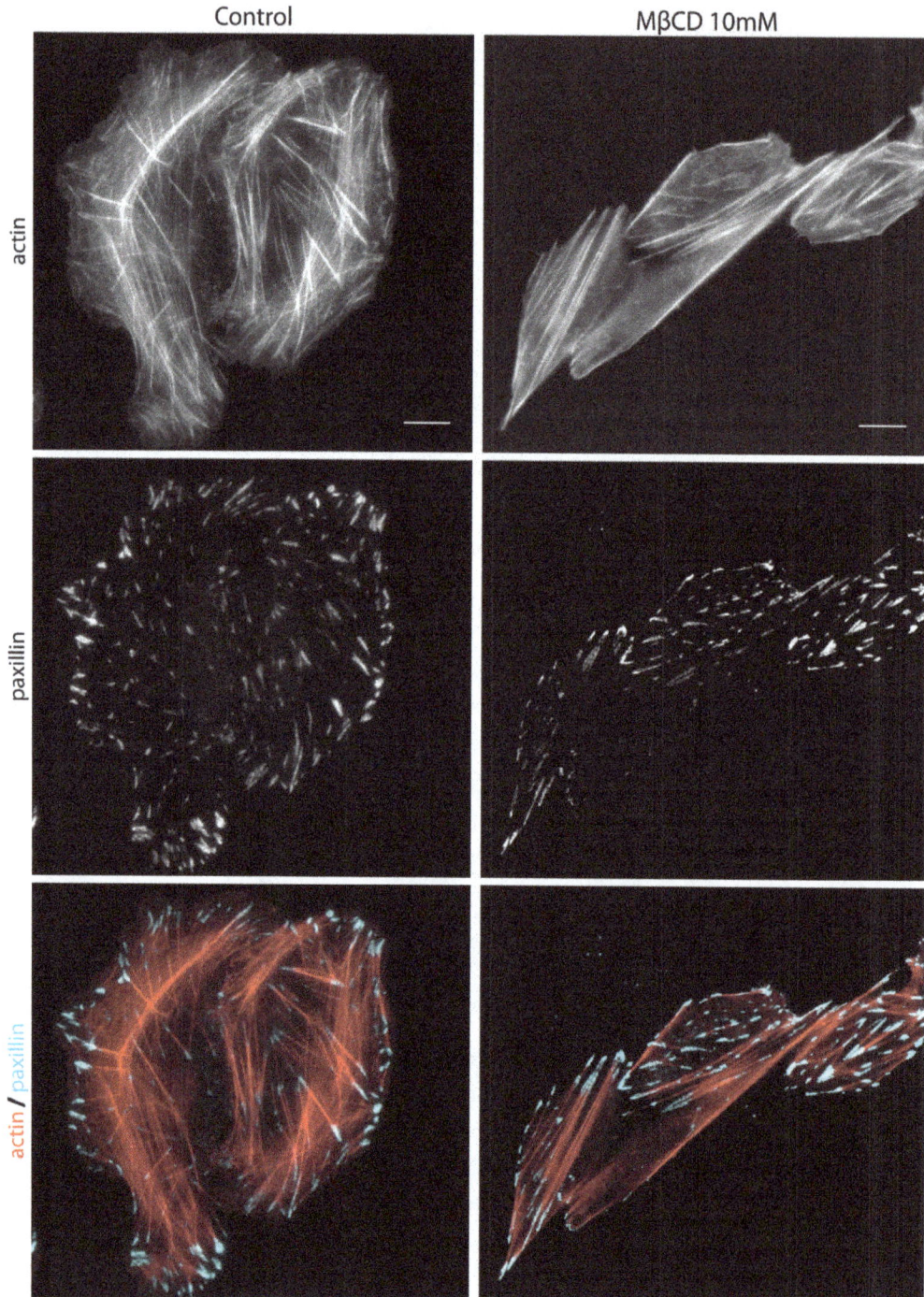

Figure 4. Fixed human osteosarcoma cell line U2OS, labeled for actin (red) paxillin (cyan), a focal adhesion protein. Notice the change in stress fibers between control and cholesterol depleted cells and how aligned the stress fibers get in the latter. Scale bar 10 m.

as well as adhesion energy between membrane and cytoskeleton, which decreased the lipid diffusion coefficient [119]. Serum starvation followed by cyclodextrin-mediated cholesterol depletion increased stress fiber formation and RhoA activation in an osteoblast cell line [120]. Later on, those results were also corroborated by our group in a murine fibroblast cell line [41]. Similar features can also be observed in an osteosarcoma cell line U2OS (**Figure 4**) in which cholesterol depletion led to stress fiber formation and reorganization of actin cytoskeleton. More studies need to be performed in order to understand why different manipulations in cholesterol content trigger opposite results regarding cellular contractility.

5. Cellular contractility in muscle cells: interplay among Ca^{2+}, sarcomeres and cholesterol

Even though statins had been shown to be relatively safe and to promote health benefits to patients with high risks of cardiac diseases, there are some side effects and risks associated with statin therapy. Myotoxicity is one of the most adverse side effects, being the most common clinical outcomes: myosite, myalgia, and rhabdomyolysis [121]. In vitro studies performed on single muscle fibers isolated from rat skeletal muscle showed that fluvastatin and pravastatin led to contractility impairment and vacuolization of the muscle after 72 h of treatment and cell death after 120 h. Those changes in cellular morphology and contraction were proven to be dependent on geranyl-geranylation of GTPases since concomitant incubation of fluvastatin and geranylgeranyl pyrophosphate attenuated the deleterious effects of statins [122]. In vivo and in vitro treatment with simvastatin also led to contractile dysfunction, actin cytoskeleton disruption and apoptosis of smooth muscle cells [123].

Regarding the effects of direct cholesterol depletion mediated by MβCD on muscle cells, our group demonstrated, using primary cell culture of neonatal rat cardiomyocytes, that a lower cholesterol content increased the contraction rate of those cells and also led to defects in cell relaxation [8]. Moreover, cholesterol depletion increased the Ca^{2+} cytoplasmic concentration and Ca^{2+} sparks during contraction. This phenotype can be attributed to changes in caveolin3 and L-type Ca^{2+} channels distribution across the plasmalemma and hyperactivation of cAMP-dependent PKA activity. Cholesterol-depleted cardiomyocytes also present aberrant myofibrils due to calpain (a Ca^{2+} sensitive protease) activation. By using high-quality confocal microscopy and quantitative data analysis, this work has set in stone the role of cholesterol in regulating cardiomyocyte contractile behavior [8]. Other groups have also shown, for adult rat cardiomyocytes, that cholesterol depletion due to MβCD incubation changed localization of caveolin-3 from a raft to a nonraft membrane fraction changing MAPK signaling and increasing contractility and intracellular Ca^{2+} concentration [124]. Adult murine cardiomyocytes treated with MβCD also presented impairment in the T-tubule system and intercalated discs, which reinforces the role of cholesterol in regulating cardiac contractility [125]. More studies need to be performed in order to understand why MβCD-driven cholesterol depletion in nonmuscle cells increase contractile behavior whereas in muscle cells the same treatment tend to abrogate cellular contractility in several levels.

6. Conclusions

Cholesterol is a very important lipid that controls several cellular processes. This chapter describes how cholesterol is organized in cellular membranes and how it regulates and orchestrates the contractile machinery in muscle and nonmuscle cells. Cholesterol and RhoA protein prenylation share the same synthetic route: the mevalonate pathway. By lowering cholesterol concentration, using either chelating agents, such as MβCD, or inhibitors of HMG-CoA reductase, such as statins, one can observe opposite effects on actin cytoskeleton organization and contractile behavior. Cellular treatments with statins lead to a less-contractile profile, since this drug depletes the amount of prenylated RhoA, which, in turn, is the main upstream regulator of contractility in nonmuscle cells. On the other hand, MβCD-mediated cholesterol depletion induces RhoA activation, stress fiber formation, and increase in cortical stiffness pointing toward a more contractile behavior. In muscle cells, the results are even more intriguing: treatments with either statins or MβCD lead to myofibril disorganization, increase of contraction rate and defects in cell relaxation and in the ability of cells to handle intracellular Ca^{2+}. The reason why muscle and nonmuscle cells behave differently regarding cholesterol depletion is not completely understood and further investigation needs to be performed in order to elucidate this paradigm.

Acknowledgements

This work was supported by the Brazilian agencies Conselho Nacional de Desenvolvimento Científico e Tecnológico (CNPq), Coordenação de Aperfeiçoamento de Pessoal de Nível Superior (CAPES), and Fundação de Amparo à Pesquisa do Rio de Janeiro (FAPERJ).

Author details

Barbara Hissa[1*†] and Bruno Pontes[2*†]

*Address all correspondence to: barbarahissa@uchicago.edu and bpontes@icb.ufrj.br

1 The University of Chicago, James Franck Institute, Institute for Biophysical Dynamics and Physics Department, Chicago, IL, USA

2 LPO-COPEA, Federal University of Rio de Janeiro, Institute of Biomedical Sciences, Rio de Janeiro, Brazil

†Both authors contributed equally to the chapter.

References

[1] Pirillo A, Bonacina F, Norata GD, Catapano AL. The interplay of lipids lipoproteins, and immunity in atherosclerosis. Current Atherosclerosis Reports. Springer Nature. 2018;**20**: 12-21. DOI: 10.1007/s11883-018-0715-0

[2] Murrell M, Oakes PW, Lenz M, Gardel ML. Forcing cells into shape: The mechanics of actomyosin contractility. Nature Reviews Molecular Cell Biology. Springer Nature. 2015;**16**:486-498. DOI: 10.1038/nrm4012

[3] Breidigan JM, Krzyzanowski N, Liu Y, Porcar L, Perez-Salas U. Influence of the membrane environment on cholesterol transfer. Journal of Lipid Research. American Society for Biochemistry and Molecular Biology (ASBMB). 2017;**58**:2255-2263. DOI: 10.1194/jlr. m077909

[4] Simons K, Sampaio JL. Membrane organization and lipid rafts. Cold Spring Harbor Perspectives in Biology. Cold Spring Harbor Laboratory. 2011;**3**:a004697-a004697. DOI: 10.1101/cshperspect.a004697

[5] Quest AFG, Leyton L, Párraga M. Caveolins caveolae, and lipid rafts in cellular transport, signaling, and disease. Biochemistry and Cell Biology. Canadian Science Publishing. 2004;**82**:129-144. DOI: 10.1139/o03-071

[6] Head BP, Patel HH, Insel PA. Interaction of membrane/lipid rafts with the cytoskeleton: Impact on signaling and function. Biochimica et Biophysica Acta (BBA)—Biomembranes. Elsevier BV. 2014;**1838**:532-545. DOI: 10.1016/j.bbamem.2013.07.018

[7] López CA, Vries AH de, Marrink SJ. Molecular mechanism of cyclodextrin mediated cholesterol extraction. In: Berkowitz M, editor. PLoS Computational Biology. Public Library of Science (PLoS). 2011;**7**:e1002020. DOI: 10.1371/journal.pcbi.1002020

[8] Hissa B, Oakes PW, Pontes B, Juan GR-S, Gardel ML. Cholesterol depletion impairs contractile machinery in neonatal rat cardiomyocytes. Scientific Reports. Springer Nature. 2017;**7**:43764. DOI: 10.1038/srep43764

[9] Hissa B, Pontes B, Roma PM, Alves AP, Rocha CD, Valverde TM, et al. Membrane cholesterol removal changes mechanical properties of cells and induces secretion of a specific pool of lysosomes. PLoS One. 2013;**8**:e82988

[10] Lombard J. Once upon a time the cell membranes: 175 years of cell boundary research. Biology Direct. Springer Nature. 2014;**9**:32-67. DOI: 10.1186/s13062-014-0032-7

[11] Gorter E, FJEM G. ON bimolecular layers of lipoids on the chromocytes of the blood. Journal of Experimental Medicine. Rockefeller University Press. 1925;**41**:439-443. DOI: 10.1084/jem.41.4.439

[12] Danielli JF. The thickness of the wall of the red blood corpuscle. The Journal of General Physiology. Rockefeller University Press. 1935;**19**:19-22. DOI: 10.1085/jgp.19.1.19

[13] Cole KS. Surface forces of the arbacia egg. Journal of Cellular and Comparative Physiology. Wiley-Blackwell. 1932;**1**:1-9. DOI: 10.1002/jcp.1030010102

[14] Fricke H. The electric capacity of suspensions with special reference to blood. The Journal of General Physiology. Rockefeller University Press. 1925;**9**:137-152. DOI: 10.1085/jgp.9.2.137

[15] Woodhouse DL, Pickworth FA. Permeability of vital membranes. Biochemical Journal. Portland Press Ltd. 1932;**26**:309-316. DOI: 10.1042/bj0260309

[16] Danielli JF, Harvey EN. The tension at the surface of mackerel egg oil with remarks on the nature of the cell surface. Journal of Cellular and Comparative Physiology. Wiley-Blackwell. 1935;**5**:483-494. DOI: 10.1002/jcp.1030050408

[17] Danielli JF, Davson H. A contribution to the theory of permeability of thin films. Journal of Cellular and Comparative Physiology, Wiley-Blackwell. 1935;**5**:495-508. DOI: 10.1002/jcp.1030050409

[18] Singer SJ, Nicolson GL. The fluid mosaic model of the structure of cell membranes. Science. 1972;**175**:720-731

[19] Bretscher MS. Membrane structure: Some general principles. Science. American Association for the Advancement of Science (AAAS). 1973;**181**:622-629. DOI: 10.1126/science.181.4100.622

[20] Yu J, Fischman DA, Steck TL. Selective solubilization of proteins and phospholipids from red blood cell membranes by nonionic detergents. Journal of Supramolecular Structure. Wiley-Blackwell. 1973;**1**:233-248. DOI: 10.1002/jss.400010308

[21] Stier A, Sackmann E. Spin labels as enzyme substrates heterogeneous lipid distribution in liver microsomal membranes. Biochimica et Biophysica Acta (BBA)—Biomembranes, Elsevier BV. 1973;**311**:400-408. DOI: 10.1016/0005-2736(73)90320-9

[22] Karnovsky MJ. The concept of lipid domains in membranes. The Journal of Cell Biology. Rockefeller University Press. 1982;**94**:1-6. DOI: 10.1083/jcb.94.1.1

[23] Estep TN, Mountcastle DB, Barenholz Y, Biltonen RL, Thompson TE. Thermal behavior of synthetic sphingomyelin-cholesterol dispersions. Biochemistry. American Chemical Society (ACS). 1979;**18**:2112-2117. DOI: 10.1021/bi00577a042

[24] Goodsaid-Zalduondo F, Rintoul DA, Carlson JC, Hansel W. Luteolysis-induced changes in phase composition and fluidity of bovine luteal cell membranes. Proceedings of the National Academy of Sciences of the United States of America. 1982;**79**:4332-4336

[25] Simons K, Meer GV. Lipid sorting in epithelial cells. Biochemistry. American Chemical Society (ACS). 1988;**27**:6197-6202. DOI: 10.1021/bi00417a001

[26] Sezgin E, Levental I, Mayor S, Eggeling C. The mystery of membrane organization: Composition regulation and roles of lipid rafts. Nature Reviews Molecular Cell Biology. Springer Nature. 2017;**18**:361-374. DOI: 10.1038/nrm.2017.16

[27] Anchisi L, Dessì S, Pani A, Mandas A. Cholesterol homeostasis: A key to prevent or slow down neurodegeneration. Frontiers in Physiology. Frontiers Media SA. 2013;**3**:486-498. DOI: 10.3389/fphys.2012.00486

[28] Pike LJ. The challenge of lipid rafts. Journal of Lipid Research. American Society for Biochemistry and Molecular Biology (ASBMB). 2008;**50**:S323-S328. DOI: 10.1194/jlr.r800040-jlr200

[29] Korade Z, Kenworthy AK. Lipid rafts cholesterol, and the brain. Neuropharmacology. Elsevier BV. 2008;**55**:1265-1273. DOI: 10.1016/j.neuropharm.2008.02.019

[30] Fantini J, Garmy N, Mahfoud R, Yahi N. Lipid rafts: Structure function and role in HIV Alzheimers and prion diseases. Expert Reviews in Molecular Medicine. Cambridge University Press (CUP). 2002;**4**:1-22. DOI: 10.1017/s1462399402005392

[31] Fivaz M, Abrami L, Goot FG van der. Landing on lipid rafts. Trends in Cell Biology. Elsevier BV; 1999;**9**:212-213. DOI: 10.1016/s0962-8924(99)01567-6

[32] Heerklotz H. Triton promotes domain formation in lipid raft mixtures. Biophysical Journal. Elsevier BV. 2002;**83**:2693-2701. DOI: 10.1016/s0006-3495(02)75278-8

[33] Honigmann A, Sadeghi S, Keller J, Hell SW, Eggeling C, Vink R. A lipid bound actin meshwork organizes liquid phase separation in model membranes. eLife. 2014;**3**:e01671

[34] Mueller V, Ringemann C, Honigmann A, Schwarzmann G, Medda R, Leutenegger M, et al. STED nanoscopy reveals molecular details of cholesterol- and cytoskeleton-modulated lipid interactions in living cells. The Biophysical Journal. 2011;**101**:1651-1660

[35] Klymchenko AS, Kreder R. Fluorescent probes for lipid rafts: From model membranes to living cells. Chemical Biology. 2014;**21**:97-113

[36] Contreras F-X, Sánchez-Magraner L, Alonso A, Goñi FM. Transbilayer (flip-flop) lipid motion and lipid scrambling in membranes. FEBS Letters. Wiley-Blackwell. 2009;**584**: 1779-1786. DOI: 10.1016/j.febslet.2009.12.049

[37] Caroni P. Actin cytoskeleton regulation through modulation of PI(4,5)P2 rafts. The EMBO Journal. Wiley-Blackwell. 2001;**20**:4332-4336. DOI: 10.1093/emboj/20.16.4332

[38] Ritchie K, Shan X-Y, Kondo J, Iwasawa K, Fujiwara T, Kusumi A. Detection of non-brownian diffusion in the cell membrane in single molecule tracking. Biophysical Journal. Elsevier BV. 2005;**88**:2266-2277. DOI: 10.1529/biophysj.104.054106

[39] Macháň R, Wohland T. Recent applications of fluorescence correlation spectroscopy in live systems. FEBS Letters. 2014;**588**:3571-3584

[40] Martinac B. Single-molecule FRET studies of ion channels. Progress in Biophysics and Molecular Biology. 2017;**130**:192-197

[41] Hissa B, Pontes B, Roma PMS, Alves AP, Rocha CD, Valverde TM, et al. Membrane cholesterol removal changes mechanical properties of cells and induces secretion of a specific pool of lysosomes. In: Seaman M, editor. PLoS ONE. Public Library of Science (PLoS). 2013;**8**:e82988. DOI: 10.1371/journal.pone.0082988

[42] Eggeling C, Ringemann C, Medda R, Schwarzmann G, Sandhoff K, Polyakova S, et al. Direct observation of the nanoscale dynamics of membrane lipids in a living cell. Nature. Springer Nature. 2008;**457**:1159-1162. DOI: 10.1038/nature07596

[43] Allen JA, Halverson-Tamboli RA, Rasenick MM. Lipid raft microdomains and neurotransmitter signalling. Nature Reviews Neuroscience. Springer Nature. 2006;**8**:128-140. DOI: 10.1038/nrn2059

[44] Classic Pages. Circulation research. Ovid Technologies (Wolters Kluwer Health). 1970;**27**: 482-482. DOI: 10.1161/01.res.27.3.482

[45] Parton RG, Simons K. The multiple faces of caveolae. Nature Reviews Molecular Cell Biology. Springer Nature. 2007;**8**:185-194. DOI: 10.1038/nrm2122

[46] Rothberg KG, Heuser JE, Donzell WC, Ying YS, Glenney JR, Anderson RG. Caveolin, a protein component of caveolae membrane coats. Cell. 1992;**68**:673-682

[47] Scherer PE, Okamoto T, Chun M, Nishimoto I, Lodish HF, Lisanti MP. Identification, sequence, and expression of caveolin-2 defines a caveolin gene family. Proceedings of the National Academy of Sciences of the United States of America. 1996;**93**:131-135

[48] Tang Z, Scherer PE, Okamoto T, Song K, Chu C, Kohtz DS, et al. Molecular cloning of caveolin-3, a novel member of the caveolin gene family expressed predominantly in muscle. The Journal of Biological Chemistry. 1996;**271**:2255-2261

[49] Pol A, Martin S, Fernández MA, Ingelmo-Torres M, Ferguson C, Enrich C, et al. Cholesterol and fatty acids regulate dynamic caveolin trafficking through the Golgi complex and between the cell surface and lipid bodies. Molecular Biology of the Cell. 2005;**16**:2091-2105

[50] Ren X, Ostermeyer AG, Ramcharan LT, Zeng Y, Lublin DM, Brown DA. Conformational defects slow Golgi exit, block oligomerization, and reduce raft affinity of caveolin-1 mutant proteins. Molecular Biology of the Cell. 2004;**15**:4556-4567

[51] Parton RG, Hanzal-Bayer M, Hancock JF. Biogenesis of caveolae: A structural model for caveolin-induced domain formation. The Journal of Cell Science. 2006;**119**:787-796

[52] Fujimoto T, Kogo H, Ishiguro K, Tauchi K, Nomura R. Caveolin-2 is targeted to lipid droplets, a new membrane domain in the cell. The Journal of Cell Science. 2001;**152**:1079-1085

[53] Drab M, Verkade P, Elger M, Kasper M, Lohn M, Lauterbach B, et al. Loss of caveolae, vascular dysfunction, and pulmonary defects in caveolin-1 gene-disrupted mice. Science. 2001;**293**:2449-2452

[54] Galbiati F, Volonte D, Chu JB, Li M, Fine SW, Fu M, et al. Transgenic overexpression of caveolin-3 in skeletal muscle fibers induces a Duchenne-like muscular dystrophy phenotype. Proceedings of the National Academy of Sciences of the United States of America. 2000;**97**:9689-9694

[55] Minetti C, Sotgia F, Bruno C, Scartezzini P, Broda P, Bado M, et al. Mutations in the caveolin-3 gene cause autosomal dominant limb-girdle muscular dystrophy. Nature Genetics. 1998;**18**:365-368

[56] Hailstones D, Sleer LS, Parton RG, Stanley KK. Regulation of caveolin and caveolae by cholesterol in MDCK cells. The Journal of Lipid Research. 1998;**39**:369-379

[57] Hill MM, Bastiani M, Luetterforst R, Kirkham M, Kirkham A, Nixon SJ, et al. PTRF-Cavin, a conserved cytoplasmic protein required for caveola formation and function. Cell. 2008;**132**:113-124

[58] Hansen CG, Bright NA, Howard G, Nichols BJ. SDPR induces membrane curvature and functions in the formation of caveolae. Nature Cell Biology. 2009;**11**:807-814

[59] McMahon KA, Zajicek H, Li WP, Peyton MJ, Minna JD, Hernandez VJ, et al. SRBC/cavin-3 is a caveolin adapter protein that regulates caveolae function. EMBO Journal. 2009;**28**:1001-1015

[60] Bastiani M, Liu L, Hill MM, Jedrychowski MP, Nixon SJ, Lo HP, et al. MURC/Cavin-4 and cavin family members form tissue-specific caveolar complexes. Journal of Cell Biology. 2009;**185**:1259-1273

[61] Stoeber M, Schellenberger P, Siebert CA, Leyrat C, Helenius A, Grünewald K. Model for the architecture of caveolae based on a flexible net-like assembly of Cavin1 and Caveolin discs. Proceedings of the National Academy of Sciences. 2016;**113**:E8069-E8078. DOI: 10.1073/pnas.1616838113

[62] Ludwig A, Nichols BJ, Sandin S. Architecture of the caveolar coat complex. Journal of Cell Biology. 2016;**129**:3077-3083

[63] Lajoie P, Kojic LD, Nim S, Li L, Dennis JW, Nabi IR. Caveolin-1 regulation of dynamin-dependent, raft-mediated endocytosis of cholera toxin-B sub-unit occurs independently of caveolae. Journal of Cellular and Molecular Medicine. 2009;**13**:3218-3225

[64] Alberts B, Johnson A, Lewis J, Raff M, Roberts K, Walter P. Molecular Biology of the Cell. 5th ed. New York: Taylor & Francis Group; 2007

[65] Tojkander S, Gateva G, Lappalainen P. Actin stress fibers-assembly, dynamics and biological roles. The Journal of Cell Science. 2012;**125**:1855-1864

[66] Heissler SM, Manstein DJ. Nonmuscle myosin-2: Mix and match. Cellular and Molecular Life Sciences. 2013;**70**:1-21

[67] Verkhovsky AB, Svitkina TM, Borisy GG. Myosin II filament assemblies in the active lamella of fibroblasts: Their morphogenesis and role in the formation of actin filament bundles. Journal of Cell Biology. 1995;**131**:989-1002

[68] Svitkina TM, Verkhovsky AB, McQuade KM, Borisy GG. Analysis of the actin-myosin II system in fish epidermal keratocytes: Mechanism of cell body translocation. Journal of Cell Biology. 1997;**139**:397-415

[69] Hotulainen P, Lappalainen P. Stress fibers are generated by two distinct actin assembly mechanisms in motile cells. Journal of Cell Biology. 2006;**173**:383-394

[70] Burnette DT, Manley S, Sengupta P, Sougrat R, Davidson MW, Kachar B, et al. A role for actin arcs in the leading-edge advance of migrating cells. Nature Cell Biology. 2011 **13**:371-381

[71] Pasapera AM, Plotnikov SV, Fischer RS, Case LB, Egelhoff TT, Waterman CM. Rac1-dependent phosphorylation and focal adhesion recruitment of myosin IIA regulates migration and mechanosensing. Current Biology. 2015;**25**:175-186

[72] Tojkander S, Gateva G, Husain A, Krishnan R, Lappalainen P. Generation of contractile actomyosin bundles depends on mechanosensitive actin filament assembly and disassembly. eLife. 2015;**4**:e06126

[73] Luo W, Yu CH, Lieu ZZ, Allard J, Mogilner A, Sheetz MP, et al. Analysis of the local organization and dynamics of cellular actin networks. Journal of Cell Biology. 2013;**202**: 1057-1073

[74] Wilson CA, Tsuchida MA, Allen GM, Barnhart EL, Applegate KT, Yam PT, et al. Myosin II contributes to cell-scale actin network treadmilling through network disassembly. Nature. 2010;**465**:373-377

[75] Livne A, Geiger B. The inner workings of stress fibers-from contractile machinery to focal adhesions and back. Journal of Cell Science. The Company of Biologists. 2016;**129**:1293-1304. DOI: 10.1242/jcs.180927

[76] Huxley HE. The mechanism of muscular contraction. Science. American Association for the Advancement of Science (AAAS). 1969;**164**:1356-1366. DOI: 10.1126/science. 164.3886.1356

[77] Trichet L, Le DJ, Hawkins RJ, Vedula SR, Gupta M, Ribrault C, et al. Evidence of a large-scale mechanosensing mechanism for cellular adaptation to substrate stiffness. Proceedings of the National Academy of Sciences of the United States of America. 2012;**109**:6933-6938

[78] Wood AW. Physiology, Biophysics and Biomedical Engineering. Boca Raton, FL: CRC Press, Taylor & Francis Group; 2012. p. 782

[79] Salbreux G, Charras G, Paluch E. Actin cortex mechanics and cellular morphogenesis. Trends in Cell Biology. Elsevier BV. 2012;**22**:536-545. DOI: 10.1016/j.tcb.2012.07.001

[80] Tooley AJ, Gilden J, Jacobelli J, Beemiller P, Trimble WS, Kinoshita M, et al. Amoeboid T lymphocytes require the septin cytoskeleton for cortical integrity and persistent motility. Nature Cell Biology. 2009;**11**:17-26

[81] Kunda P, Baum B. The actin cytoskeleton in spindle assembly and positioning. Trends in Cell Biology. 2009;**19**:174-179

[82] Wolf K, Mazo I, Leung H, Engelke K, von AUH, Deryugina EI, et al. Compensation mechanism in tumor cell migration: Mesenchymal-amoeboid transition after blocking of pericellular proteolysis. Journal of Cell Biology. 2003;**160**:267-277

[83] Morone N, Fujiwara T, Murase K, Kasai RS, Ike H, Yuasa S, et al. Three-dimensional reconstruction of the membrane skeleton at the plasma membrane interface by electron tomography. Journal of Cell Biology. 2006;**174**:851-862

[84] Charras GT, Hu CK, Coughlin M, Mitchison TJ. Reassembly of contractile actin cortex in cell blebs. Journal of Cell Biology. 2006;**175**:477-490

[85] Moeendarbary E, Harris AR. Cell mechanics: Principles, practices, and prospects. Wiley Interdisciplinary Reviews: Systems Biology and Medicine. 2014;**6**:371-388

[86] Pontes B, Monzo P, Gauthier NC. Membrane tension: A challenging but universal physical parameter in cell biology. Seminars in Cell and Developmental Biology. Elsevier BV. 2017;**71**:30-41. DOI: 10.1016/j.semcdb.2017.08.030

[87] Nussenzveig HM. Cell membrane biophysics with optical tweezers. The European Biophysics Journal. 2017;**46**:1-16

[88] Charras GT, Coughlin M, Mitchison TJ, Mahadevan L. Life and times of a cellular bleb. The Biophysical Journal. 2008;**94**:1836-1853

[89] Dai J, Sheetz MP. Membrane tether formation from blebbing cells. The Biophysical Journal. 1999;**77**:3363-3370

[90] Pontes B, Ayala Y, Fonseca AC, Romão LF, Amaral RF, Salgado LT, et al. Membrane elastic properties and cell function. PLoS One. 2013;**8**:e67708

[91] Liu Y, Belkina NV, Park C, Nambiar R, Loughhead SM, Patino-Lopez G, et al. Constitutively active ezrin increases membrane tension, slows migration, and impedes endothelial transmigration of lymphocytes in vivo in mice. Blood. 2012;**119**:445-453

[92] Rouven BB, Pietuch A, Nehls S, Rother J, Janshoff A. Ezrin is a major regulator of membrane tension in epithelial cells. Scientific Reports. 2015;**5**:14700

[93] Nambiar R, McConnell RE, Tyska MJ. Control of cell membrane tension by myosin-I. Proceedings of the National Academy of Sciences of the United States of America. 2009;**106**:11972-11977

[94] Gérard A, Patino-Lopez G, Beemiller P, Nambiar R, Ben-Aissa K, Liu Y, et al. Detection of rare antigen-presenting cells through T cell-intrinsic meandering motility, mediated by Myo1g. Cell. 2014;**158**:492-505

[95] Pontes B, Viana NB, Salgado LT, Farina M, Moura NV, Nussenzveig HM. Cell cytoskeleton and tether extraction. The Biophysical Journal. 2011;**101**:43-52

[96] Chen C, Tao T, Wen C, He WQ, Qiao YN, Gao YQ, et al. Myosin light chain kinase (MLCK) regulates cell migration in a myosin regulatory light chain phosphorylation-independent mechanism. The Journal of Biological Chemistry. 2014;**289**:28478-28488

[97] Ayala YA, Pontes B, Hissa B, Monteiro AC, Farina M, Moura-Neto V, et al. Effects of cytoskeletal drugs on actin cortex elasticity. Experimental Cell Research. 2017;**351**:173-181

[98] Khatibzadeh N, Gupta S, Farrell B, Brownell WE, Anvari B. Effects of cholesterol on nanomechanical properties of the living cell plasma membrane. Soft Matter. 2012;**8**:8350-8360

[99] Hissa B, Oakes PW, Pontes B, Ramírez-San JG, Gardel ML. Cholesterol depletion impairs contractile machinery in neonatal rat cardiomyocytes. Science Reports. 2017;**7**:43764e

[100] Citi S, Kendrick-Jones J. Regulation of non-muscle myosin structure and function. BioEssays. Wiley-Blackwell. 1987;**7**:155-159. DOI: 10.1002/bies.950070404

[101] Chrzanowska-Wodnicka M. Rho-stimulated contractility drives the formation of stress fibers and focal adhesions. The Journal of Cell Biology. Rockefeller University Press. 1996;**133**:1403-1415. DOI: 10.1083/jcb.133.6.1403

[102] Madaule P, Axel R. A novel ras-related gene family. Cell. Elsevier BV. 1985;**41**:31-40. DOI: 10.1016/0092-8674(85)90058-3

[103] Paterson HF. Microinjection of recombinant p21rho induces rapid changes in cell morphology. The Journal of Cell Biology. Rockefeller University Press. 1990;**111**:1001-1007. DOI: 10.1083/jcb.111.3.1001

[104] Ridley AJ, Hall A. The small GTP-binding protein rho regulates the assembly of focal adhesions and actin stress fibers in response to growth factors. Cell. Elsevier BV. 1992;**70**:389-399. DOI: 10.1016/0092-8674(92)90163-7

[105] Etienne-Manneville S, Hall A. Rho GTPases in cell biology. Nature. Springer Nature. 2002;**420**:629-635. DOI: 10.1038/nature01148

[106] Maltese WA. Posttranslational modification of proteins by isoprenoids in mammalian cells. The FASEB Journal. FASEB. 1990;**4**:3319-3328. DOI: 10.1096/fasebj.4.15.2123808

[107] Rowell CA, Kowalczyk JJ, Lewis MD, Garcia AM. Direct demonstration of geranylgeranylation and farnesylation of Ki-Ras in vivo. Journal of Biological Chemistry. American Society for Biochemistry and Molecular Biology (ASBMB). 1997;**272**:14093-14097. DOI: 10.1074/jbc.272.22.14093

[108] Katayama M, Kawata M, Yoshida Y, Horiuchi H, Yamamoto T, Matsuura Y, et al. The posttranslationally modified C-terminal structure of bovine aortic smooth muscle rhoA p21. The Journal of Biological Chemistry. 1991;**266**:12639-12645

[109] Waiczies S, Bendix I, Prozorovski T, Ratner M, Nazarenko I, Pfueller CF, et al. Geranylgeranylation but not GTP loading determines rho migratory function in T cells. The Journal of Immunology. The American Association of Immunologists. 2007;**179**:6024-6032. DOI: 10.4049/jimmunol.179.9.6024

[110] Goldstein JL, Brown MS. Regulation of the mevalonate pathway. Nature. Springer Nature. 1990;**343**:425-430. DOI: 10.1038/343425a0

[111] Siperstein MD, Fagan VM. Feedback control of mevalonate synthesis by dietary cholesterol. The Journal of Biological Chemistr. 1966;**241**:602-609

[112] Lowering blood cholesterol to prevent heart disease. NIH Consensus Development Conference statement. Arteriosclerosis, Thrombosis, and Vascular Biology. 1985;**5**:404-412. Originally published July 1, 1985. DOI: 10.1161/01.atv.5.4.404

[113] Tobert JA. Lovastatin and beyond: The history of the HMG-CoA reductase inhibitors. Nature Reviews Drug Discovery. Springer Nature. 2003;**2**:517-526. DOI: 10.1038/nrd1112

[114] Oesterle A, Laufs U, Liao JK. Pleiotropic effects of statins on the cardiovascular system. Circulation Research. Ovid Technologies (Wolters Kluwer Health). 2017;**120**:229-243. DOI: 10.1161/circresaha.116.308537

[115] Dick M, Jonak P, Leask RL. Statin therapy influences endothelial cell morphology and F-actin cytoskeleton structure when exposed to static and laminar shear stress conditions. Life Sciences. Elsevier BV. 2013;**92**:859-865. DOI: 10.1016/j.lfs.2013.03.002

[116] Lampi MC, Faber CJ, Huynh J, Bordeleau F, Zanotelli MR, Reinhart-King CA. Simvastatin ameliorates matrix stiffness-mediated endothelial monolayer disruption. In: Komarova Y, editor. Plos ONE. Public Library of Science (PLoS). 2016;**11**:e0147033. DOI: 10.1371/journal.pone.0147033

[117] Kwik J, Boyle S, Fooksman D, Margolis L, Sheetz MP, Edidin M. Membrane cholesterol lateral mobility, and the phosphatidylinositol 4,5-bisphosphate-dependent organization of cell actin. Proceedings of the National Academy of Sciences. 2003;**100**:13964-13969. DOI: 10.1073/pnas.2336102100

[118] Byfield FJ, Aranda-Espinoza H, Romanenko VG, Rothblat GH, Levitan I. Cholesterol depletion increases membrane stiffness of aortic endothelial cells. Biophysical Journal. Elsevier BV. 2004;**87**:3336-3343. DOI: 10.1529/biophysj.104.040634

[119] Sun M, Northup N, Marga F, Huber T, Byfield FJ, Levitan I, et al. The effect of cellular cholesterol on membrane-cytoskeleton adhesion. Journal of Cell Science. The Company of Biologists. 2007;**120**:2223-2231. DOI: 10.1242/jcs.001370

[120] Qi M, Liu Y, Freeman MR, Solomon KR. Cholesterol-regulated stress fiber formation. Journal of Cellular Biochemistry. Wiley-Blackwell. 2009;**106**:1031-1040. DOI: 10.1002/jcb.22081

[121] Hilton-Jones D. Statin-related myopathies. Practical Neurology. British Medical Journal. 2018;**18**(2):97-105. DOI: 10.1136/practneurol-2017-001738

[122] Sakamoto K, Honda T, Yokoya S, Waguri S, Kimura J. Rab-small GTPases are involved in fluvastatin and pravastatin-induced vacuolation in rat skeletal myofibers. The FASEB Journal. 2007;**21**:4087-4094

[123] Kang S, Kim K, Noh JY, Jung Y, Bae ON, Lim KM, et al. Simvastatin induces the apoptosis of normal vascular smooth muscle through the disruption of actin integrity via the impairment of RhoA/Rac-1 activity. The Journal of Thrombosis and Haemostasis. 2016;**116**:496-505

[124] Haque MZ, McIntosh VJ, Samra ABA, Mohammad RM, Lasley RD. Cholesterol depletion alters cardiomyocyte subcellular signaling and increases contractility. In: Hsieh YH, editor. Plos One. Public Library of Science (PLoS). 2016;**11**:e0154151. DOI: 10.1371/journal.pone.0154151

[125] Zhu Y, Zhang C, Chen B, Chen R, Guo A, Hong J, et al. Cholesterol is required for maintaining T-tubule integrity and intercellular connections at intercalated discs in cardiomyocytes. Journal of Molecular and Cellular Cardiology. Elsevier BV. 2016;**97**:204-212. DOI: 10.1016/j.yjmcc.2016.05.013

11

Intracellular Cholesterol Lowering as Novel Target for Anti-Atherosclerotic Therapy

Alexander N. Orekhov and Ekaterina A. Ivanova

Abstract

Atherosclerosis and disorders associated with cardiovascular system remain the major problem of modern medicine and the leading cause of mortality in developed countries. According to the current knowledge, atherosclerosis development can begin early in life. Clinically silent early-stage lesions can be detected in a large population of young adults. Despite substantial progress in the recent years, therapy of atherosclerosis mostly remains limited to plasma lipid profile correction. Moreover, no therapy is currently available for the treatment of asymptomatic early stages of the disease. The existing synthetic drugs could not be used for this purpose, because of the unfavourable risk/benefit ratio and high cost of treatment, which has to be long-lasting. In this regard, medications based on natural agents with anti-atherosclerotic activity may offer interesting possibilities. Current research should focus on detection and evaluation of such agents. One of the important tools for anti-atherosclerotic drug evaluation is a cell-based model, which allows measurement of intracellular lipid accumulation. Anti-atherosclerotic activity of various substances can therefore be evaluated by the decrease of intracellular lipid storage. In this chapter, we will discuss the development and application of cellular models based on primary culture of human arterial wall cells that are suitable for detection and measurement of anti-atherosclerotic activity of various substances. Using these models, several natural agents have been successfully evaluated, which led to the development of pharmaceutical products with anti-atherosclerotic activity based on botanicals.

Keywords: atherosclerosis, arteries, cholesterol accumulation, cellular models, anti-atherosclerotic drugs

1. Introduction

Atherosclerosis remains one of the most challenging problems of modern medicine. Epidemiological data on atherosclerosis and cardiovascular diseases are frequently updated and demonstrate an increase in overall mortality, partly because of the ageing of human population, especially in favourable economic conditions [1]. In developed countries, cardiovascular diseases remain the primary cause of overall morbidity and mortality [2]. Atherosclerotic lesions develop in the walls of large arteries and cause occlusion of blood vessels as a result of either arterial wall thickening or thrombus formation on the surface of unstable plaques. This latter condition is especially dangerous, since it can lead to a sudden and often fatal thromboembolia, which represents the first clinical manifestation of atherosclerosis in many patients. By contrast, early stages of the disease usually pass unnoticed. Recent studies have demonstrated that asymptomatic atherosclerosis is, in fact, a widespread condition among young adults [2–5]. In this cohort of subjects, the incidence of atherosclerotic lesions reaches 100%, although no clinical manifestations can be observed [3–5].

The development of atherosclerosis is a complex process, which, despite the significant progress made during the last decade, still remains to be fully understood. Atherosclerosis and related cardiovascular disorders are associated with several known risk factors, including elevated plasma cholesterol level, diabetes, tobacco smoking and others [6, 7].

Modern atherosclerosis prevention strategies are largely based on elimination or attenuation of relevant risk factors, which slows down the atherosclerotic plaque progression in an indirect way [8]. For instance, statins are commonly used for plasma cholesterol reduction and attenuation of atherosclerosis progression. However, limited indications and serious side effects make statins unsuitable for preventive therapy of atherosclerosis, which has to be long-term. Currently, there exists no widespread "direct" anti-atherosclerotic therapy that could be suitable for treatment of the early, subclinical stages of the disease. Such therapy should target the molecular and cellular mechanisms of atherogenesis at the level of blood vessel wall and should result in prevention of *de novo* lesion formation or regression of existing plaques [8–10]. Natural agents appear to be attractive candidates for preventive anti-atherosclerosis therapy because of their favourable safety profile and low cost. Because of their complex composition, biologically active substances of botanical origin and their combinations may have a wider range of effects than synthetic drugs, targeting several atherosclerosis risk factors simultaneously. It is therefore possible that the botanical substances can possess both direct and indirect anti-atherosclerotic effects, such as protective activity at the cellular level combined with cholesterol lowering and hypotensive activity. Current knowledge of cardioprotective effects of natural agents and nutraceuticals is rather limited, although they have been actively studied by several groups during the recent years [11–17]. It is important to establish novel anti-atherosclerotic preventive therapies based on natural products and confirm their effectiveness by clinical studies.

The search for potential anti-atherosclerotic agents and evaluation of their activity requires adequate test models. Lipid accumulation is one of the most prominent features of atherosclerotic lesions. Lipid uptake and storage are performed by several cell types of the arterial wall. Both resident cells and inflammatory cells that are recruited to the lesion site can participate in the process. Increased lipid content can be observed already at the earliest stages of the plaque development. The main source of cholesterol deposit in the arterial wall is low-density lipoprotein (LDL), especially its modified, atherogenic forms. The risk of atherosclerosis development has been demonstrated to be associated with unfavourable plasma lipid profile and the increased contents of atherogenic LDL types, such as small dense LDL [18]. The ability of the blood plasma to cause lipid accumulation in the arterial wall cells is referred to as blood serum atherogenicity [19]. Anti-atherosclerotic effect of a substance can be evaluated by its ability to prevent lipid accumulation in cultured arterial wall cells induced by the exposure to atherogenic LDL. Importantly, lipid profile in cells with or without treatment can precisely be measured to quantitatively evaluate anti-atherosclerotic potential.

In this chapter, we will give an overview of current knowledge on atherosclerotic lesion progression and discuss the development and application of models based on primary culture of human arterial wall cells.

2. Atherosclerotic plaque development

According to the classic lipid theory of atherogenesis, atherosclerotic lesion development is caused by extracellular and intracellular lipid accumulation in the intimal layer of the arterial wall [20, 21]. It has been shown that the major source of lipid accumulation in the intimal cells is circulating LDL, especially its atherogenic forms, such as chemically modified and aggregated LDL. Chemical modification of lipoprotein particles appears to be necessary for the atherogenic effect, since native (non-modified) LDL added to cultured cells could not induce significant lipid accumulation. Atherogenic modifications of LDL in the bloodstream include desialylation, acquisition of negative charge and increase of the particle hydrated density (small dense LDL formation). All these modifications can be accompanied by oxidation [22–25]. Study of the atherogenic LDL modification in the bloodstream currently remains challenging. Different laboratory methods of LDL isolation, quantification and analysis deliver different results, which hinders direct comparison of studies employing different methods and protocols. For instance, analysing LDL size and density by ultracentrifugation in different buffers will give slightly different outcome. Moreover, no consensus has been reached so far on the classification of LDL subfractions [22]. It is likely that LDL particles undergo multiple atherogenic modification in human plasma, but the resulting products are differently evaluated by different methods from several laboratories [26–28]. One of the earliest atherogenic modifications demonstrated to occur in human bloodstream is desialylation. The removal of sialic acid residues from the carbohydrate components of LDL particles is performed by trans-sialidase, which is active in the bloodstream. Increased level of circulating modified LDL leads to aggregation of the particles, which is facilitated by increased surface charge. The resulting large complexes have especially high atherogenic potential. Moreover, modified forms of LDL can induce formation of autoantibodies triggering inflammatory response and giving rise to circulating immune complexes. Another feature that can significantly increase atherogenic potential of modified LDL is its ability to associate with the components of extracellular matrix proteins in the subendothelial space of the arterial wall, which prolongs its residence time and facilitates lipid accumulation. Unlike native LDL, which is internalized by cells via receptor-mediated uptake, modified LDL complexes enter the cells through uncontrolled phagocytosis and follow a distinct metabolic pathway [29]. This can explain the rapid accumulation of atherogenic modified LDL in cellular cytoplasm, mostly in the form of lipid droplets. Cells containing large amounts of lipid inclusions in the cytoplasm are called "foam cells" because of their microscopic appearance. Such cells commonly occur in atherosclerotic lesions.

Figure 1 shows the development of atherosclerotic lesions and the main stages of the athero-genesis [30]. According to the current knowledge, atherosclerotic lesion initiation is dependent on two conditions: the presence of modified atherogenic LDL in the bloodstream in sufficient quantities and the internalization of LDL by the arterial wall cells. The latter is usually triggered by local disturbance of endothelial function that causes increased permeability of the endo-thelial lining allowing modified LDL to penetrate into the intimal layer of the arterial wall. Atherogenic modification of LDL may also occur in the intimal layer, after the particles have crossed the endothelial barrier. Local disturbances of endothelial function frequently take place in certain parts of the vascular system, such as branching points and bends, where laminar blood flow is altered [31]. Sites of the arterial wall that are especially vulnerable are marked by altered morphology of endothelial cells and presence of enlarged multinucleated cells. The pre-existent mosaicism of the endothelial lining may explain the focal development of atherosclerotic lesions. However, more studies are needed to determine the mechanisms of endothelial dysfunction leading to atherosclerosis.

Focal lipid infiltration into the arterial wall intima marks the early stages of atherosclerotic lesion development. Apparently, several cell types of the arterial wall participate in lipid accumulation. Cells populating the intimal layer can be either resident mesenchymal cells,

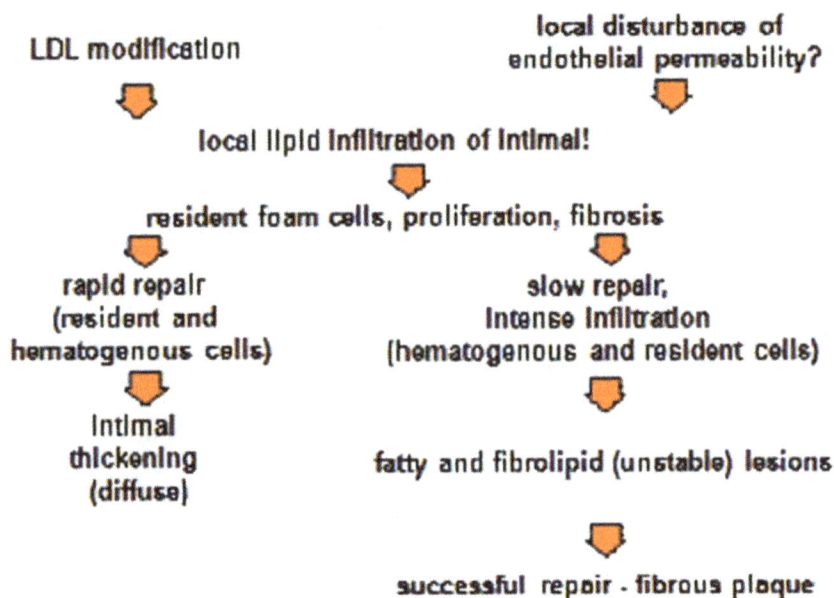

Figure 1. Scheme showing the consecutive events in the development of atherosclerotic lesions. Reproduced with permission from [30].

such as smooth muscle cells, or inflammatory cells, such as monocytes/macrophages, that can be recruited from the bloodstream in large numbers by a local inflammatory response. Along with macrophages, smooth muscular cells also take part in lipid uptake and can be transformed into foam cells. While native LDL particles are metabolized by intimal cells through a well-developed and controlled receptor-mediated endocytosis, it is likely that the LDL associations are recognized by macrophages as pathogens that have to be cleared by phagocytosis [32]. Such clearance is accompanied by secretion of signalling molecules that attract immune cells to the developing lesion site and therefore initiation of the inflammatory process [33]. Phago-cytosis-mediated lipid accumulation in atherosclerosis can therefore be regarded as a variation of innate immune response. Enhanced phagocytosis followed by lipid accumulation and foam cell formation contributes to lesion development. Lipid accumulation affects intercellular contacts that are essential for proper function of intimal wall resident cells [34]. On the other hand, lipid accumulation also triggers processes that are typical for the reparative phase of inflammation, such as proliferation and extracellular matrix synthesis leading to the fibrosis. In favourable conditions, these reparation processes rapidly lead to formation of areas with increased cellularity and extracellular matrix deposition. Gradual development of such focal lesion areas leads to a diffuse intimal thickening, which is frequently observed in adult arteries. However, the inflammatory response can become chronic, with continuous local lipid infiltration, increased cellularity due to the proliferation of cells in the lesion site and enhanced fibrosis.

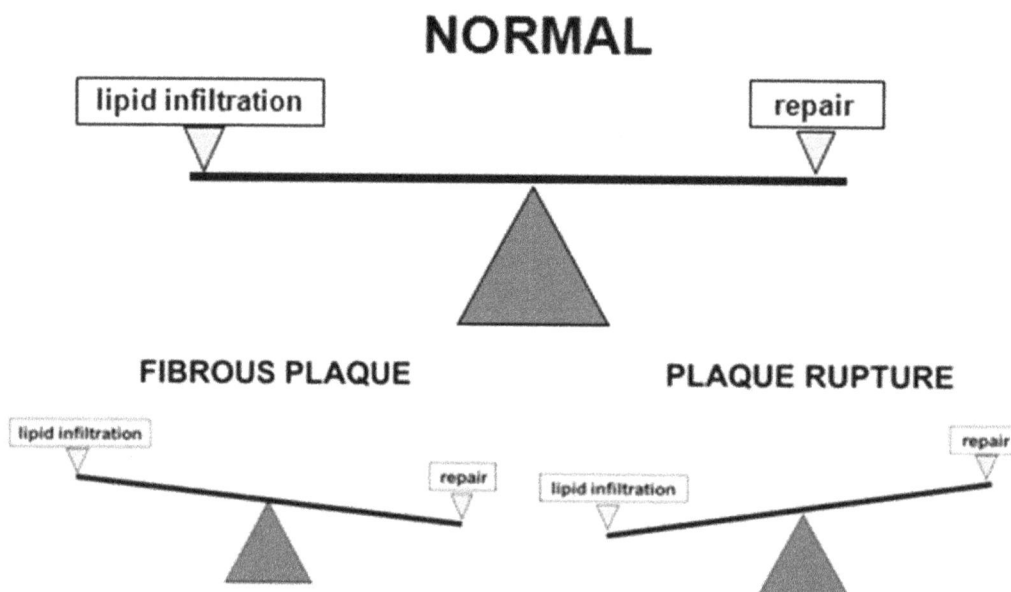

NORMAL

lipid infiltration   repair

FIBROUS PLAQUE   **PLAQUE RUPTURE**

lipid infiltration   repair   lipid infiltration   repair

Figure 2. Scheme showing the delicate balance between infiltrative and reparative phases in fatty atherosclerotic lesion. Reproduced with permission from [30].

Atherosclerotic plaques can be protected from the bloodstream by formation of a fibrous cap, which serves as a barrier for lipoproteins and inflammatory cells. Such isolation of the local inflammatory site has a protective role, suppressing the inflammatory response and restoring the tissue functions. On the other hand, formation of fibrolipid plaques predisposed to rupture (unstable plaques) can have fatal consequences because of thrombus formation.

In fibrolipid plaques, two opposing processes are likely to take place: infiltration and reparation that exist in a state of unstable equilibrium (**Figure 2**). Shifting the balance towards reparation leads to the formation of fibrous plaques, which is a favourable outcome from the clinical point of view. Inefficient reparation and continuous lipid infiltration cause plaque rupture with possible thrombus formation. Lipidosis plays therefore a crucial role in atherosclerotic lesion development at cellular and tissue levels and represents an important target for the development of anti-atherosclerotic therapy.

3. Evaluation of substances' anti-atherosclerotic activity using cellular models

Preventive anti-atherosclerotic therapy should be aimed at reduction of intracellular lipid accumulation [35]. Such reduction can be achieved by different approaches [36]. First, the therapy may decrease the level of circulating modified LDL. Second, it can target atherogenic modification of LDL in the bloodstream. Third, it can reduce lipid uptake and storage by the arterial wall cells. Finally, the therapy can be aimed at depletion of the existing intracellular lipid stores. All these approaches can be evaluated by measuring the reduction of intracellular lipid accumulation and the decrease of the intracellular pool of cholesterol esters [9, 37, 38]. A number of available medications can be used to decrease blood serum atherogenicity [9, 36, 38, 39], which is defined as the ability of blood serum to induce cholesterol accumulation in cultured cells. Blood serum from patients with coronary atherosclerosis usually has high atherogenicity [19]. Changes of blood serum atherogenicity reflect lipid accumulation in the arterial wall and are therefore relevant for the development of preventive therapy. Such changes can be detected using cultured cells as models of early stages of human atherogenesis [9, 38, 40]. Cellular models can be used for evaluation of anti-atherosclerotic potential of different drugs and active substances, for screening of potential anti-atherosclerotic agents and for evaluation of potential clinical efficacy of various molecules.

4. *In vitro* model

In vitro model based on primary culture of human aortic wall cells was developed for screening of potential anti-atherosclerotic substances. Cells were isolated from the subendothelial layer of healthy human aortic intima, the layer of the arterial wall, which is most severely affected in atherosclerosis [41]. The process of cell isolation from autopsy material using collagenase and elastase treatment has been described previously [9, 42–44]. The obtained cell population has been characterized using immunocytochemistry methods and was found to be heterogeneous and containing smooth muscle cells (20–50%), pericytes (30–70%) and inflammatory cells and tissue macrophages (10%) (**Table 1**) [9, 43, 44].

Smooth muscle α-actin⁺	3G5⁺	2A7⁺	CD45⁺	CD68⁺
89.6 ± 6.7%	45.8 ± 10.9%	24.1 ± 9.9%	3.6 ± 0.4%	5.2 ± 1.3%

Table 1. Proportion of cell types in primary culture cells isolated from human aortic subendothelial intima (% of positive cells for each marker).

Substance	References
Anti-atherosclerotic	
Cyclic AMP	[9, 44, 46–49]
Prostacyclin	[9, 50–54]
Prostaglandin E₂	[9, 52, 55]
Artificial HDL*	[56]
Antioxidants	[9]
Calcium antagonists	[9, 51, 57–59]
Trapidil and its derivatives	[60, 61]
Lipoxygenase inhibitors	[55]
Lipostabil	[9]
Mushroom extracts	[62]
Pro-atherogenic	
Beta blockers	[58, 63]
Thromboxane A₂	[51, 55]
Phenothiazine	[58]
Indifferent	
Nitrates	[58]
Cholestyramine	[58]
Sulfonylureas	[64]

ᵃ HDL, high-density lipoprotein.

Table 2. Substances that have been tested *in vitro* cell model.

Smooth muscle cells and pericytes were positive for smooth muscle α-actin. Pericytes had a distinct stellate shape and were identified using antibodies to 3G5 and 2A7 that are expressed by resting and activated pericytes, respectively. Together, smooth muscle cells and pericytes represented the majority of cell population in the obtained primary cultures. A smaller population consisted of the inflammatory cells that could be detected using antibodies to leukocyte-specific marker CD45 and macrophage marker CD68 [45]. Cellular lipid accumulation was induced by incubation of cells with atherogenic serum obtained from patients with confirmed atherosclerosis. The increase of cellular cholesterol content reached as high as two folds after a 24-h incubation with atherogenic serum.

Potential anti-atherogenic substances were evaluated by concomitant incubation of cells with atherogenic serum and aqueous solutions of tested substances. Anti-atherosclerotic effect was measured as a decrease in the levels of intracellular cholesterol in the cells with test substances compared to the control cells (treated with atherogenic serum only). The described model allowed evaluating a number of different drugs and substances and detecting several novel active molecules with anti-atherosclerotic potential. Some substances were demonstrated to possess a pro-atherogenic effect, enhancing intracellular cholesterol accumulation induced by atherogenic serum (**Table 2**).

5. *Ex vivo* model

Ex vivo model is based on primary culture of cells from unaffected human aortic intima that are incubated with blood serum from patients treated with the substance of interest. Therefore, potential anti-atherogenic properties of substances are evaluated based on their pharmacodynamic properties, or the influence on blood serum atherogenicity after digestion and possible metabolic modifications in patient's body. Blood samples are drawn before and after administration of single doses of tested substances, and serum obtained from the samples is added to cultured primary cells. *Ex vivo* model can be used for testing drugs with known safety profiles, as well as various natural products.

Several studies have demonstrated successful application of this model for evaluation of anti-atherogenic properties of botanicals. Screening studies were performed on volunteers (groups of 4–8 men and women 45–60 years old) with high blood serum atherogenicity. One of the tested natural products with anti-atherosclerotic properties was encapsulated onion (*Allium cepa*) bulb powder (300 mg) (**Figure 3**). Administration of a single dose of the product resulted in a moderate decrease of blood serum atherogenicity by 12, 28, and 24% from the baseline after 2, 4, and 6 h, respectively. Another tested natural product with anti-atherosclerotic properties was preparation of wheat seedlings (*Triticum aestivum*). Administration of a single dose of 300 mg of the preparation resulted in a pronounced reduction of blood serum atherogenicity after 4 h (**Figure 4**). Moderate but prolonged anti-atherosclerotic effect was registered for dry beet (*Beta vulgaris*) juice (encapsulated preparation of 300 mg) (**Figure 5**). Garlic (*Allium sativum*) powder possessed a strong and prolonged effect (**Figure 6**). Blood serum atherogenicity was completely suppressed 4 h after administration of a single dose of 300 mg of the preparation. Several other natural products were screened for potential anti-atherosclerotic activity using the *ex vivo* model (**Table 3**). The highest activity after a single dose administration was detected for garlic powder and wheat seedlings, with garlic powder providing the strongest effect. Importantly, anti-atherosclerotic effects of garlic have been reported by several independent groups during the recent years [65–67].

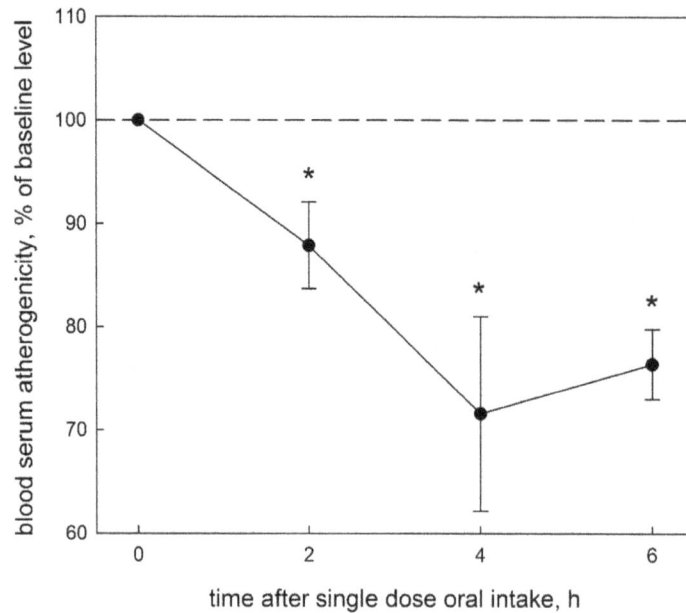

Figure 3. Anti-atherosclerotic effect of onion in *ex vivo* model.The study involved four volunteers (three males, one female, mean age 57 ± 5 years) whose blood serum induced 1.3–1.5-fold increase in cholesterol content of cells cultured from unaffected human aortic intima (the average level of serum atherogenicity was 141 ± 4%). Intracellular cholesterol in control cultures was 38.4 ± 1.1 mg/mg cell protein. Baseline serum atherogenicity was taken as 100%. The average values of changes of serum atherogenicity with indication of standard errors are presented. Reproduced with permission from [30].

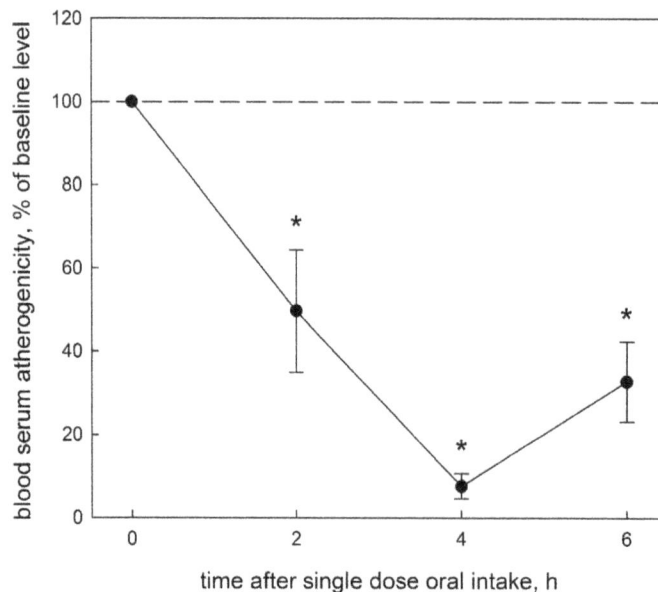

Figure 4. Anti-atherosclerotic effect of wheat seedlings in *ex vivo* model.The study involved eight volunteers (five males, three females, mean age 51 ± 2 years) whose blood serum induced 1.7–2.3-fold increase in cholesterol content of cells cultured from unaffected human aortic intima (the average level of serum atherogenicity was 199 ± 6%). Intracellular cholesterol in control cultures was 28.0 ± 1.2 mg/mg cell protein. Baseline serum atherogenicity was taken as 100%. The average values of changes of serum atherogenicity with indication of standard errors are presented. *, Significant decrease of serum atherogenicity, p < 0.05. Reproduced with permission from [30].

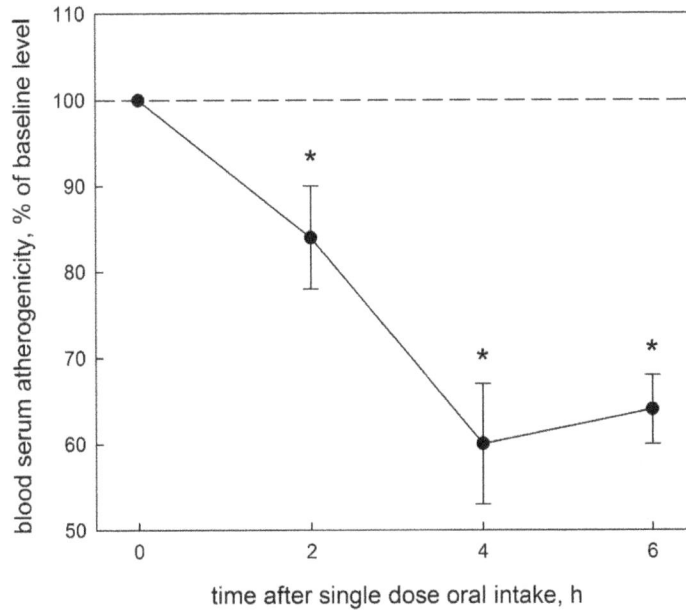

Figure 5. Anti-atherosclerotic effect of beet juice in *ex vivo* model. The study involved eight volunteers (six males, two females, mean age 53 ± 5 years) whose blood serum induced 1.3–2.2-fold increase in cholesterol content of cells cultured from unaffected human aortic intima (the average level of serum atherogenicity was $161 \pm 8\%$). Intracellular cholesterol in control cultures was 37.0 ± 3.6 mg/mg cell protein. Baseline serum atherogenicity was taken as 100%. The average values of changes of serum atherogenicity with indication of standard errors are presented. *, Significant decrease of serum atherogenicity, $p < 0.05$. Reproduced with permission from [30].

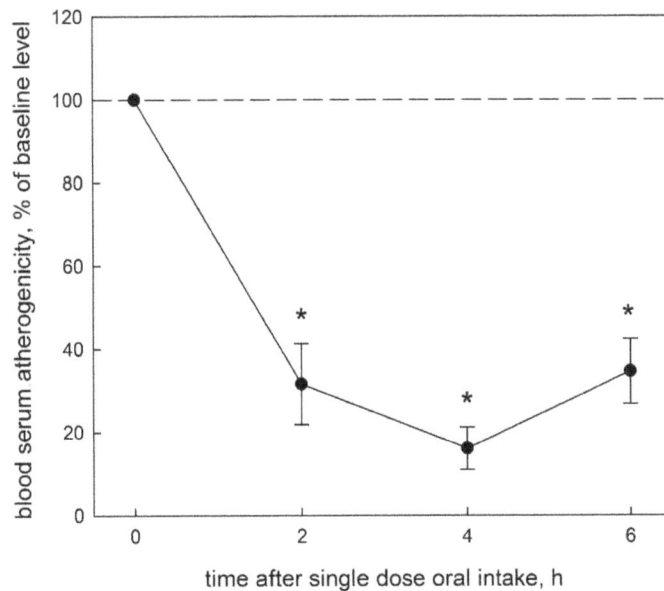

Figure 6. Anti-atherosclerotic effect of garlic powder in the *ex vivo* model. The study involved eight volunteers (six males, two females, mean age 53 ± 5 years) whose blood serum induced 1.3–2.7-fold increase in cholesterol content of cells cultured from unaffected human aortic intima (the average level of serum atherogenicity was $164 \pm 9\%$). Intracellular cholesterol in control cultures was 39.0 ± 4.2 mg/mg cell protein. Baseline serum atherogenicity was taken as 100%. The average values of changes of serum atherogenicity with indication of standard errors are presented. *, Significant decrease of serum atherogenicity, $p < 0.05$. Reproduced with permission from [30].

Botanical and its source	The mean efficiency of atherogenic reduction (%)	Maximum effect (%)
Spirulina platensis powder	50.7	61
Onion (*Allium cepa*) bulb powder	21.4	28
Beet (*Beta vulgaris*) juice powder	30.7	40
Wheat (*Triticum vulgaris*) seedlings powder	70.0	100
Licorice (*Glycyrrhiza glabra*) root powder	54.6	32
Salsola collina leaf powder	10.9	28
Garlic (*Allium sativum*) bulbs powder	76.6	100
Pine (*Pinus sylvestris*) needles extract	52.1	62

*The integrated effect was calculated as a mean reduction in serum atherogenicity for 6 h after a single oral dose.

Table 3. Integral estimation of anti-atherogenic actions of natural products*.

The described *ex vivo* model could be used for establishing the effective dose and posology of the potential anti-atherosclerotic natural products. For this purpose, blood samples were drawn before and after (2 and 4 h) administration of a single dose to patients with high blood serum atherogenicity. Dose dependency was tested by comparison of the effect of two different doses. Each dose was evaluated on at least six different study participants. It was demonstrated that the anti-atherosclerotic effect of garlic powder was present in the dose range from 50 to 300 mg with half-maximal effect observed at a dose of 100 mg, and maximal effect—at 150 mg. Therefore, natural products of botanical origin can be regarded as an important source of agents with anti-atherosclerotic activity that can be used for the development of direct anti-atherosclerotic therapy. Based on the obtained results, several dietary supplements were registered and further evaluated in clinical studies presented below.

As any model, cellular models for studying atherosclerosis development have their limitations [68–71]. Limitations of the experimental models used for atherosclerosis research have been discussed in a number of comprehensive reviews [72–77]. However, the described test system allows performing the initial screening for anti-atherosclerotic activity that can be further studied and confirmed in pre-clinical and clinical studies.

6. Clinical studies

Tests on cellular models demonstrated that garlic powder preparations possessed a pronounced anti-atherosclerotic activity. Based on the obtained results, a garlic-based dietary supplement (Allicor, INAT-Farma, Russia) was developed. The effect of the supplement on carotid intima-media thickness (cIMT) was evaluated in an open-label prospective pilot study conducted on 28 men (46–58 years old, mean age 52.0, SD = 9.0). The study participants had no signs of coronary heart disease, no chronic diseases requiring treatment with vasoactive drugs, diuretics, lipid-lowering or antidiabetic drugs and were normolipidemic or mildly hyperlipidemic. Study subjects were analysed for presence of diffuse intimal thickening by ultrasound imaging of common carotid arteries [65]. The cut-off cIMT value of 0.7 mm in the distal segment of at least one common carotid artery was set up to diagnose diffuse intimal thickening. The mean cIMT value at the baseline was 0.832 ± 0.024 mm. Study participants were divided into two groups. Subjects from Allicor group (n = 16) received 600 mg of Allicor daily, and subjects from the control group (n = 12) received no treatment. The total duration of the study was 12 months, with interviews and ultrasound assessment of cIMT every 3 months. No adverse effects were observed during the follow-up period, and the product was demonstrated to have good tolerability. The results of cIMT assessments are presented on **Figure 7**.

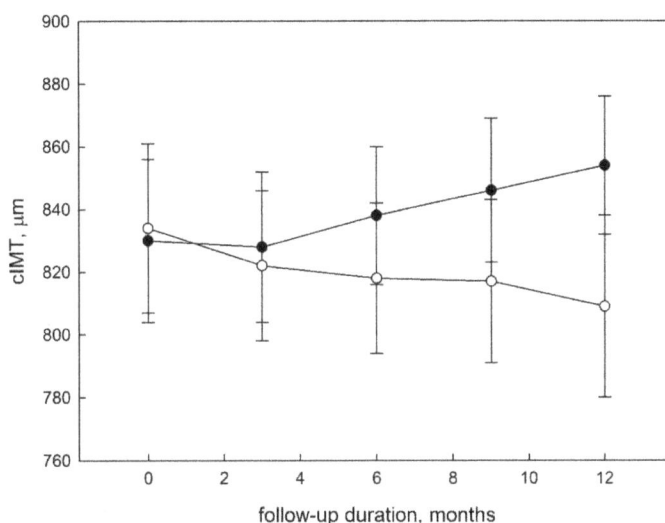

Figure 7. The effects of garlic-based drug Allicor on atherosclerosis determined by cIMT. Open circles, Allicor recipients; solid circles, control subjects. Presented are mean values ±S.E.M. Reproduced from [30].

No statistically significant changes of cIMT were observed after 12 months, and the value was not significantly different between the two groups. However, regression analysis revealed a significant difference between the trends of cIMT dynamics (p < 0.05). In the control group, a tendency to cIMT increase was detected, which was significantly different from that of null hypothesis of no change (F-test, 31.72; p = 0.011). In the Allicor-treated group, the tendency to cIMT decrease was revealed, which was also significantly different from that of null hypothesis (F-test, 28.81; p = 0.013). These results indicate that treatment with Allicor may potentially halter the development and induce the regression of subclinical atherosclerosis. The statistical power of this pilot study was insufficient to avoid type 2 error. Therefore, the pilot study was followed by a larger prospective clinical study, in which a number of clinical and biochemical parameters associated with atherogenesis were taken into account. The dynamic of serum atherogenicity was also assessed. This double-blind placebo-controlled clinical study evaluated the effect of garlic powder tablets Allicor on the progression of cIMT in 211 men (40–74 years old) with no symptoms of atherosclerosis (ClinicalTrials.gov identifier, NCT01734707). The primary outcome was the progression of subclinical atherosclerosis evaluated by B-mode ultrasonography as the increase of cIMT. By the end of the first 12-month follow-up period, a decrease of cIMT by 0.028 ± 0.008 mm was observed in the Allicor group. At the same time, moderate increase of 0.014 ± 0.009 mm was observed in the placebo group (p = 0.002). Serum atherogenicity was decreased in the Allicor group by 45% from the baseline and remained unaltered in the placebo group. Therefore, long-term treatment with Allicor had a direct anti-atherosclerotic effect in patients with subclinical atherosclerosis associated with decreased serum atherogenicity [78]. By the end of the 24-month follow-up period, the mean rate of cIMT was decreased in the Allicor group by 0.022 ± 0.007 mm per year, which was significantly different (p = 0.002) from the placebo group, in which there was a moderate but statistically significant progression of 0.015 ± 0.008 mm at the overall mean baseline cIMT of 0.931 ± 0.009 mm [37, 39]. A significant reduction of cIMT was observed in 47.3% of study subjects from the Allicor group vs 30.1% in the placebo group (p < 0.05). Further significant increase of cIMT was registered in 32.2% study participants in Allicor-treated group vs 47.3% in placebo group (p < 0.05). Study of blood serum atherogenicity demonstrated a 1.56-fold increase of intracellular cholesterol accumulation in the cellular test at the baseline. Study participants from Allicor group had an average 30% decrease of blood serum atherogenicity, while in the placebo group, this parameter remained unaltered during the study. A significant correlation was observed between changes of blood serum atherogenicity and intima-media thickness of common carotid arteries (r = 0.144, p = 0.045) (**Figures 8** and **9**). Therefore, it was demonstrated that garlic-based food supplement Allicor possessed a direct anti-atherosclerotic effect at the subclinical stage of the disease, which could be attributed to the decrease of blood serum atherogenicity [37, 39].

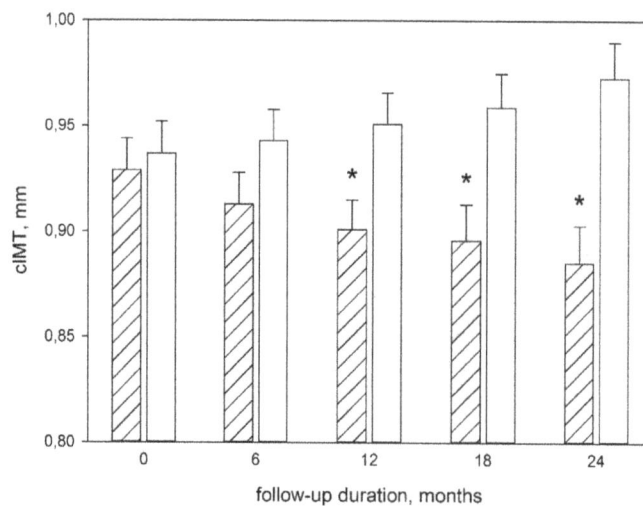

Figure 8. The dynamics of cIMT in double-blind placebo-controlled study on anti-atherosclerotic effects of garlic-based drug Allicor. Hatched bars, Allicor recipients; open bars, placebo recipients. Presented are mean values ±S.E.M. *, significant difference between groups, p < 0.05. Reproduced with permission from [30].

Another clinical study was focused on the evaluation of potential anti-atherosclerotic activity of herbal products with anti–inflammatory effects. Atherosclerosis is tightly associated with the inflammatory process at all stages of the disease development [79, 80]. Substances with systemic anti-inflammatory properties can therefore be regarded as potential therapeutic agents for treatment and prevention of atherosclerosis.

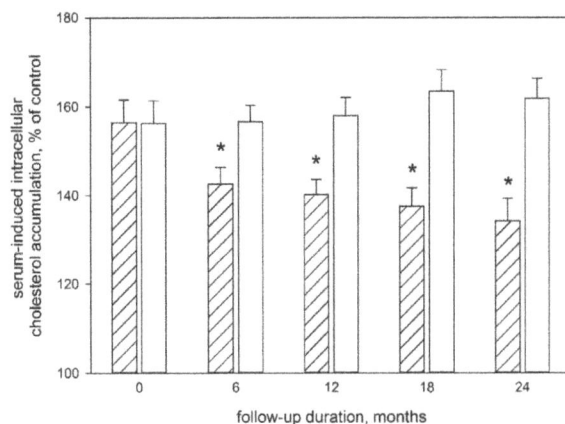

Figure 9. The dynamics of serum atherogenicity in double-blind placebo-controlled study on anti-atherosclerotic effects of garlic-based drug Allicor. Hatched bars, Allicor recipients; open bars, placebo recipients. Presented are mean values ±S.E.M. *, significant difference between groups, $p < 0.05$. Reproduced with permission from [30].

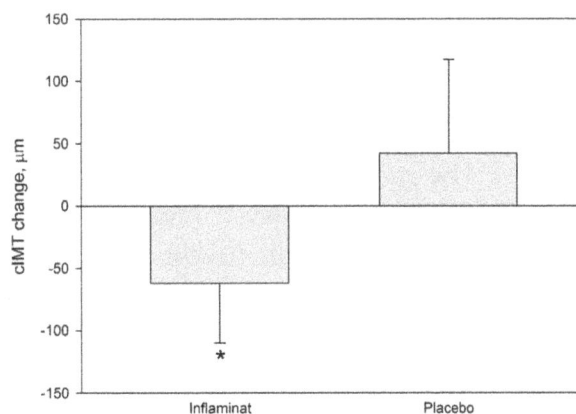

Figure 10. The changes of cIMT in double-masked placebo-controlled study on anti-atherosclerotic effects of Inflaminat. Presented are mean values ±S.E.M. *, significant difference between groups, $p < 0.05$. Reproduced with permission from [30].

Several natural compounds, such as calendula (*Calendula officinalis*), elder (*Sambucus nigra*) and violet (*Viola* sp.), were demonstrated to possess not only anti-inflammatory, but also anti-atherosclerotic effects [81–83]. The combination of these herbs was used for the development of a novel dietary supplement (Inflaminat, INAT-Farma, Russia) [84]. The effect of Inflaminat on cIMT dynamics was evaluated in a pilot placebo-controlled double-blinded study performed on 67 asymptomatic men (ClinicalTrials.gov Identifier, NCT01743404) [39, 85]. The protocol of the 12-month study was similar to that described for Allicor food supplement. Administration of Inflaminat induced cIMT regression in subclinical atherosclerosis, with statistically significant difference between the baseline as the placebo group (**Figure 10**). Therefore, Inflaminat was demonstrated to possess anti-inflammatory and anti-atherosclerotic effects at the cellular level and to induce regression of subclinical atherosclerotic lesions in asymptomatic men.

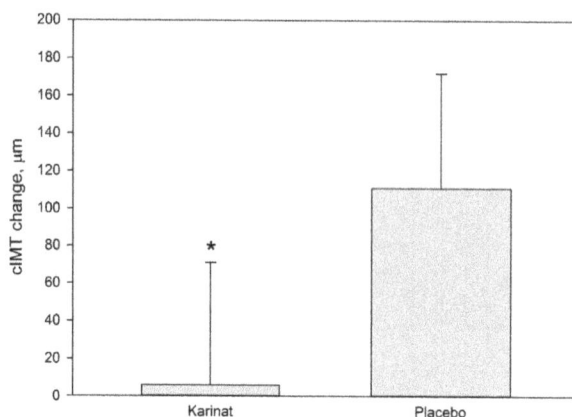

Figure 11. The changes of cIMT in double-masked placebo-controlled study on anti-atherosclerotic effects of Karinat. The data are presented in the terms of means and S.D. *, significant difference between groups, p < 0.05. Reproduced with permission from [30].

Finally, several phytoestrogen-rich natural substances were evaluated for potential anti-atherosclerotic activity using the described *in vitro* and an *ex vivo* models [86–88]. The most promising of these compounds were garlic powder, extract of grape seeds, green tea leaf and hop cones. All these substances possessed a significant anti-atherogenic effect. A combination of these compounds was used for development of a novel isoflavonoid-rich dietary supplement (Karinat, INAT-Farma, Russia). The resulting supplement is a source of biologically active polyphenols, including resveratrol, genisteine and daidzeine that are claimed to produce beneficial effects on atherosclerosis development. The efficiency of Karinat was evaluated in a randomized double-blind placebo-controlled 12-month clinical study conducted on 157 asymptomatic postmenopausal women (ClinicalTrials.gov Identifier, NCT01742000) [89, 90]. The primary endpoint was the annual rate of cIMT change. The protocol of the study was similar to that reported above. An annual increase of mean cIMT of more than 100 μm (13% per year) was observed in the placebo group, indicative of a high rate of cIMT progression in postmenopausal women. Growth of atherosclerotic plaques was estimated to be 40% per year. In the Karinat group, mean cIMT value remained unaltered, with a statistically insignificant increase of 6 μm per year, *that is* <1% (**Figure 11**). Therefore, phytoestrogen-rich substances were proven to possess beneficial effects on the dynamics of subclinical atherosclerosis progression in postmenopausal women [39, 91].

7. Conclusions

Introduction of the concept of blood serum atherogenicity allowed creating cell model suitable for screening of substances with potential anti-atherosclerotic activity. Such models helped revealing several novel compounds of botanical origin that could be used for the development of dietary supplements for treatment of subclinical (asymptomatic) atherosclerosis. The effect of "direct" anti-atherosclerotic therapy can be observed at the level of the arterial wall cells by a decrease of intracellular lipid accumulation. Therapy of patients with established atherosclerosis should induce regression of the existing plaques or hinder the progression of novel lesions. Introduction of food supplements from botanicals with anti-atherosclerotic properties and suitable for long-term consumption is an important step toward the improvement of the preventive treatment of atherosclerosis. Further studies will help revealing natural products with anti-atherogenic and anti-atherosclerotic effects that can be used for the development of novel cardiovascular drugs possessing mechanistic mode of action. Despite the unavoidable limitations of the described models, the obtained results have demonstrated that cultured arterial wall cells offer a suitable instrument for initial analysis of drug effects. The discovery of anti-atherosclerotic activity of natural products opens great opportunities for prevention and treatment of atherosclerotic disease, reducing cardiovascular morbidity and mortality.

Acknowledgements

The work was supported by Ministry of Education and Sciences, Russia (Project # RFME-FI61614X0010).

Author details

Alexander N. Orekhov[1,2,3] and Ekaterina A. Ivanova[4*]

*Address all correspondence to: kate.ivanov@gmail.com

1 Department of Biophysics, Faculty of Biology, Lomonosov Moscow State University, Moscow, Russia

2 Laboratory of Angiopathology, Institute of General Pathology and Pathophysiology, Moscow, Russia

3 Institute for Atherosclerosis Research, Skolkovo Innovative Center, Moscow, Russia

4 KU Leuven, Department of Development and Regeneration, Leuven, Belgium

References

[1] Barquera S, Pedroza-Tobias A, Medina C, Hernandez-Barrera L, Bibbins-Domingo K, Lozano R, Moran AE. Global overview of the epidemiology of atherosclerotic cardiovascular disease. Arch Med Res 2015; 46: 328–38.

[2]   Simmons A, Steffen K, Sanders S. Medical therapy for peripheral arterial disease. Curr Opin Cardiol 2012; 27: 592–7.

[3]   Berenson GS, Srinivasan SR, Bao W, Newman WP 3rd, Tracy RE, Wattigney WA. Association between multiple cardiovascular risk factors and atherosclerosis in children and young adults. The Bogalusa Heart Study. N Engl J Med 1998; 338: 1650–6.

[4]   McGill HC Jr, Herderick EE, McMahan CA, Zieske AW, Malcolm GT, Tracy RE, Strong JP. Atherosclerosis in youth. Minerva Pediatr 2002; 54: 437–47.

[5]   Tuzcu EM, Kapadia SR, Tutar E, Ziada KM, Hobbs RE, McCarthy PM, Young JB, Nissen SE. High prevalence of coronary atherosclerosis in asymptomatic teenagers and young adults: evidence from intravascular ultrasound. Circulation 2001; 103: 2705–10.

[6]   Anderson KM, Wilson PW, Odell PM, Kannel WB. An updated coronary risk profile. A statement for health professionals. Circulation 1991; 83: 356–62.

[7]   Fowkes FG, Rudan D, Rudan I, Aboyans V, Denenberg JO, McDermott MM, Norman PE, Sampson UK, Williams LJ, Mensah GA, Criqui MH. Comparison of global estimates of prevalence and risk factors for peripheral artery disease in 2000 and 2010: a systematic review and analysis. Lancet 2013; 382: 1329–40.

[8]   Orekhov AN, Tertov VV. *In vitro* effect of garlic powder extract on lipid content in normal and atherosclerotic human aortic cells. Lipids 1997; 32: 1055–60.

[9]   Orekhov AN, Tertov VV, Kudryashov SA, Khashimov KhA, Smirnov VN. Primary culture of human aortic intima cells as a model for testing antiatherosclerotic drugs. Effects of cyclic AMP, prostaglandins, calcium antagonists, antioxidants, and lipid-lowering agents. Atherosclerosis 1986; 60: 101–10.

[10] Sazonova M, Budnikov E, Khasanova Z, Sobenin I, Postnov A, Orekhov A. Studies of the human aortic intima by a direct quantitative assay of mutant alleles in the mitochondrial genome. Atherosclerosis 2009; 204: 184–90.

[11] Rai AK, Debetto P, Sala FD. Molecular regulation of cholesterol metabolism: HDL-based intervention through drugs and diet. Indian J Exp Biol 2013; 51: 885–94.

[12] Al-Waili N, Salom K, Al-Ghamdi A, Ansari MJ, Al-Waili A, Al-Waili T. Honey and cardiovascular risk factors, in normal individuals and in patients with diabetes mellitus or dyslipidemia. J Med Food 2013; 16: 1063–78.

[13] Ried K, Toben C, Fakler P. Effect of garlic on serum lipids: an updated meta-analysis. Nutr Rev 2013; 71: 282–99.

[14] Hopkins AL, Lamm MG, Funk JL, Ritenbaugh C. Hibiscus sabdariffa L. In the treatment of hypertension and hyperlipidemia: a comprehensive review of animal and human studies. Fitoterapia 2013; 85: 84–94.

[15] Sobenin IA, Nedosugova LV, Filatova LV, Balabolkin MI, Gorchakova TV, Orekhov AN. Metabolic effects of time-released garlic powder tablets in type 2 diabetes mellitus: the results of double-blinded placebo-controlled study. Acta Diabetol 2008; 45: 1–6.

[16] Sobenin IA, Pryanishnikov VV, Kunnova LM, Rabinovich YA, Martirosyan DM, Orekhov AN. The effects of time-released garlic powder tablets on multifunctional cardiovascular risk in patients with coronary artery disease. Lipids Health Dis 2010; 9: 119.

[17] Sobenin IA, Andrianova IV, Fomchenkov IV, Gorchakova TV, Orekhov AN. Time-released garlic powder tablets lower systolic and diastolic blood pressure in men with mild and moderate arterial hypertension. Hypertens Res 2009; 32: 433–7.

[18] Diffenderfer MR, Schaefer EJ. The composition and metabolism of large and small LDL. Curr Opin Lipidol. 2014; 25: 221–6.

[19] Chazov EI, Tertov VV, Orekhov AN, Lyakishev AA, Perova NV, Kurdanov KA, Khashimov KA, Novikov ID, Smirnov VN. Atherogenicity of blood serum from patients with coronary heart disease. Lancet 1986; 2: 595–8.

[20] Schönfelder M. Ortologie und patologie der Langhans-zellen der aortenintima des menschen. Pathol Microbiol (Basel) 1969; 33: 129–45.

[21] Konstantinov IE, Mejevoi N, Anichkov NM. Nikolai N. Anichkov and his theory of atherosclerosis. Tex Heart Inst J 2006; 33: 417–23.

[22] Jaakkola O, Solakivi T, Tertov VV, Orekhov AN, Miettinen TA, Nikkari T. Characteristics of low-density lipoprotein subfractions from patients with coronary artery disease. Coron Artery Dis 1993; 4: 379–85.

[23] Sobenin IA, Tertov VV, Orekhov AN. Optimization of the assay for sialic acid determination in low density lipoprotein. J Lipid Res 1998; 39: 2293–9.

[24] Tertov VV, Sobenin IA, Gabbasov ZA, Popov EG, Jaakkola O, Solakivi T, Nikkari T, Smirnov VN, Orekhov AN. Multiple-modified desialylated low density lipoproteins that cause intracellular lipid accumulation. Isolation, fractionation and characterization. Lab Invest 1992 67: 665–75.

[25] Tertov VV, Sobenin IA, Orekhov AN. Modified (desialylated) low-density lipoprotein measured in serum by lectin-sorbent assay. Clin Chem 1995; 41: 1018–21.

[26] Tertov VV, Bittolo-Bon G, Sobenin IA, Cazzolato G, Orekhov AN, Avogaro P. Naturally occurring modified low density lipoproteins are similar if not identical: more electronegative and desialylated lipoprotein subfractions. Exp Mol Pathol 1995; 62: 166–72.

[27] Tertov VV, Sobenin IA, Orekhov AN. Similarity between naturally occurring modified desialylated, electronegative and aortic low density lipoprotein. Free Radic Res 1996; 25: 313–319.

[28] Tertov VV, Sobenin IA, Gabbasov ZA, Popov EG, Yaroslavov AA, Jauhiainen M, Ehnholm C, Smirnov VN, Orekhov AN. Three types of naturally occurring modified lipoproteins induce intracellular lipid accumulation in human aortic intimal cells – the role of lipoprotein aggregation. Eur J Clin Chem Clin Biochem 1992; 30: 171–8.

[29] Goldstein JL, Brown MS. Regulation of low-density lipoprotein receptors: implications for pathogenesis and therapy of hypercholesterolemia and athero-sclerosis. Circulation 1987; 76: 504–7.

[30] Orekhov AN, Sobenin IA, Revin VV, Bobryshev YV. Development of antiatherosclerotic drugs on the basis of natural products using cell model approach. Oxid Med Cell Longev 2015; 2015: 46379, doi:10.1155/2015/463797.

[31] Vanhoutte PM. How we learned to say NO. Arterioscler Thromb Vasc Biol. 2009; 29: 1156–1160.

[32] Kruth HS. Sequestration of aggregated low-density lipoproteins by macrophages. Curr Opin Lipidol. 2002; 13: 483–488.

[33] Gratchev A, Sobenin I, Orekhov A, Kzhyshkowska J. Monocytes as a diagnostic marker of cardiovascular diseases. Immunobiology 2012; 217: 476–82.

[34] Andreeva ER, Pugach IM, Orekhov AN. Collagen-synthesizing cells in initial and advanced atherosclerotic lesions of human aorta. Atherosclerosis 1997; 130: 133–42.

[35] Orekhov AN, Andreeva ER, Bobryshev YV. Cellular mechanisms of human athero-sclerosis: role of cell-to-cell communications in subendothelial cell functions. Tissue Cell. 2016; 48: 25–34.

 36] Orekhov AN. Direct anti-atherosclerotic therapy; development of natural anti-atherosclerotic drugs preventing cellular cholesterol retention. Curr Pharm Des 2013; 1 : 5 0 –28.

[37] Sobenin IA, Chistiakov DA, Bobryshev YV, Orekhov AN. Blood atherogenicity as a target for anti-atherosclerotic therapy. Curr Pharm Des 2013; 19: 5954–5962.

[38] Orekhov AN, Tertov VV, Lyakishev AA, Ruda MY. Use of cultured atherosclerotic cells for investigation of antiatherosclerotic effects of anipamil and other calcium antago-nists. J Hum Hypertens. 1991; 5: 425–430.

[39] Orekhov AN, Sobenin IA, Korneev NV, Kirichenko TV, Myasoedova VA, Melnichenko AA, Balcells M, Edelman ER, Bobryshev YV. Anti-atherosclerotic therapy based on botanicals. Recent Pat Cardiovasc Drug Discov 2013; 8: 56–66.

[40] Orekhov AN, Tertov VV, Kudryashov SA, Smirnov VN. Triggerlike stimulation of cholesterol accumulation and DNA and extracellular matrix synthesis induced by atherogenic serum or low density lipoprotein in cultured cells. Circ Res 1990; 66: 311–320.

[41] Rekhter MD, Andreeva ER, Mironov AA, Orekhov AN. Three-dimensional cytoarchitecture of normal and atherosclerotic intima of human aorta. Am J Pathol 1991; 138: 569–580.

[42] Orekhov AN, Andreeva ER, Krushinsky AV, Smirnov VN. Primary cultures of enzyme-isolated cells from normal and atherosclerotic human aorta. Med Biol 1984; 62: 255–259.

[43] Orekhov AN, Tertov VV, Novikov ID, Krushinsky AV, Andreeva ER, Lankin VZ, Smirnov VN. Lipids in cells of atherosclerotic and uninvolved human aorta. I. Lipid composition of aortic tissue and enzyme-isolated and cultured cells. Exp Mol Pathol 1985; 42: 117–137.

[44] Orekhov AN, Krushinsky AV, Andreeva ER, Repin VS, Smirnov VN. Adult human aortic cells in primary culture: heterogeneity in shape. Heart Vessels 1986; 2: 193–201.

[45] Andreeva ER, Pugach IM, Orekhov AN. Subendothelial smooth muscle cells of human aorta express macrophage antigen *in situ* and *in vitro*. Atherosclerosis. 1997; 135: 19–27.

[46] Tertov VV, Orekhov AN, Repin VS, Smirnov VN. Dibutyryl cyclic AMP decrease proliferative activity and the cholesteryl ester content in cultured cells of atherosclerotic human aorta. Biochem Biophys Res Commun 1982; 109: 1228–33.

[47] Tertov VV, Orekhov AN, Smirnov VN. Agents that increase cellular cyclic AMP inhibit proliferative activity and decrease lipid content in cells cultured from atherosclerotic human aorta. Artery 1986; 13: 365–372.

[48] Tertov VV, Orekhov AN, Smirnov VN. Effect of cyclic AMP on lipid accumulation and metabolism in human atherosclerotic aortic cells. Atherosclerosis 1986; 62: 55–64.

[49] Tertov VV, Orekhov AN, Grigorian GYu, Kurennaya GS, Kudryashov SA, Tkachuk VA, Smirnov VN. Disorders in the system of cyclic nucleotides in atherosclerosis: cyclic AMP and cyclic GMP content and activity of related enzymes in human aorta. Tissue Cell 1987; 19: 21–28.

[50] Akopov SE, Orekhov AN, Tertov VV, Khashimov KA, Gabrielyan ES, Smirnov VN. Stable analogues of prostacyclin and thromboxane A2 display contradictory influences on atherosclerotic properties of cells cultured from human aorta. The effect of calcium antagonists. Atherosclerosis 1988; 72: 245–248.

[51] Baldenkov GN, Akopov SE, Ryong LH, Orekhov AN. Prostacyclin, thromboxane A2 and calcium antagonists: effects on atherosclerotic characteristics of vascular cells. Biomed Biochim Acta 1988; 47: S324–327.

[52] Kudryashov SA, Tertov VV, Orekhov AN, Geling NG, Smirnov VN. Regression of atherosclerotic manifestations in primary culture of human aortic cells: effects of prostaglandins. Biomed Biochim Acta 1984; 43: S284–286.

[53] Orekhov AN, Tertov VV, Smirnov VN. Prostacyclin analogues as anti-atherosclerotic drugs. Lancet 1983; 2: 521.

[54] Orekhov AN, Tertov VV, Mazurov AV, Andreeva ER, Repin VS, Smirnov VN. "Regression" of atherosclerosis in cell culture: effects of stable prostacyclin analogues. Drug Develop Res 1986; 9: 189–201.

[55] Tertov VV, Panosyan AG, Akopov SE, Orekhov AN. The effects of eicozanoids and lipoxygenase inhibitors on the lipid metabolism of aortic cells. Biomed Biochim Acta 1988; 47: S286–288.

[56] Orekhov AN, Misharin AYu, Tertov VV, Khashimov KhA, Pokrovsky SN, Repin VS, Smirnov VN. Artificial HDL as an anti-atherosclerotic drug. Lancet 1984; 2: 1149–1150.

[57] Orekhov AN, Tertov VV, Khashimov KA, Kudryashov SS, Smirnov VN. Evidence of antiatherosclerotic action of verapamil from direct effects on arterial cells. Am J Cardiol 1987; 59: 495–496.

[58] Orekhov AN, Baldenkov GN, Tertov VV, Ryong LH, Kozlov SG, Lyakishev AA, Tkachuk VA, Ruda MYa, Smirnov VN. Cardiovascular drugs and atherosclerosis: effects of calcium antagonists, beta-blockers, and nitrates on atherosclerotic characteristics of human aortic cells. J Cardiovasc Pharmacol 1988; 12 (Suppl 6): S66–68.

[59] Orekhov AN, Baldenkov GN, Tertov VV, Ruda MYa, Khashimov KA, Kudryashov SA, Ryong LH, Kozlov SG, Lyakishev AA, Tkachuk VA, Smirnov VN. Antiatherosclerotic effects of calcium antagonists. Study in human aortic cell culture. Herz 1990; 15: 139–145.

[60] Giessler C, Fahr A, Tertov VV, Kudryashov SA, Orekhov AN, Smirnov VN, Mest HJ. Trapidil derivatives as potential anti-atherosclerotic drugs. Arzneimittelforschung 1987; 37: 538–541.

[61] Heinroth-Hoffmann I, Kruger J, Tertov VV, Orekhov AN, Mest HJ. Influence of trapidil and trapidil derivatives on the content of cyclic nucleotides in human intima cells cultured from atherosclerotic plaques. Drug Develop Res 1990; 19: 321–327.

[62] Li HR, Tertov VV, Vasil'ev AV, Tutel'yan VA, Orekhov AN. Anti-atherogenic and antiatherosclerotic effects of mushroom extracts revealed in human aortic intima cell culture. Drug Develop Res 1989; 17: 109–117.

[63] Orekhov AN, Ruda MYa, Baldenkov GN, Tertov VV, Khashimov KA, Ryong LH, Lyakishev AA, Kozlov SG, Tkachuk VA, Smirnov VN. Atherogenic effects of beta blockers on cells cultured from normal and atherosclerotic aorta. Am J Cardiol 1988; 61: 1116–1117.

[64] Sobenin IA, Maksumova MA, Slavina ES, Balabolkin MI, Orekhov AN. Sulfonylureas induce cholesterol accumulation in cultured human intimal cells and macrophages. Atherosclerosis 1994; 105: 159–163.

[65] Karagodin VP, Sobenin IA, Orekhov AN. Antiatherosclerotic and cardioprotective effects of time-released garlic powder pills. Curr Pharm Des. 2015; 22: 196–213.

[66] Sung J, Harfouche Y, De La Cruz M, Zamora MP, Liu Y, Rego JA, Buckley NE. Garlic (*Allium sativum*) stimulates lipopolysaccharide-induced tumor necrosis factor-alpha production from J774A.1 murine macrophages. Phytother Res. 2015; 29: 288–294.

[67] Koscielny J, Klüssendorf D, Latza R, Schmitt R, Radtke H, Siegel G, Kiesewetter H. The antiatherosclerotic effect of *Allium sativum*. Atherosclerosis. 1999; 144: 237–249.

[68] Hartung T, Daston G. Are *in vitro* tests suitable for regulatory use? Toxicol Sci 2009; 111: 233–237.

[69] Hill BT. *In vitro* human tumour model systems for investigating drug resistance. Cancer Surv 1986; 5: 129–149.

[70] Camenisch G, Folkers G, van de Waterbeemd H. Review of theoretical passive drug absorption models: historical background, recent developments and limitations. Pharm Acta Helv 1996; 71: 309–327.

[71] Bocan TM. Animal models of atherosclerosis and interpretation of drug intervention studies. Curr Pharm Des 1998; 4: 37–52.

[72] Carmeliet P, Moons L, Collen D. Mouse models of angiogenesis, arterial stenosis, atherosclerosis and hemostasis. Cardiovasc Res 1998; 39: 8–33.

[73] Johnson GJ, Griggs TR, Badimon L. The utility of animal models in the preclinical study of interventions to prevent human coronary artery restenosis: analysis and recommendations. On behalf of the Subcommittee on Animal, Cellular and Molecular Models of Thrombosis and Haemostasis of the Scientific and Standardization Committee of the International Society on Thrombosis and Haemostasis. Thromb Haemost 1999; 81: 835–843.

[74] Moghadasian MH, Frohlich JJ, McManus BM. Advances in experimental dyslipidemia and atherosclerosis. Lab Invest 2001; 81: 1173–1183.

[75] Kones R. Primary prevention of coronary heart disease: integration of new data, evolving views, revised goals, and role of rosuvastatin in management. A comprehensive survey. Drug Des Devel Ther 2011; 5: 325–380.

[76] Peng X. Transgenic rabbit models for studying human cardiovascular diseases. Comp Med 2012; 62: 472–479.

[77] Getz GS, Reardon CA. Animal models of atherosclerosis. Arterioscler Thromb Vasc Biol. 2012; 32: 1104–1115.

[78] Sobenin IA, Korneev NV, Romanov IV, Shutikhina IV, Kuntsevich GI, Romanenko EB, Myasoedova VA, Revin VV, Orekhov AN. The effects of garlic powder tablets in subclinical carotid atherosclerosis. Exp Clin Cardiol 2014; 20: 629–638.

[79] Libby P. Inflammation in atherosclerosis. Arterioscler Thromb Vasc Biol 2012; 32: 2045–2051.

[80] Wolf D, Stachon P, Bode C, Zirlik A. Inflammatory mechanisms in atherosclerosis. Hamostaseologie 2014; 34: 63–71.

[81] Gorchakova T, Suprun I, Sobenin I, Orekhov A. The suppression of the inflammatory cytokines expression by natural substances. Atherosclerosis 2005; 6: 66–67.

[82] Gorchakova TV, Suprun IV, Sobenin IA, Orekhov AN. Use of natural products in anticytokine therapy. Bull Exp Biol Med 2007; 143: 316–319.

[83] Gorchakova TV, Sobenin IA, Orekhov AN. The reduction of proinflammatory cytokine expression by natural components: a new approach to the prevention and treatment of atherosclerosis at the cellular level. J Clin Lipidol 2007; 1: 492.

[84] Gorchakova TV, Suprun IV, Sobenin IA, Orekhov AN. Combined anti-inflammatory and anti-atherogenic activity of natural drug Inflaminat – a perspective for long-term atherosclerosis prevention and treatment. Atherosclerosis Suppl 2007; 8: 224.

[85] Gorchakova T, Myasoedova, Sobenin I, Orekhov A. Atherosclerosis prevention with the anti-inflammatory dietary supplement Inflaminat. Atherosclerosis Suppl 2009; 10: 387.

[86] Sobenin IA, Nikitina NA, Myasoedova VA, Korennaya VV, Khalilov EG, Orekhov AN. Antiatherogenic properties of isoflavones from phytoestrogen-rich botanicals. Atherosclerosis Suppl 2003; 4: 339.

[87] Korennaya VV, Myasoedova VA, Nikitina NA, Sobenin IA, Orekhov AN. Bioflavonoid-rich botanicals reduce blood serum atherogenicity in perimenopausal women. Atherosclerosis Suppl 2006; 7: 444.

[88] Nikitina NA, Sobenin IA, Myasoedova VA, Korennaya VV, Mel'nichenko AA, Khalilov EM, Orekhov AN. Antiatherogenic effect of grape flavonoids in an *ex vivo* model. Bull Exp Biol Med. 2006; 141: 712–715.

[89]   Sobenin IA, Myasoedova VA, Orekhov AN. Antiatherogenic action of isoflavonoid-rich botanicals: an implementation for atherosclerosis prevention in postmenopausal women. J Clin Lipidol 2007; 491.

[90]   Myasoedova VA, Sobenin IA. Background, rationale and design of clinical study of the effect of isoflavonoid-rich botanicals on natural history of atherosclerosis in women. Atherosclerosis Suppl 2008; 9: 171.

[91]   Sobenin I, Myasoedova V, Orekhov A. Atherosclerosis prevention in postmenopausal women with the isoflavonoid-rich dietary supplement Karinat. J Clin Lipidol 2008; 2: S26–27.

12

Role of Pleural Fluid Cholesterol in Pleural Effusion

Achyut Bikram Hamal

Abstract

Pleural effusion occurs when formation and accumulation of pleural fluid exceeds its absorption. It indicates an imbalance between pleural fluid formation and its removal. Pleural fluid accumulates in settings of increased hydrostatic pressure, increased vascular permeability, decreased oncotic pressure, increased intrapleural negative pressure and decreased lymphatic drainage. On the basis of pathophysiology, pleural effusion can be transudates or exudates. It is important to establish an accurate etiological diagnosis so that the patient may be treated in a rational manner. Using Light's criteria may need other extra investigations to differentiate transudates and exudates but using pleural fluid cholesterol (pCHOL) will help to diagnose them with only the pleural fluid analysis. Moreover the albumin or protein gradient will need serum as well as the pleural fluid investigations and will have more financial burden than just investigating pleural fluid cholesterol. Pleural cholesterol is thought to be derived from degenerating cells and vascular leakage from increased permeability. Thus pleural fluid cholesterol is one of the important investigations that can distinguish exudates from transudates. Routine use of pleural fluid cholesterol for classifying pleural effusion should be encouraged to improve the accuracy, sensitivity and specificity.

Keywords: pleural effusion (PE), pleural fluid cholesterol (pCHOL), transudates, exudates, pleural fluid lactate dehydrogenase (pLDH), serum lactate dehydrogenase (sLDH), congestive heart failure (CHF)

1. Introduction

Pleurae are the continuous membranes of the serous pleural sac that invest and enclose the lungs. They are called parietal and visceral pleura. The visceral pleura is also called the pulmonary pleura that closely covers the lung and is adherent to its surfaces. The parietal pleura adhere to the diaphragm, mediastinum and the wall of the thorax. It consists of costal

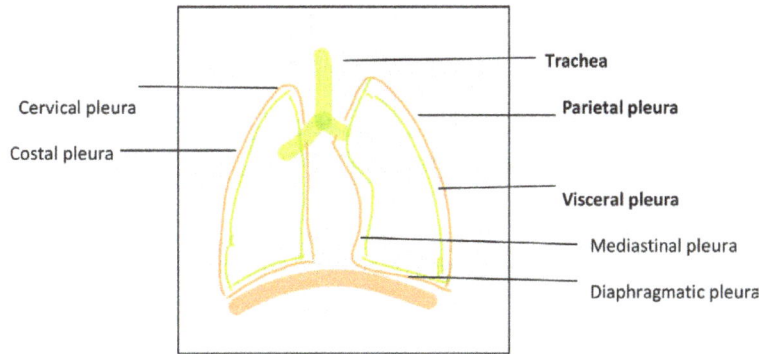

Figure 1. Schematic diagram of pleura and pleural cavity.

pleura, mediastinal pleura, diaphragmatic pleura and cervical pleura. The pleural space lies between the lung and the chest wall and is bounded by the parietal and visceral membranes. It contains a thin layer of fluid that serves as a coupling system called pleural fluid. A pleural effusion (PE) is present when there is an excess fluid in the pleural space. It indicates an imbalance between pleural fluid formation and its removal. It is important to establish an accurate etiological diagnosis so that the patient may be treated in a rational manner.

The pleural space is a real, not potential, space that is approximately 10–20 μm wide and extends completely around the lung to the hilar root [1, 2]. When air or fluid collects between the two layers, the pleural cavity expands. The schematic diagram for pleural cavity and pleurae is in **Figure 1**.

Pleural fluid is formed from the systemic vessels of the pleural membranes at an approximate rate of 0.6 ml/h and is absorbed at a similar rate by the parietal pleural lymphatic system. Normally, the pleural spaces contain approximately 0.25 ml/kg of low protein liquid. Disturbances in either formation or absorption result in the accumulation of excess pleural fluid [3].

The volume of pleural fluid is small, approximately 0.1–0.2 ml/kg in different studies. From parietal pleural capillaries, there is constant movement of fluid into the pleural space at a rate of 0.01 ml/kg bodyweight/h. There is a balance of the formation (entry) and absorption (exit) of the pleural fluid. The resultant homeostasis leaves 5–15 ml of fluid in the normal pleural space [4]. For pleural effusion to be there must be an increase in entry rate or a reduction in exit rate.

The parietal pleura has a hydrostatic pressure similar to that of the systemic circulation (30 cm H_2O), whereas that of the visceral pleura depends on the pulmonary circulation (10 cm H_2O). Oncotic pressure is similar in both (25 cm H_2O), but the pressure within the pleural cavity is affected by the gravity gradient. Thus, the pleural space is heterogeneous with a nondependent portion in which Starling forces favor outpouring of fluid into the cavity and the parenchymal capillaries [5].

2. Pathophysiology

The mechanism of pleural liquid formation is that the liquid originates from the systemic vessels of the pleural membranes, not from the pulmonary vessels [6]. It means that pleural liquid is interstitial fluid of the systemic pleural microvessels. There are three major considerations that support this hypothesis [7]:

i.   The systemic vessels (of both parietal and visceral pleural membranes) are adjacent to the pleural space and are much closer to the pleural space than are the pulmonary vessels.

ii. The low pleural liquid protein concentration (1 g/dl) and ratio to the plasma protein concentration (0.15 g/dl) are consistent with a filtrate from high-pressure systemic vessels. Large particles will be sieved and relatively restrained compared to the liquid if liquid and protein are filtered at high-pressure and high flow across a semi permeable membrane. Thus, plasma proteins, being large, will be retarded much more than the liquid in their movement across a membrane, and the protein concentration of the resultant filtrate will be low. On the other hand, if liquid and protein are filtered at low pressure and low flow, proteins are retarded less, and the protein concentration of the resultant filtrate is higher. Filtrates from low-pressure pulmonary vessels, e.g., lung lymph, have a high protein concentration (4.5 g/dl) and ratio (0.7) compared to filtrates from systemic vessels and to pleural liquid. Of note in this argument, pleural liquid formation is described as high flow, whereas its measured rate is relatively slow (0.01 ml/kg/h). However, it is the filtration at the systemic microvessels that is described as high as or at least higher than filtration across pulmonary microvessels. Some of that filtrate is reabsorbed into the low-pressure post capillary venules, and some is removed by bulk flow via the local lymphatic vessels. It is only the remainder that then moves into the low-pressure pleural space.

iii. In situations where systemic pressure varies, the pleural liquid protein concentration varies in concert. For example, systemic hypertensive rats have a lower pleural liquid protein-to-plasma protein concentration ratio than do normotensive rats (0.42 versus 0.55), even though their pulmonary pressures are the same [8]. During development from the fetus to the adult, systemic blood pressure generally rises and pulmonary pressure falls. In a study in sheep, the pleural protein ratio decreased with development, as would be expected if the pleural liquid originated from the high-pressure systemic vessels [9].

2.1. Increased fluid entry

Excess liquid filters out of microvessels based on a balance of hydrostatic and osmotic forces across a semi permeable membrane [1, 6]. These forces are well described in the Starling equation, in which the hydrostatic forces that filter water out of the vessel are balanced by osmotic forces that reabsorb water back into the vessel [10, 11].

$$\text{Flow} = k \times \left[(P_{mv} - P_{pmv}) - s\,(\pi_{mv} - \pi_{pmv})\right]. \tag{1}$$

In this equation, k is liquid conductance of the microvascular barrier, P_{mv} and P_{pmv} represent hydrostatic pressure in the microvascular and perimicrovascular compartments, respectively, is the reflection coefficient for total protein and ranges from 0 (completely permeable) to 1 (completely impermeable), and π_{mv} and π_{pmv} represent protein osmotic pressure in microvascular and perimicrovascular liquids, respectively and s is Staverman's reflection coefficient. In normal micro vessels, there is ongoing filtration of a small amount of low protein liquid. The flow can increase with changes in various parameters of the Starling equation.

Increase in permeability: An increase in flow can be due to increases in either liquid conductance (an increase in k) or protein permeability (a decrease in reflection coefficient). If the endothelial barrier becomes more permeable to liquid and protein, for example, there will be an increase in flow of a higher protein liquid. Because absorption does not alter the protein concentration of pleural liquid, pleural liquid with a high protein concentration indicates its origin from a circulation across an area of increased permeability.

Increase in microvascular pressure: An elevation in venous outflow pressure induces the elevation of microvascular pressure (Pmv). Increases in arterial pressure are less likely to be transmitted to the microvessels because of the high precapillary resistance and autoregulation of arteriolar tone.

Elevations in either systemic venous pressure (affecting the parietal pleura) or pulmonary venous pressure (affecting the visceral pleura) can lead to an increase in pleural liquid formation and the development of a pleural effusion. As vascular permeability is unchanged in this setting, the increased flow is associated with a greater sieving of proteins, leading to a filtrate with a lower protein concentration than normal (with a pleural liquid-to-plasma protein ratio of less than 0.15). Of course, most effusions formed due to increased microvascular pressures, i.e., transudative effusions, have a pleural liquid-to-plasma protein ratio much higher than this, between 0.4 and 0.5. This fact demonstrates that most liquid must arise from a source other than the systemic circulation of the pleural membranes. The likely source is the large non-systemic circulation adjacent to the pleural space, namely the pulmonary circulation of the nearby lung. In the normal state, lung interstitial liquid, e.g., lymph, filtered from the low-pressure pulmonary circulation has a protein concentration ratio [12] (lung to plasma protein concentration ratio) of 0.7, but with increased flow due to increased pulmonary microvascular pressures, this ratio falls to 0.4–0.5. This lung interstitial oedema liquid then is the likely source of the majority of the hydrostatic pleural effusion [13].

The way lung liquid reach the pleural space is that when the rate of filtrate formation exceeds the absorptive capacity of the lung lymphatics, the filtrate accumulates in the peribronchovascular spaces ("cuffs") [14]. Once in these interstitial spaces, the liquid is not accessible to lung lymphatics [15].

Thus, although the lymphatics are undeniably important in removing liquid as it is filtered from the pulmonary circulation, they cannot account for the clearance of already established oedema from the lung [16]. This interstitial oedema probably leaves the lung by flowing down pressure gradients along the interstitial spaces (interlobular septae, peribronchovascular bundles and visceral pleura) of the lung toward either the mediastinum or the pleural space. The entry of large amounts of lung interstitial liquid into the pleural space will elevate the overall protein concentration of the pleural liquid, giving a ratio of 0.40–0.50, the expected range for a transudative effusion [16].

Decrease in pleural pressure: A decrease in pleural pressure, as seen with significant atelectasis, may alter the balance of forces described in the Starling equation by reducing the pressures surrounding the nearby micro vessels. This decrease in perimicrovascular pressures

(Ppmv) can enhance filtration across the microvascular barrier of a low protein liquid (with a pleural liquid-to-plasma protein ratio of less than 0.15).

Decrease in plasma osmotic pressure: Hypoproteinemia (due to hypoalbuminemia) will decrease the plasma oncotic pressure (πmv), thereby increasing the forces favoring filtration until the balance is restored. By itself, hypoproteinemia can probably induce small effusions with a low protein concentration. In addition, hypoproteinemia can lower the threshold for effusion formation when other Starling forces are changed. In a study of hospitalized patients with AIDS, for example, hypoproteinemia alone was the apparent cause of 19% of all pleural effusions [17]. Together with other factors, a lower plasma protein concentration may have contributed to effusion formation in many more patients, because, in general, all patients with effusions had a lower plasma albumin concentration than those without effusion (2.5 versus 3.4 g/dl).

2.2. Decreased fluid exit

A decrease in exit rate reflects a reduction in lymphatic function. Because lymphatic function is poorly understood, much of this discussion is speculative. Unlike blood vessels, lymphatic vessels have one-way valves and propel lymph using both their own rhythmic contractions and the respiratory motions of the chest wall. In addition, flow is affected by lymphatic patency, availability of liquid, and the pressures influencing filling (pleural pressure) and emptying (systemic venous pressure) of lymphatics [18–20].

Intrinsic factors: A number of factors can interfere with or inhibit the ability of lymphatic's to contract, including:

- Cytokines and products of inflammation (e.g., endotoxins)
- Endocrine abnormalities (e.g., hypothyroidism)
- Injury due to radiation or drugs (e.g., chemotherapeutic agents)
- Infiltration of lymphatics by cancer
- Anatomic abnormalities (e.g., yellow nail syndrome)

Extrinsic factors: Multiple extrinsic factors can inhibit lymphatic function although the lymphatics themselves are normal. These include:

- Limitation of respiratory motion (e.g., diaphragm paralysis, lung collapse and pneumothorax)
- Extrinsic compression of lymphatics (e.g., pleural fibrosis and pleural granulomas)
- Blockage of lymphatic stomata (e.g., fibrin deposition on pleural surface and pleural malignancy)
- Decreased intrapleural pressure (e.g., trapped lung caused by a fibrous rind on the visceral pleura)

Normal pleural fluid resembles water in appearance and clarity, and is odorless [20]. Its chemical composition is summarized in **Table 1**.

Pleural effusion is present when there is excess accumulation of pleural fluid due to its exceeding formation on pleural fluid absorption. At normal circumstances, pleural fluid entering the pleural space from the capillaries in the parietal pleura is removed by the lymphatics which can absorb 20 times more fluid than is formed.

Fluid can enter the pleural space from the interstitial spaces in the visceral pleura or through the diaphragmatic pores from the peritoneal cavity. So pleural effusion will develop in two circumstances:

1. When there is excess formation of pleural fluid from parietal pleura, interstitial spaces from the lung and peritoneal cavity.

2. When there is inability of removal of pleural fluid by the lymphatics.

Local factors: There is change in the pleural surface permeability due to which the exudative pleural effusion occurs.

Systemic factors: There is increase in pulmonary capillary wedge pressure (PCWP) or decrease in oncotic pressure that result in alteration of formation and absorption of pleural fluid as in transudative pleural effusion.

Translocation of fluid: Small pores in diaphragm act as pathways for peritoneal fluid to enter into the pleural cavity as in hepatic hydrothorax. It may be massive even without marked ascites.

Parameters	Value
Volume	0.1-0.2ml/kg
Cells	1000-5000/mm3
Mesothelial cells	3- 70%
Monocytes	30-75%
lymphocytes	2-30%
Granulocytes	10%
Protein	1-2gm/dl
Albumin /protein	50-70%
Glucose	as in plasma
Lactate Dehydrogenase	< 50% of plasma

Table 1. Normal composition of pleural fluid.

The basis in which accumulation of pleural fluid occurs are: increased hydrostatic pressure, increased vascular permeability, decreased oncotic pressure, increased intrapleural negative pressure and decreased lymphatic drainage.

Pleural effusion may be of two types depending upon the underlying pathology, i.e., transudative and exudative. The causes of transudative and exudative pleural effusion are summarized in **Tables 2** and **3**, respectively.

Transudate will be clear fluid with low protein while exudates will have cloudy fluid with high protein. Exudates have a ratio of protein in pleural fluid and serum >0.5; ratio of LDH in pleural fluid and serum >0.6 and pleural fluid LDH > 2/3rd of upper limit of serum LDH. Protein in transudate is less than 2.5 g/dl while exudates have higher values [21].

Transudative pleural effusion is usually due to the increased hydrostatic pressure that is caused by congestion in the capillaries, e.g., in heart failure and there is formation of pleural fluid from the increased venous pressure of the pleural membranes. However in case of exudates, there is vascular leakage of fluid due to increased permeability as a result of inflammation.

1.	Increased hydrostatic pressure	Congestive Heart Failure
		Superior vena cava syndrome
		Pericardial effusion
		Constrictive cardiomyopathy
		Massive pulmonary embolism
2.	Decreased capillary Oncotic pressure	Cirrhosis of Liver
		Nephrotic syndrome
		Malnutrition
		Protein losing enteropathy
		Small Bowel disease
3.	Transmission from Peritoneum	Any cause of ascites
		Peritoneal Dialysis
4.	Increased capillary permeability	Small pulmonary emboli
		Myxoedema
5.	Miscellaneous	Urinothorax
		Acute atelectasis
		Wet Beriberi
		Idiopathic

Table 2. Transudative pleural effusion.

1. Respiratory causes	Parapneumonic effusion
	Tuberculosis
	sarcoidosis
	Parasitic infections
	Pulmonary embolism
	Trapped lung
2. Gastrointestinal causes	Pancreatitis
	Postoperative
	Intrabdominal abscesses
	Posttransplant of liver
	Esophageal perforation
	Endoscopic variceal sclerotherapy
3. Cardiac causes	Post Myocardial Infarction
	Constrictive pericarditis
	PostPericardiotomy
4. Occupational	Asbestosis
5. Traumatic	Hemothorax
6. Post surgical	Coronary artery bypass surgery
7. Autoimmune causes	Systemic lupus erythematosus
	Rhematoid pleurisy
	Drug induced lupus
	Sjogren syndrome
	Wegener's granulomatosis
	Chrug strauss Syndrome
8. Endocrine causes	Hypothyroidism
	Ovarian hyperstimulation syndrome
9. Renal related	Uremia
	Peritoneal dialysis
10. Malignancies and complications	Mesothelioma
	Metastases
	Superior vena caval obstruction
11. Drug induced	Bromocriptine,Dantrolene, Nitrofurantoin, Amiodarone,etc
12. Lymphatic cause	Chylothorax

13. MISCELLANEOUS	Amyloidosis
	Iatrogenic injury
	Radiation therapy
	Yellow nail syndrome

Table 3. Exudative pleural effusion.

3. Clinical features

The clinical features of pleural effusion depend on the amount, the rate of accumulation of fluid and the underlying cause. In acute cases, the symptoms appear suddenly. Patients may present with shortness of breath, pleuritic pain, cough and constitutional symptoms. Dyspnea may result from compression of lung tissue and from mechanical alterations in the respiratory muscles as the fluid changes their length-tension relationship. There will be associated symptoms related to the etiology of the pleural effusion. So careful elicitation of history in cases of pleural effusion may streamline the physician toward the etiological aspect of pleural effusion.

Physical examination reveals decreased respiratory movements on the affected side and displacement of mediastinum to the opposite side. If there is an associated collapse of lung or fibrosis, the trachea may be central or may even be pulled to the same side depending on the degree of collapse or fibrosis. Tactile fremitus may be decreased to absent but may also be increased toward the top of large effusion. Percussion reveals dull to flat note over the fluid.

Auscultation reveals decreased to absent breath sounds but bronchial breath sounds may be heard near top of large effusion. Pleural rub can also be heard and sometimes crackles above the level of effusion. Frequently, there are E to A changes (egobronchophony) at the upper fluid border where underlying lung parenchyma is compressed.

4. Diagnostic clues for exudates from transudates

Light et al. in 1972 found a criteria to have sensitivity and specificity of 99% and 98%, respectively, for differentiating transudative and exudative PE (ratio of protein in pleural fluid and serum >0.5; ratio of LDH in pleural fluid and serum >0.6 and pleural fluid LDH > 2/3rd of upper limit of serum LDH) [21]. But the other investigators could only reproduce specificities of 70–86% using light's criteria. Also it is found that 25% of patients with transudates pleural effusion are mistakenly identified as having exudative effusion by Light's criteria.

Most transudates have absolute total protein concentrations below 3.0 g/dl (30 g/l), although acute diuresis in heart failure can elevate protein levels into the exudative range [22–24].

If one or more of the exudative criteria are met and the patient is clinically thought to have a condition producing a transudative effusion, the difference between the protein levels in the serum and the pleural fluid should be measured. If this gradient is >31 g/l (3.1 g/dl), the exudative categorization by these criteria can be ignored because almost all such patients have a transudative pleural effusion [25]. About only 75% of cases, the etiology of pleural effusion can be established with the clinical presentation, biochemical parameters and fluid cytology. Despite extensive diagnostic work up in about 20% of pleural effusion, the etiology remains unknown [26].

From meta-analysis, Heffner et al. has identified pleural effusion of exudative type with at least one of the following condition [27]:

- Pleural fluid protein >2.9g/dl

- Pleural fluid cholesterol >45 mg/dl (1.16 mmol/l)

- Pleural fluid LDH > 2/3rd of upper limit of serum

Roth et al. [28] found that despite the high sensitivity of Light's criteria (100%), these criteria had a low specificity (72%). Using an albumin gradient of 1.2 g/dl or less to indicate exudates and greater than 1.2 g/dl to indicate transudates, 57 of the 59 patients (41 exudates; 18 transudates) were correctly classified. Two patients with malignant effusions were misclassified as having transudates.

In 2003 National medical journal of India, one article published by Guleria R of AIIMS, New Delhi [29] found that for exudative pleural effusion, pleural fluid cholesterol ≥60 mg/dl has 92% accuracy, 88% sensitivity and 100% specificity; however, Light's criteria was 98% sensitive and 80% specific.

Evaluation through pleural fluid cholesterol only can avoid the financial burden and double pricks (serum and pleural fluid) in anxious patients to go through the series of tests to confirm the exudative pleural effusion.

In a study done in Nepal by Hamal et al. [30], pleural fluid cholesterol (pCHOL) is highly correlated than protein ratio (pleural fluid protein/serum protein) with clinical diagnosis for exudates. It is found that in transudates, parapneumonic, tubercular and neoplastic pleural effusion, pCHOL levels were 0.53 ± 0.28, 1.81 ± 0.59, 2.08 ± 0.58 and 1.58 ± 0.65 mmol/l, respectively. With a classifying threshold of 1.16 mmol/L, pCHOL has a sensitivity of 97.7% and specificity of 100% for diagnosis of exudates with accuracy of 98.3%.

Pleural cholesterol is thought to be derived from degenerating cells and vascular leakage from increased permeability. Though the cause of the rise in cholesterol levels in pleural exudates is unknown, two possible explanations have been put forward.

According to the first, the cholesterol is synthesized by pleural cells themselves for their own needs [31] (extrahepatic synthesis of cholesterol is now known to be much greater than was once thought, depends on the metabolic needs of cells, and is in dynamic equilibrium with cholesterol supply by LDL and cholesterol removal by HDL) [32] and the concentration of cholesterol in pleural cavity is increased by the degeneration of leukocytes and erythrocytes, which contain large quantities.

The second possible explanation is that pleural cholesterol derives from plasma; some 70% of plasma cholesterol is bound to low density, high molecular weight lipoproteins (LDL) and the rest to HDL or very low density lipoproteins (VLDL) and the increased permeability of pleural capillaries in pleural exudate patients would allow plasma cholesterol to enter the pleural cavity.

The cause of the increased cholesterol concentration is unknown, but two hypotheses are available [33, 34]: (A) cholesterol production by different cells has been recognized and it is possible that destruction of white and red blood cells in pleural effusion can cause an increase in the fluid cholesterol level. (B) Increased pleural permeability causes cholesterol concentrations to increase.

Measurement of pleural cholesterol >45 mg/dl has been used to improve the accuracy of differentiating transudative and exudative effusion [35].

Another study done in Catholic University hospital, Santiago, Chile [36] Marina Costa found sensitivity and specificity of following parameters for exudative pleural effusion as 98 and 82% (criteria by Light et al.), 90 and 100% (pCHOL >45 mg/dl) and 99 and 98% (by pCHOL+ pLDH >200 IU/l), respectively.

A study done by Hamm et al., mean cholesterol level in malignant effusions was 94 mg/dl, 76 mg/dl in inflammatory effusions and 30 mg/dl in the transudates. Using a dividing line of 60 mg/dl to separate the exudates from transudates, only 5% were incorrectly classified. Elevated cholesterol levels in exudates seem to be independent of serum levels [34].

Using pleural fluid, cholesterol levels at a cut-off point of greater than 60 mg/dl and/or total protein at a cut-off point of greater than 3 g/dl for distinguishing transudates and exudates, the sensitivity, specificity, positive predictive value (PPV) and negative predictive value (NPV), were 100% in a study done by Patel and Choudhury [37].

Brett reviewing Eid et al. CHEST 2002 Nov, most but not all, exudative effusions in CHF patients have causes other than heart failure. The authors believe that, in some cases with no apparent cause other than CHF, transudates might be 'converted' into exudates by traumatic taps (which lead to increased pleural fluid lactate dehydrogenase—itself a criterion for an exudate) or by aggressive dieresis (which might transiently increase protein and LDL cholesterol concentrations in pleural fluid). In patients with previous bypass surgery, persistent impairment of lymphatic clearance might predispose to exudative effusions [38].

Pleural fluid cholesterol is better than Light's criteria for the differentiation of transudates and exudates and is less cumbersome as it does not require a simultaneous blood sampling. Cut-off value of pleural fluid cholesterol for differentiating transudates and exudates should be 45 mg/dl [39]. In this study, the sensitivity, specificity, positive predictive value and negative predictive value of the pleural fluid cholesterol (cut-off >45 mg/dl) were 97.06, 94.74, 97.06 and 94.74%, respectively, for identifying exudates.

NT-proBNP has been shown to correctly diagnose congestive heart failure as a cause of most effusions that have been misclassified as exudates by Light's criteria. Use of this test may therefore avoid repeated invasive investigations in patients where there is a strong clinical suspicion of cardiac failure. The cut-off value however, varied widely from 600 to 4000 pg/ml (with 1500 pg/ml being most commonly used), and most studies excluded patients with more than one possible etiology for their effusion [40].

The findings in a study done by Mehdi Kashmiri showed taking a value of pleural cholesterol >55 mg/dl and pleural/serum cholesterol >0.3 to define exudative effusion resulted in less erroneous classification with a sensitivity of 93%, a specificity of 100%, a positive predictive value (PPV) of 100% and an accuracy of 95.2%. Using Light's criteria gave a sensitivity of 95%, a specificity of 95%, a PPV of 97.6% and an accuracy of 95.2%. Using cholesterol in differentiating exudate from transudate was especially useful in patients with congestive heart failure who received diuretics [41].

There are other biochemical parameters other than pleural fluid cholesterol to identify the exudative pleural effusions. The difficulties in classifying pleural fluid effusion are wiped away with few parameters other than cholesterol.

It has been observed that increase in uric acid level was present in pleural fluid of transudative pleural effusion than exudative pleural effusion. The optimum cut-off level for pleural fluid uric acid was 5.35 mg/dl with sensitivity of 89.32% and specificity of 92.60% [42]. Increase in uric acid in pleural fluid can be regarded to be a manifestation of tissue hypoxia [43]. Most of the patients with reasons to produce transudative effusion had oxidative stress or hypoxemia to explain the increased uric acid synthesis. The respiratory tract, indeed, remains a major target of oxidative damage caused by both endogenous and exogenous processes [44, 45]. The major causes of tissue damage associated with chronic inflammatory lung disease are the reactive species produced by phagocytes.

Metintas et al. [46] stated that the binding of uric acid is minimal to plasma protein and it is diffuse freely to different compartments. They suggested that the increase permeability, due to change in pleural-capillary pressure in formation of transudate, is the cause of the increase of uric acid levels in pleural fluid. So all these factors explains why uric acid level increases in transudative condition than exudative one.

In cases where no cause for an exudative effusion can be identified or CHF suspected, the sequential application of the fluid LDH, followed by the serum to pleural fluid protein (SF-P) and then the serum to pleural fluid albumin (SF-A) gradients, may assist in reclassifying pleural effusions as transudates [47].

Leers Mathie P.G. from Netherlands [48] found that combination of the parameters: pleural cholesterol and pleural LDH had accuracy of 98%, sensitivity of 98% and 95% specificity for diagnosing exudative pleural effusion compared that calculated by light's criteria being accuracy of 93%, sensitivity 100% and specificity 73%.

5. Conclusion

A pleural effusion (PE) is present when there is an excess fluid in the pleural space. It indicates an imbalance between pleural fluid formation and its removal. Pleural fluid is formed from the systemic vessels of the pleural membranes at an approximate rate of 0.6 ml/h and is absorbed at a similar rate by the parietal pleural lymphatic system [6]. Pleural fluid accumulates due to local factors, systemic factors or translocation of fluid. At normal circumstances, pleural fluid entering the pleural space from the capillaries in the parietal pleura is removed by the lymphatics which can absorb 20 times more fluid than is formed.

Pleural fluid accumulates in settings of increased hydrostatic pressure, increased vascular permeability, decreased oncotic pressure, increased intrapleural negative pressure and decreased lymphatic drainage. On the basis of pathophysiology, pleural effusion can be transudates or exudates. It is important to classify the pleural fluid for diagnosis and appropriate management. Transudates occur when the mechanical factors influencing the formation or reabsorption of pleural fluid are altered, like a decrease in plasma or elevated systemic or pulmonary hydrostatic pressure. Exudates results from inflammation or irritation or other disease processes involving pleura resulting in increased permeability.

Light et al. found criteria to have sensitivity and specificity of 99 and 98%, respectively, for differentiating transudative and exudative PEs (ratio of protein in pleural fluid and serum >0.5; ratio of LDH in pleural fluid and serum >0.6 and pleural fluid LDH >2/3rd of upper limit of serum LDH) [20]. It is found that 25% of patients with transudates pleural effusion are mistakenly identified as having exudative effusion by Light's criteria. In cases of heart failure on diuretic therapy, the transudative pleural effusions have high protein. Pleural cholesterol is thought to be derived from degenerating cells and vascular leakage from increased permeability. The cause of the increased cholesterol concentration is unknown, but two hypotheses are available: one states that cholesterol production by different cells has been recognized and it is possible that destruction of white and red blood cells in pleural effusion can cause an increase in the fluid cholesterol level and second relates with increased pleural permeability that causes cholesterol concentrations to increase.

Pleural fluid cholesterol as proposed by Heffner's meta-analysis can diagnose exudative pleural effusion without need of serum values. This can avoid the financial burden and double pricks (serum and pleural fluid) in anxious patients to go through the series of tests to confirm the exudative pleural effusion. With a classifying threshold of 1.16 mmol/l, pCHOL has a sensitivity of 97.7% and specificity of 100% for diagnosis of exudates with accuracy of 98.3% compared to Light's criteria (98% sensitivity and 82% specificity). pCHOL is highly correlated than protein ratio with clinical diagnosis for exudates [29]. Moreover in pleural effusion with etiologies as transudates, parapneumonic, tubercular and neoplastic pleural effusion, pCHOL levels were 0.53 ± 0.28, 1.81 ± 0.59, 2.08 ± 0.58 and 1.58 ± 0.65 mmol/L, respectively.

Study done by Leers Mathie PG, it was found that pleural cholesterol and pleural LDH had accuracy of 98%, sensitivity of 98% and 95% specificity for diagnosing exudative pleural effusion compared that calculated by light's criteria being accuracy of 93%, sensitivity 100% and specificity 73% [47].

It is concluded that pCHOL has a better sensitivity, specificity and accuracy in differentiating transudates and exudates than the parameters of Light's criteria. This also avoids the plasma protein and gradients, sLDH, pleural fluid protein and LDH. Therefore it is more efficient, easier and more cost effective method to differentiate exudates from transudates. This study also suggests that determination of pCHOL should be in routine practice in cases of pleural effusion.

Author details

Achyut Bikram Hamal

Address all correspondence to: abhamal@gmail.com

Nepal Police Hospital, Maharajgunj, Kathmandu, Nepal

References

[1] Lai-Fook SJ. Pleural mechanics and fluid exchange. Physiological Reviews. 2004;**84**:385

[2] Albertine KH, Wiener-Kronish JP, Bastacky J, Staub NC. No evidence for mesothelial cell contact across the costal pleural space of sheep. Journal of Applied Physiology. 1991;**70**:123

[3] Broaddus VC. Fluid and solute exchange in normal physiological states. In: Light RW, Lee YGC, editors. Textbook of Pleural Diseases. 2nd ed. London: Hodder, Arnold; 2008. p. 43

[4] Stephen J, Maxine A. Pleural effusion. Current Medical Diagnosis and Treatment. 2011:306

[5] Bickley LS. Physical findings in selected chest disorders. In: BATES' Guide to Physical Examination and History Taking. 10th ed. 2011. p. 32

[6] Staub NC, Wiener-Kronish JP, Albertine KH. Transport through the Pleura: Physiology of Normal Liquid and Solute Exchange in the Pleural Space. New York: Marcel Dekker; 1985

[7] Courtney Broaddus V. Mechanism of pleural liquid accumulation in normal state. Uptodate. Jan 2013;**21**:6

[8] Lai-Fook SJ, Kaplowitz MR. Pleural protein concentration and liquid volume in spontaneously hypertensive rats. Microvascular Research. 1988;**35**:101

[9] Broaddus VC, Araya M, Carlton DP, Bland RD. Developmental changes in pleural liquid protein concentration in sheep. The American Review of Respiratory Disease. 1991;**143**:38

[10] Starling EH. On the absorption of fluids from the connective tissue spaces. The Journal of Physiology. 1896;**19**:312

[11] Staub NC. Pulmonary oedema. Physiological Reviews. 1974;**54**:678

[12] Erdmann AJ, Vaughan TR, Brigham KL, et al. Effect of increased vascular pressure on lung fluid balance in unanesthetized sheep. Circulation Research. 1975;**37**:271

[13] Broaddus VC, Wiener-Kronish JP, Staub NC. Clearance of lung edema into the pleral space of volume-loaded anesthetized sheep. Journal of Applied Physiology. 1990; **68**(6):2623

[14] Staub NC, Nagano H, Pearce ML. Pulmonary edema in dogs, especially the sequence of fluid accumulation in lungs. Journal of Applied Physiology. 1967;**22**:227

[15] Gee MH, Havill AM. The relationship between pulmonary perivascular cuff fluid and lung lymph in dogs with edema. Microvascular Research. 1980;**19**:209

[16] Mackersie RC, Christensen J, Lewis FR. The role of pulmonary lymphatics in the clearance of hydrostatic pulmonary edema. The Journal of Surgical Research. 1987;**43**(6):495

[17] Joseph J, Strange C, Sahn SA. Pleural effusions in hospitalized patients with AIDS. Annals of Internal Medicine. 1993;**118**(11):856

[18] Quick CM, Venugopal AM, Dongaonkar RM, Laine GA, Stewart RH. First-order approximation for the pressure-flow relationship of spontaneously contracting lymphangions. American Journal of Physiology. Heart and Circulatory Physiology. 2008;**294**(5):H2144

[19] Hosking B, Makinen T. Lymphatic vasculature: A molecular perspective. BioEssays. 2007;**29**(12):1192-1202

[20] Miserechi G, Agostini E. Content of pleural space. Journal of Applied Physiology. 1972;**30**:208-213

[21] Light RW, Macgregor MI, Lucshsinger PC, Ball WC Jr. Pleural effusion; the diagnostic separation of transudates and exudates. Annals of Internal Medicine. 1972;**77**:507-513

[22] Chakko SC, Caldwell SH, Sforza PP. Treatment of congestive heart failure: Its effect on pleural fluid chemistry. Chest. 1989;**95**(4):798

[23] Shinto RA, Light RW. Effects of diuresis on characteristics of pleural fluid in patients with congestive heart failure. The American Journal of Medicine. 1990;**88**(3):230

[24] Romero-Candeira S, Femaindez C, Marfa-n C, Sainchez-Paya J. Influence of diuretics on the concentration of proteins and other components of pleural exudates in patients with heart failure. The American Journal of Medicine. 2001;**110**(9):681

[25] Light RW. Disorders of pleura and mediastinum: Pleural effusion. In: Harrison's Principles of Internal Medicine. 18th ed. 2012. pp. 2178-2180

[26] Collins TR, Sahn SA. Thoracocentesis: Clinical value, complications, technical problems and patient experience. Chest. 1987;**91**:817-822

[27] Heffner JE, Sahn SA, Brown LK. Multilevel likelihood ratios for identifying exudative pleural effusion. Chest. 2002;**121**(6):1916-1920

[28] Roth BJ, O'Meara TF, Cragun WH. The serum-effusion albumin gradient in the evaluation of pleural effusions. Chest. 1990;**98**(3):546-549

[29] Guelaria R. Role of pleural fluid cholesterol in differentiating transudates from exudative pleural effusion. National Medical Journal of India. 2003;**16**(2):64-69

[30] Hamal AB et al. Pleural fluid cholesterol in differentiating exudative and transudative pleural effusions. Pulmonary Medicine. 2012;**2013**:135036

[31] Spady DK, Dietschy JM. Sterol synthesis in vivo in 18 tissues of squirrel, monkey, Guinea pig, rabbit, hamster and rat. Journal of Lipid Research. 1983;**24**:303-315

[32] Brown MS, Goldstein JL. Receptor mediated control of cholesterol metabolism. Science. 1976;**63**:695-702

[33] Valdes L et al. Cholesterol: A useful parameter for distinguishing between pleural exudates and transudates. Chest. 1991;**99**:1097-1102

[34] Hamm H et al. Cholesterol in pleural effusions-a diagnostic aid. Chest. 1987;**92**:296-302

[35] Heffner JE, Brown LK, Barbiere CA. Diagnostic value of tests that discriminate between exudative and transudative pleural effusions. Chest. 1997;**111**(4):970

[36] Costa M, Quiroga T, Cruz E. Measurement of pleural fluid cholesterol and lactate dehydrogenase: A simple and accurate set of indicators for separating exudates from transudates. Chest. 1995;**108**:1260-1263

[37] Patel AK, Choudhury S. Pleural fluid cholesterol and total protein in differentiation of exudates and transudates. The Indian Journal of Chest Diseases & Allied Sciences. 2013;**55**:21-24

[38] Eid AA et al. Exudative effusions in congestive heart failure. Chest. 2002;**122**:1518-1523

[39] Dhandapani et al. Differentiating pleural effusions: Criteria based on pleural fluid cholesterol. Eurasian Journal of Pulmonology. 2016;**18**:76-79

[40] Hooper C et al. Investigation of a unilateral pleural effusion in adults: British Thoracic Society Pleural Disease Guideline 2010. Thorax. 2010 Aug;**65**(Suppl 2):ii4-17

[41] Mehdi Keshmiri, Mojtaba Hashemzadeh. Use of cholesterol in the differentiation of exudative and transudative pleural effusion. Medical Journal of Islamic Republic of Iran. 1997;**11**(3):187-190

[42] Hazarika B et al. Role of pleural fluid uric acid estimation in differentiation between transudative and exudative pleural effusion. The Pulmo-Face. Nov 2015;**XV**(2)

[43] Uzun K, Vural H, Ozer F, Imecik O. Diagnostic value of uric acid to differentiate transudates and exudates. Clinical Chemistry and Laboratory Medicine. 2000;**38**:661-665

[44] Rajendrasozhan S, Yang SR, Edirisinghe I, Yao H, Adenuga D, Rahman I. Deacetylases and NF-κB in redox regulation of cigarette smoke-induced lung inflammation: Epigenetics in pathogenesis of COPD. Antioxidants and Redox Signaling. 2008;**10**(4):799-811

[45] Park TJ, Kim JY, Oh SP, et al. TIS21 negatively regulates hepatocarcinogenesis by disruption of cyclin B1-forkhead box M1 regulation loop. Hepatology. 2008;**47**(5):1533-1543

[46] Muzaffer M, Ozkan A, et al. Comparative analysis of biochemical parameters for differentiation of pleural exudates from transudates Light's criteria, cholesterol, bilirubin, albumin gradient, alkaline phosphatase, creatine kinase, and uric acid. Clinica Chimica Acta. 1997;**264**:149-162

[47] Kummerfeldt CE et al. Improving the predictive accuracy of identifying exudative effusions. Chest; **145**(3):586-592

[48] Leers MPG, Kleinveld HA, Schamhorst V. Differentiating transudative from exudative pleural effusion: Should we measure effusion cholesterol dehydrogenase? Clinical Chemical Laboratory Medicine. 2007;**45**(10):1332-1338

Permissions

All chapters in this book were first published in CHOLESTEROL&CLTD, by InTech Open; hereby published with permission under the Creative Commons Attribution License or equivalent. Every chapter published in this book has been scrutinized by our experts. Their significance has been extensively debated. The topics covered herein carry significant findings which will fuel the growth of the discipline. They may even be implemented as practical applications or may be referred to as a beginning point for another development.

The contributors of this book come from diverse backgrounds, making this book a truly international effort. This book will bring forth new frontiers with its revolutionizing research information and detailed analysis of the nascent developments around the world.

We would like to thank all the contributing authors for lending their expertise to make the book truly unique. They have played a crucial role in the development of this book. Without their invaluable contributions this book wouldn't have been possible. They have made vital efforts to compile up to date information on the varied aspects of this subject to make this book a valuable addition to the collection of many professionals and students.

This book was conceptualized with the vision of imparting up-to-date information and advanced data in this field. To ensure the same, a matchless editorial board was set up. Every individual on the board went through rigorous rounds of assessment to prove their worth. After which they invested a large part of their time researching and compiling the most relevant data for our readers.

The editorial board has been involved in producing this book since its inception. They have spent rigorous hours researching and exploring the diverse topics which have resulted in the successful publishing of this book. They have passed on their knowledge of decades through this book. To expedite this challenging task, the publisher supported the team at every step. A small team of assistant editors was also appointed to further simplify the editing procedure and attain best results for the readers.

Apart from the editorial board, the designing team has also invested a significant amount of their time in understanding the subject and creating the most relevant covers. They scrutinized every image to scout for the most suitable representation of the subject and create an appropriate cover for the book.

The publishing team has been an ardent support to the editorial, designing and production team. Their endless efforts to recruit the best for this project, has resulted in the accomplishment of this book. They are a veteran in the field of academics and their pool of knowledge is as vast as their experience in printing. Their expertise and guidance has proved useful at every step. Their uncompromising quality standards have made this book an exceptional effort. Their encouragement from time to time has been an inspiration for everyone.

The publisher and the editorial board hope that this book will prove to be a valuable piece of knowledge for researchers, students, practitioners and scholars across the globe.

List of Contributors

Chunfa Huang and Carl E. Freter
Division of Hematology and Oncology, Department of Internal Medicine, and Cancer Center, Saint Louis University, Saint Louis, Missouri, United States of America

Dongxiao Hao, Yizhuo Che, Lei Zhang and Shengli Zhang
Department of Applied Physics, School of Science, Xi'an Jiaotong University, Xi'an, Shaanxi, China

Zhiwei Yang
Department of Applied Physics, School of Science, Xi'an Jiaotong University, Xi'an, Shaanxi, China
Department of Applied Chemistry, School of Science, Xi'an Jiaotong University, Xi'an, China
School of Life Science and Technology, Xi'an Jiaotong University, Xi'an, China

Zaid Almarzooq and Parmanand Singh
Weill Cornell Medical College, New York Presbyterian Hospital, New York, NY, USA

Zhuo Mao, Jinghui Li and Weizhen Zhang
Department of Physiology, Center for Diabetes, Obesity and Metabolism, University Health Science Center, Shenzhen, Guangdong Province, China

Gamaleldin I. Harisa
Kayyali Chair for Pharmaceutical Industry, College of Pharmacy, King Saud University, Riyadh, Saudi Arabia
Department of Biochemistry, College of Pharmacy, Al-Azhar University (Boys), Nasr City, Cairo, Egypt

Sabry M. Attia
Department of Pharmacology and Toxicology, College of Pharmacy, King Saud University, Riyadh, Saudi Arabia

Gamil M. Abd Allah
Department of Biochemistry, College of Pharmacy, Al-Azhar University (Boys), Nasr City, Cairo, Egypt

Min-Ji Charng
Division of Cardiology, Taipei Veterans General Hospital and National Yang-Ming University, Taipei, Taiwan, R.O.C

Zeynep Banu Gungor
Department of Medical Biochemistry, Cerrahpasa Medical School, University of Istanbul, Istanbul, Turkey

Eyup Avci and Didar Elif Akgun
Faculty of Medicine, Department of Cardiology, Balikesir University, Turkey

Ahmet Dolapoglu
Cardiovascular Surgery Clinic, Balikesir Ataturk State Hospital, Turkey

Yuan Yuan and Tamie Nakajima
College of Life and Health Sciences, Chubu University, Kasugai, Japan

Hisao Naito
Department of Public Health, Fujita Health University School of Medicine, Toyoake, Japan

Barbara Hissa
The University of Chicago, James Franck Institute, Institute for Biophysical Dynamics and Physics Department, Chicago, IL, USA

Bruno Pontes
LPO-COPEA, Federal University of Rio de Janeiro, Institute of Biomedical Sciences, Rio de Janeiro, Brazil

Alexander N. Orekhov
Department of Biophysics, Faculty of Biology, Lomonosov Moscow State University, Moscow, Russia
Laboratory of Angiopathology, Institute of General Pathology and Pathophysiology, Moscow, Russia
Institute for Atherosclerosis Research, Skolkovo Innovative Center, Moscow, Russia

Ekaterina A. Ivanova
KU Leuven, Department of Development and Regeneration, Leuven, Belgium

Achyut Bikram Hamal
Nepal Police Hospital, Maharajgunj, Kathmandu, Nepal

Index